Emerging Therapeutic
ULTRASOUND

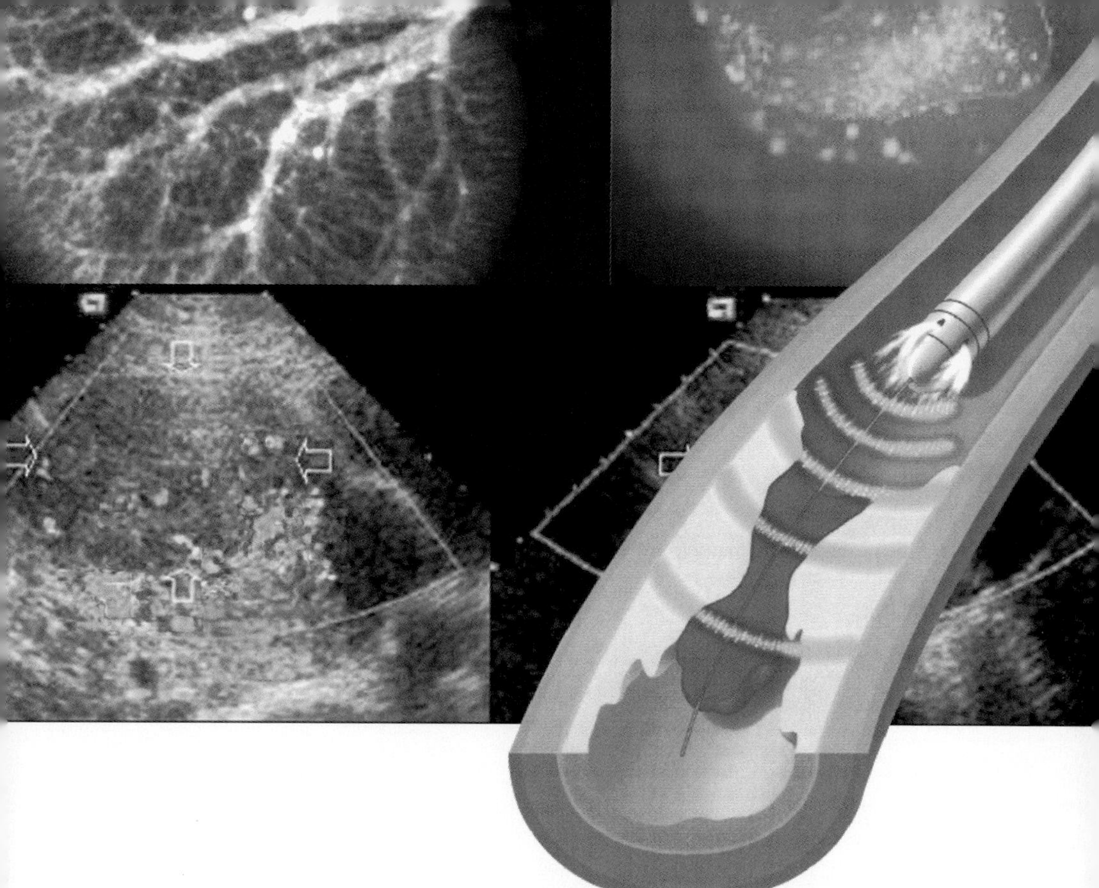

Emerging Therapeutic
ULTRASOUND

editors

Junru Wu
Wesley Nyborg

University of Vermont, USA

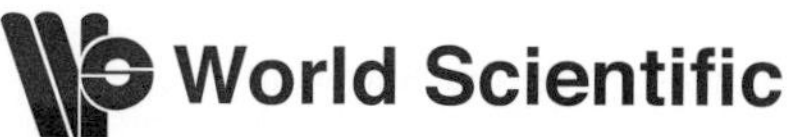 **World Scientific**

NEW JERSEY · LONDON · SINGAPORE · BEIJING · SHANGHAI · HONG KONG · TAIPEI · CHENNAI

Published by

World Scientific Publishing Co. Pte. Ltd.

5 Toh Tuck Link, Singapore 596224

USA office: 27 Warren Street, Suite 401-402, Hackensack, NJ 07601

UK office: 57 Shelton Street, Covent Garden, London WC2H 9HE

British Library Cataloguing-in-Publication Data
A catalogue record for this book is available from the British Library.

EMERGING THERAPEUTIC ULTRASOUND

ISBN 981-256-685-6

Printed by FuIsland Offset Printing (S) Pte Ltd, Singapore

Contents

3.   Ultrasound-Mediated Gene Therapy   **69**

D L Miller

K Tachibana and S Tachibana

5. MRI-guided Focused Ultrasound for Local Tissue Ablation and Other Image-guided Interventions   167

K Hynynen and N McDannold

**8.   Clinical Applications of High Intensity Focused
       Ultrasound in the Treatment of Patients
       with Solid Malignancy**   **279**

F Wu

Contents

Contributors

Kullervo Hynynen
Professor,
Department of Radiology,
Brigham and Women's
Hospital and Harvard
Medical School,
Boston, MA, USA

Nathan McDannold
Doctor,
The Brigham and
Women's Hospital,
Harvard Medical School,
Boston, MA, USA

Douglas L. Miller
Professor,
Department of Radiology,
University of Michigan,
Ann Arbor, MI, USA

Samir Mitragotri
Professor,
Department of Chemical
Engineering,
The University of California,
Santa Barbara, USA

Wesley Nyborg
Professor Emeritus,
Department of Physics,
The University of Vermont,
Burlington VT 05405

Katsuro Tachibana
Professor,
Department of Anatomy,
School of Medicine,
Fukuoka University, Japan

Shunro Tachibana
Doctor,
Sasaguri Hospital,
Fukuoka, Japan

Feng Wu
Professor,
Clinical Center for Tumor
Therapy of 2nd Affiliated
Hospital and Institute of
Ultrasonic Engineering
in Medicine,
Chongqing University of
Medical Sciences, China

Junru Wu
Professor and Chair,
Department of Physics,
The University of Vermont,
Burlington VT 05405

Preface

With enthusiasm, I accepted the invitation of editors Wu and Nyborg to prepare this short Preface. These editors are extraordinarily prescient in preparing this volume. Recent scientific and engineering developments are reaching the point where it is possible to foresee the educational preparation necessary for the next generation to participate in the future developments a decade henceforth.

It is not accidental that Wu and Nyborg, both physicists, have contributed significantly to the biomedical ultrasound field which has been endowed with abundant participation of physical scientists, since its very beginnings. For example, one can point to the officership of the American Institute of Ultrasound in Medicine, of which five of its twenty-five presidents have been physicists or engineers. Beyond that, there are the beginnings of the ultrasound field in the 1920s by Wood and Loomis involving biological specimens (Wood and Loomis, 1927) and the prodigious work led by W.J. Fry in the 1950s and 1960s, University of Illinois, which studied in great detail, the effects of high intensity ultrasound in laboratory studies and initiated the field of neurosonicsurgery (Fry *et al.*, 1958; Meyers *et al.*, 1959; Hickey *et al.*, 1961; Fry and Meyers, 1962).

This monograph provides both enlightenment in the newer areas as well as textual details for becoming well informed on their practice. Thus, it is far more than simply a glimpse into the future. Wu and Nyborg are to be commended for their acumen regarding the future of biomedical ultrasound and their effort in producing this, expected to be, long lasting treatise.

Floyd Dunn
Professor Emeritus, University of Illinois
Member, National Academy of Sciences
Member, National Academy of Engineering

References

Fry WJ, Meyers R, Fry FJ, Schultz DF, Dreyer LL, Noyes RF. Topical differentia of pathogenetic mechanisms underlying Parkinsonian tremor and rigidity as indicated by ultrasonic irradiation of the human brain. *Trans Am Neurol Assoc* (1958) **16**.

Fry WJ, Meyers R. Ultrasonic method of modifying brain structures. *Confin Neurol* (1962) **22**: 315–327.

Hickey RC, Fry WJ, Meyers R, Fry FJ, Bradbury JT. Human pituitary irradiation with focused ultrasound. *AMA Arch Surg* (1961) **83**: 620–633.

Meyers R, Fry WJ, Fry FJ, Dreyer LL, Schultz DF, Noyes RF. Early experiences with ultrasound irradiation of the pallidofugal and nigral complexes in hyperkinetic and hypertonic disorder. *J Neurosurg* (1959) **16**: 32–54.

Wood RW, Loomis AL. The physical and biological effects of high-frequency sound-waves of great intensity. *Phil Mag* (1927) **6**: 417–436.

I

PREAMBLE

Junru Wu and Wesley Nyborg

Ultrasound has been commonly used as a diagnostic real time imaging modality in medicine for decades because it is relatively safe, inexpensive and noninvasive. Long before it became a diagnostic modality, ultrasound had been applied as a therapeutic tool. Unfocused ultrasound has been used in physical therapy since the 1930s; the development and application of techniques for this purpose was recently reviewed by Nyborg (2001). Focused ultrasound has been employed clinically since the 1950s. In a review, Fry (1958) describes both structural and functional changes produced in exposures of the central nervous system to focused ultrasound, and states that "by appropriate control of the dosage conditions, it is possible to produce either reversible or selected irreversible changes."

In the past ten years or so, therapeutic ultrasound has grown rapidly. It has been shown that several emerging ultrasonic techniques may already have or will become very powerful therapeutic tools in medicine. The purpose of this book is to bring together internationally renowned authorities and experts in this field to give our readers comprehensive reviews on basic physical principles and applications of those emerging therapeutic ultrasound techniques. The topics of this book include reviews of mechanisms for bioeffects of ultrasound relevant to therapeutic applications (Chap. II), high intensity focused ultrasound and its application in surgery (Chaps. V and VIII), ultrasound assisted target drug and gene delivery (Chaps. III, IV, VI) and transdermal drug delivery (Chap. VII). We believe that medical professionals, biomedical engineers, graduate students and others working in this multidisciplinary field will benefit by reading the exciting chapters written by our contributors, many of whom are pioneers in their fields.

Some techniques discussed in this book have already been used clinically. For example, extracorporeal ultrasound-guided high intensity focused ultrasound (HIFU) has been successfully used in treatment of patients with solid malignancy (Chap. VIII). From December 1997 to March 2004, approximately 3,500 patients received HIFU treatment of solid malignancies in 20 Chinese hospitals. The malignancies treated with HIFU include liver cancer, malignant bone tumors, breast cancer, soft tissue sarcomas, kidney cancer, pancreatic cancer, abdominal and pelvic malignant tumors, uterine fibroid, benign breast tumors, and hepatic hemangioma. When combined with MRI, an imaging modality of high resolution, HIFU may be further improved in its accuracy of locating tumors, as well as temperature monitoring and will eventually provide surgeons a "knife" of high precision without opening a patient's body (Chap. V).

Other techniques are still at the clinical trial stage. For example, professionals in several countries have shown that ultrasound can enhance the efficacy of thrombolytic agents to benefit acute stroke patients (Chap. IV). Transdermal drug delivery is another successful application of ultrasound. Clinical studies have already demonstrated that low-frequency ultrasound (20 kHz–100 kHz) can be effectively used in both transdermal drug delivery and glucose extraction applications (Chap. VII). Compared with traditional oral and injection drug administration methods, transdermal delivery can avoid gastro-intestinal side effects and can release drugs in a controlled fashion for a sustained period of time.

Gene therapy and targeted drug delivery are two promising technologies in medicine. They are evolving and will continue to change how medicine can be delivered. Although the development of ultrasound-directed drug and gene delivery is still in a research stage, their potential has already been demonstrated *in vitro* and *in vivo* (Chaps. III, IV and VI). Specificity in targeting is a unique characteristic of ultrasound techniques, compared with other delivery means such as electroporation and many viral techniques.

The ultrasonic techniques described in this book are still swiftly developing. It is our hope that this book will serve as a reference for this exciting field. Readers who are interested in learning more about techniques described in the various chapters can find further information in the comprehensive bibliographies provided.

References

Fry WJ. Intense ultrasound in investigations of the central nervous system, in Tobias CA, Lawrence JH (eds.) *Advances in Biological and Medical Physics* (1958) Academic Press: New York, pp. 281–348.

Nyborg WL. Biological effects of ultrasound: Development of safety guidelines. Part II: General review. *Ultrasound Med Biol* (2001) **27**: 301–333.

II

MECHANISMS FOR BIOEFFECTS OF ULTRASOUND RELEVANT TO THERAPEUTIC APPLICATIONS

Wesley L. Nyborg

Many studies have been made of changes that can be produced by exposure of biological systems to ultrasound (Nyborg, 2001; NCRP, 2002; Hill *et al.*, 2004). The systems include tissues and cell suspensions, as well as living plants and animals. With various medical and other applications in mind, the purpose has been to determine conditions under which biological effects occur, and to learn the mechanisms which are involved in producing them. This chapter reviews present knowledge on mechanisms, along with examples of bioeffects to which they apply, with emphasis on those which are, or may be, relevant to therapeutic applications.

1. Introduction

1.1. *General considerations*

Ultrasound is a form of sound whose frequency is higher than the natural audible range for humans; the latter is often considered to have an upper limit of about 20 kHz (For a listing of acoustical quantities and their units, see Table 1). In medical applications, the ultrasound is produced by the use of piezoelectric materials, *i.e.*, materials whose dimensions change when exposed to an electric field, or magnetostrictive materials, whose dimensions change when exposed to a magnetic field. The ultrasound generated in the piezoelectric or magnetostrictive material may pass directly to an object of interest; alternatively, it may pass through an intervening liquid

                                   W. L. Nyborg

Table 1. Acoustical quantities.

Quantity	Unit	Multiple	Conversions
Frequency (f)	hertz (Hz)	kilohertz (kHz) megahertz (MHz)	$1\,\text{kHz} = 10^3\,\text{Hz}$ $1\,\text{MHz} = 10^6\,\text{Hz}$
Time (t)	second (s)	millisecond (ms) microsecond (μs)	$1\,\text{ms} = 10^{-3}\,\text{s}$ $1\,\mu s = 10^{-6}\,\text{s}$
Displacement (ξ)	meter (m)	centimeter (cm) millimeter (mm) micrometer (μm)	$1\,\text{cm} = 10^{-2}\,\text{m}$ $1\,\text{mm} = 10^{-3}\,\text{m}$ $1\,\mu\text{m} = 10^{-6}\,\text{m}$
Particle velocity (u)	meter/second (m/s)	centimeter/ second (cm/s)	$1\,\text{cm/s} = 10^{-2}\,\text{m/s}$
Acoustic pressure (p)	pascal (Pa)	megapascal (MPa)	$1\,\text{MPa} = 10^6\,\text{Pa}$
Acoustic power (W)	watt (W)	milliwatt (mW) microwatt (μW)	$1\,\text{mW} = 10^{-3}\,\text{W}$ $1\,\mu\text{W} = 10^{-6}\,\text{W}$
Acoustic intensity (I)	watt/meter^2 (W/m^2)	watt/centimeter^2 (W/cm^2)	$1\,\text{W/cm}^2 = 10^{-4}\,(\text{W/m}^2)$

or, as another possibility, it may pass through a solid waveguide in the form of a cylinder, a tapered probe or a thin flexible rod or wire.

In discussing basic features of **ultrasound fields**, which are composed of **ultrasound waves**, it is useful to begin with simplified models and deal with the complications later. With this in mind, we represent schematically in Fig. 1 the situation involved when the object of interest is a suspension of biological cells or a region of tissue in an animal subject. Although the ultrasound may come to the object in a variety of ways, we assume, for definiteness, that it emanates from a disc of radius a with axis of symmetry along x which lies in the plane $x = 0$ when at rest. It is caused to vibrate sinusoidally in time so that its displacement ξ from its original position is given by $\xi_o \sin (2\pi ft)$; where ξ_o is the displacement amplitude, *i.e.*, the maximum value of the displacement. The velocity (u) of the surface is then given by the time derivative of the displacement, *i.e.*, by $u_o \cos(2\pi ft)$ where u_o is the velocity amplitude $2\pi f\xi_o$. For simplicity, we consider the displacement and velocity to be uniform over the disc, an approximation which is often acceptable.

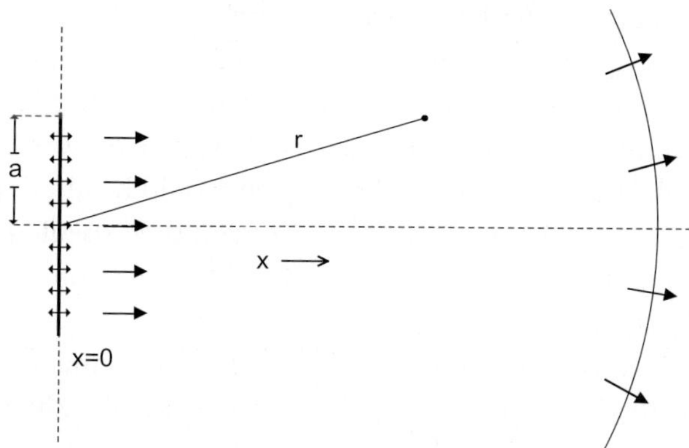

Fig. 1. Schematic of arrangement where a vibrating disc in the plane $x = 0$ produces ultrasound in the space to the right, which is filled with a medium of interest. The nature of the ultrasound field depends on the ratio of the disc radius to the acoustic wavelength. Rayleigh (1945) treated this problem, considering the disc to be one end of a vibrating piston, imposing the condition of zero motion along x in the plane $x = 0$ outside the disc; hence this situation is often described as a "piston in a baffle".

1.2. *Traveling plane wave*

Vibration of the source leads to the production of an ultrasound field in the region $x > 0$; the nature of the field depends on the ratio a/λ, where a is the source radius and λ the acoustic wavelength; the latter is equal to the ratio c/f, where c is the speed of sound in the medium (approximately 1500 m/s in water and in soft tissue). For example, at a frequency of 1 MHz in water, the wavelength λ is approximately 0.0015 m or 1.5 mm. In this subsection, we assume that the ratio a/λ is large; the ultrasound field near the source is then a beam of radius a that propagates as a plane traveling wave. We also assume that assumptions of linear acoustics prevail; consequences of nonlinearities are discussed later. In this beam, the particle velocity is only a function of x and t, being given as a solution $u(x, t)$ of the acoustical wave equation by

$$u(x, t) = u_o \cos(\omega t - kx) e^{-\alpha^* x}, \tag{1}$$

where $\omega = 2\pi f$ is the **angular frequency**, $k = 2\pi/\lambda$ is the **propagation constant** (or **wave number**) and α^* is the **attenuation coefficient**. As indicated by the quantity kx in the argument of the cosine function in Eq. (1), the particle velocity in the field varies sinusoidally with x as well as t. In plots of the velocity $u(x, t)$ *vs* the distance x at different times, the zeroes of velocity move outward from the source with exactly the speed $c = f\lambda$; if α^* is zero, the maxima and minima of velocity also move outward with exactly the same speed. If α^* is not zero, their speed would be altered somewhat, though for typical values of α^*, the change would be small. Thus, Eq. (1) represents an ultrasound wave moving outward from the source with a speed approximately equal to c.

The attenuation coefficient α^* represents processes that remove energy from the wave. In a homogeneous liquid, α^* reduces to the **absorption** coefficient α; the latter represents **absorption** processes which convert acoustic energy irreversibly into heat. In aqueous suspensions of cells or other particles, α^* includes scattering, a process whereby the particles disturb the wave and re-direct some of its energy to regions outside the beam. In water or dilute aqueous suspensions, the attenuation coefficient α^* is often negligible, and the multiplying factor $e^{-\alpha^* x}$ may be omitted from Eq. (1).

When a sound field is introduced into a liquid which is in equilibrium at atmospheric pressure P_o, the momentary (positive or negative) increase p in the pressure at any point, is defined as the local acoustic pressure there. The pressure gradient accompanying a sound field such as that represented by Eq. (1), exerts a force in the x direction per unit volume of the liquid in any locality equal to the local value of $-\partial p/\partial x$. By Newton's Law, this causes acceleration, such that the force per unit volume is equal to $\rho\, \partial u/\partial t$, where ρ is the local density. For the wave represented in Eq. (1), the acceleration can be obtained by differentiating the expression given, with respect to time. Equating the expression $\rho\, \partial u/\partial t$ so obtained to $-\partial p/\partial x$, and integrating the result with respect to x, one obtains, approximately,

$$p(x, t) = p_o \cos(\omega t - kx)e^{-\alpha^* x}, \tag{2}$$

where p_o, the pressure amplitude, is equal to $\rho c u_o$; the approximation made in the integration is appropriate if $\alpha^* \ll k$, which is usually true.

Energy is required to propagate a sound wave into a medium. Across the plane at any given distance x from the source, the medium on the near side does continuous work on, and thus transmits energy into, the medium on the far side. For the plane traveling wave represented by Eqs. (1) and (2), the time-averaged rate at which work is done across any such plane, per unit area, is the **intensity** (I) and is given by the time average of the product pu, *i.e.*, by

$$I = I_o e^{-2\alpha^* x}, \tag{3a}$$

where I_o can be written in any of the equivalent expressions:

$$I_o = 0.5 p_o u_o = 0.5 p_o^2 / \rho c = 0.5 \rho c u_o^2. \tag{3b}$$

The total work done by the source transducer per unit time is the acoustic **power** (W_o) expended; since the source is at $x = 0$ and the disc area is πa^2, one simply obtains,

$$W_o = \pi a^2 I_o. \tag{4}$$

An ultrasound wave such as is represented in Eqs. (1) and (2) is often referred to as a **continuous** (*CW*) wave. In many applications of ultrasound, the wave is pulsed, *i.e.*, delivered in segments of equal **pulse duration** (*PD*) at a fixed **pulse repetition frequency** (*PRF*). The **duty factor** (*DF*) is the fraction of time during which the ultrasound is "on" and is equal to the product $PD \times PRF$. The time-averaged acoustic power W_a delivered during a pulsed regime is equal to the product $W_o \times DF$, where W_o is the power delivered during a pulse.

In practice, another aspect of ultrasound fields makes them more complicated than the plane traveling wave represented by Eqs. (1) and (2); as discussed later, the pressure amplitude at the surface of a source transducer is not uniform over its surface, and the intensity is also nonuniform. The intensity averaged over time and over the source area is $W_a / \pi a^2$ and called I_{SATA}, the **spatial-average time-average** intensity at the source. The corresponding quantity averaged over the duration PD of a single pulse is the **spatial-average pulse-average** intensity I_{SAPA}.

In some applications, **the energy fluence** is found to be important (see Chap. VII; also, Guzmán, 2001). This quantity, designated as **F**, is defined as the total acoustic energy delivered per unit area during an application. In an exposure where CW ultrasound of intensity I_o is applied for time t, the energy fluence is just $I_o t$. If the ultrasound is pulsed, $I_o t$ is multiplied by the duty factor DF. For example, a biological effect occurs when it is exposed to an energy fluence F of 2 J/cm^2, if it occurs after an exposure to ultrasound of intensity 2 W/cm^2, pulsed with a duty factor of 0.2 for 5 s.

                               W. L. Nyborg

2. Thermal Considerations

2.1. *Temperature distributions: One dimension*

Since ultrasound can produce heat, it is not surprising that thermal mechanisms are often responsible for the biological effects of ultrasound. Pohlman (1951) was a pioneer in recognizing that ultrasound can be useful as a therapeutic agent, especially because of its capacity for producing heat in tissue. Lehmann (1990) and Michlovitz (1996) provide considerable information on the procedures followed in the applications of ultrasound as part of physical therapy programs. They also review many reports of findings from the use of ultrasound in the treatments of bursitis, back pain and other problems.

As anticipated, the attenuation of a traveling plane wave, represented by the attenuation coefficient α^*, is accompanied by heat production if it occurs partly or wholly because of absorption, represented by the absorption coefficient α, For illustrative purposes, if scattering can be ignored such that α can replace α^* in Eqs. (1)–(3), then the rate at which acoustical energy is irreversibly lost per unit volume by conversion into heat is given by $-dI/dx$, i.e., by $2\alpha I$. This is also equal to the rate q_v at which heat is produced per unit volume; thus, in a region of a traveling plane wave where the intensity is I we have

$$q_v = 2\alpha I. \tag{5}$$

[A more general expression for q_v is given in Eq. (18).] If heat is not transported into or out from this region by conduction or other means, the temperature will rise at the rate q_v/c_v, where c_v is the heat capacity per unit volume, and the temperature T after time t will be given by

$$T = (2\alpha I/c_v)t + T_o, \tag{6}$$

where T_o is the temperature at $t = 0$. For water and soft tissues c_v is approximately $4.2\,\mathrm{J\,cm^{-3}}$. For muscle fibers oriented perpendicular to ultrasound propagation, α has been measured to be $0.06\,\mathrm{Np\,cm^{-1}}$ at a frequency of 1 MHz. Hence, according to Eq. (6), when plane ultrasound waves of frequency 1 MHz and intensity $1\,\mathrm{W\,cm^{-2}}$ are transmitted through muscle, the temperature of the tissue should rise $0.029°\mathrm{C}$ in 1 s and $0.29°\mathrm{C}$ in 10 s, if no heat transport takes place.

Many experiments have been done in which tissues have been exposed to ultrasound and the temperature measured as a function of time. Examples

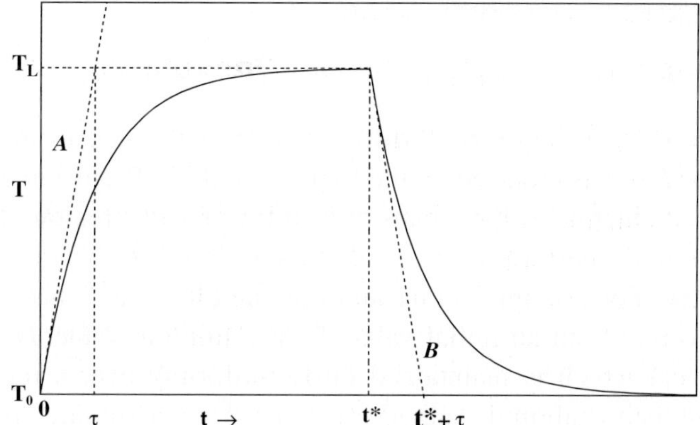

Fig. 2. Solid line shows time course of temperature (T) in a region where q_v and T are uniform spatially, so that Eqs. (8) and (9) apply. See text. The magnitude $|dT/dt|$ has the value $(T_L - T_o)/\tau$ immediately after both $t = 0$ and $t = t^*$, as indicated by dotted lines A and B, respectively.

are discussed in NCRP (1992). It is found that in a region where heat is being produced at a constant rate the temperature (T) does indeed increase linearly with time for a brief period after the exposure begins, as expected from Eq. (6) and as shown by dashed line A in Fig. 2. However, as time goes on, the region containing heat sources becomes warmer than other regions, and heat flows in the direction of decreasing temperature. The temperature T in the source region then rises at a slower rate, as indicated in Fig. 2, and Eq. (6) becomes no longer applicable.

The heat flow occurs partly because of **thermal conduction**, an inter-atomic mechanism by which heat transport will occur in any material; when this mechanism applies, the rate at which thermal energy passes across a surface per unit area is equal to the product of the temperature gradient normal to the surface and the coefficient of **thermal conductivity** K for the material. If the temperature gradient is in the x direction, the heat flow will be in the opposite direction and given by $-KdT/dx$ per unit area.

In mammalian tissue, heat is transported not only by conduction, but also by the flowing blood, a mechanism referred to as **blood perfusion** or **perfusion**. A differential equation was introduced by Pennes (1948) for analyzing situations where heat is generated and the transport of heat occurs by both conduction and perfusion. This equation, called the **bio-heat transfer equation** (BHTE), can be written for one-dimensional heat flow as

$$dT/dt = \kappa d^2T/dx^2 - (T - T_o)/\tau + q_v/c_v, \tag{7}$$

where $\kappa = K/c_v$ is the **thermal diffusivity**. (For 3-dimensional heat flow, the term d^2T/dx^2 is replaced by the Laplacian of T.) Perfusion will dominate over conduction as the means of heat transfer in a region, if the temperature is fairly uniform there, so that the term $\kappa d^2T/dx^2$ in Eq. (7) can be neglected. For example, let us suppose that ultrasound causes the temperature to rise from an initial value T_o to a limiting value T_L (equal to $T_o + q_v\tau/c_v$) which is maintained fairly uniformly over a region, until $t = t^*$ and then is abruptly turned off. For $t \geq t^*$, assuming $\kappa d^2T/dx^2$ is small, Eq. (7) then reduces to

$$dT/dt = -(T - T_o)/\tau, \tag{8}$$

of which a solution is

$$T = T_o + (T_L - T_o)e^{-(t-t^*)/\tau}. \tag{9}$$

The situation is shown in Fig. 2, where the temperature is seen to approach a limiting value T_L, then maintain a value near T_L until $t = t^*$, at which time the heat source is shut off and Eq. (9) applies. The values of $|-dT/dt|$ immediately after $t = 0$ and immediately after $t = t^*$ are both equal to $(T_L - T_o)/\tau$. In general, when the heat transport is primarily by perfusion time τ serves as a measure of the time required for perfusion to cause a change in temperature when there are changes in the heat sources,

In the formulation of the bio-heat transfer equation originally given by Pennes (1948), a quantity w based on direct measurements of blood flow was used instead of the time constant τ; the two quantities are inversely related as follows:

$$w = B/\tau, \quad B = \rho_b c_v/c_b, \tag{10}$$

where ρ_b is the blood density, while c_v/c_b is the ratio of the heat capacity of tissue to that of blood. Equation (10) is the basis of a method for determining w that was used by ter Haar and Hopewell (1983); their experiments involved exposure of pig thigh muscle to therapeutic ultrasound, while the tissue temperature was monitored with thermocouples. After the temperature elevation had reached several °C and had been maintained at this level for a brief period, the ultrasound was abruptly shut off. The initial rate of temperature decline $(-dT/dt)$ was then measured; equating this to $(T_L - T_o)/\tau$, it was possible to determine τ and hence w. Their values of w varied from 3.3 to 5.5 kg m^{-3}s^{-1}, corresponding to τ values varying from 320 to 190 s.

In a region where a steady-state temperature field is generated by heat sources outside the region, and heat is transported by a combination of perfusion and thermal conduction, the terms dT/dt and q_v/c_v in Eq. (7) are zero and the remaining equation can be written

$$d^2T/dx^2 = L^{-2}(T - T_o); \tag{11}$$

T_o is the temperature in the region when heat sources are absent, and $L = (\kappa\tau)^{0.5}$ is the **perfusion length constant**. A solution of Eq. (11) is

$$T = T_o + (T_1 - T_o)e^{-x/L}. \tag{12}$$

Equation (12) applies to a steady-state situation where heat flows in the x direction from a heated surface at $x = 0$ whose temperature is maintained at a constant value T_1. According to Eq. (12), the temperature falls off exponentially with distance, the gradient near the heated surface being given in magnitude by $(T_1 - T_o)/L$. See Fig. 3.

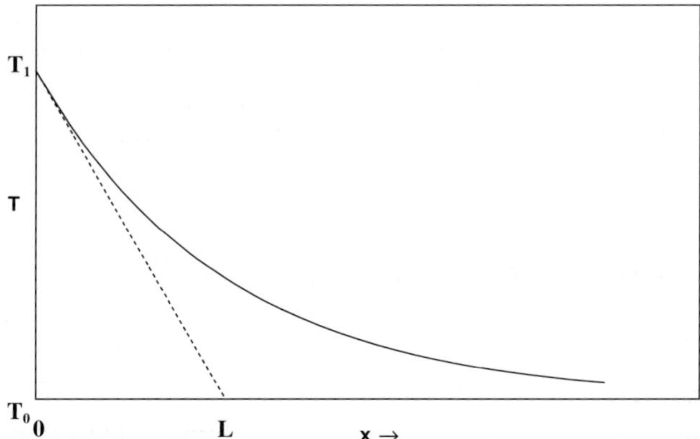

Fig. 3. Solid line shows steady-state temperature (T) in tissue with perfusion length (L) near heated surface at $x = 0$. Temperature gradient at this surface is $(T_1 - T_o)/L$. See Eq. (12).

The discussion above [Eqs. (11) and (12) together with Fig. 3] is relevant to the topic of transducer **self-heating**. A number of investigators have shown that the surfaces of transducers used to produce medical ultrasound become warm during applications (Williams *et al.*, 1987; Nyborg, 1988; Duck *et al.*, 1989; NCRP, 1992, 2002; Wu *et al.*, 1992, 1995); this self-heating comes about because of internal processes which convert some of the incoming electrical energy into heat. Hence consideration of the temperature fields produced during applications of ultrasound must include contributions from transducer self-heating. If a heated surface is in contact with tissue, the temperature of the adjoining tissue itself will be elevated throughout a layer of representative thickness L. For muscle in the forearm or thigh, L has been given as 16–18 mm (NCRP, 1992).

Among the various tissues of the body, bone has the highest value for the absorption coefficeient α and hence is given special attention when thermal effects of ultrasound are considered. Carstensen *et al.* (1990) did *in vivo* experiments in which 3.6 MHz ultrasound was focused on a portion of mouse skull into which a thermocouple had been inserted. Plots of the temperature *vs* time showed the temperature rising rapidly at first, then leveling off to a limiting value. The results agreed well with theory based on a solution of Eq. (7). A simplified form of the theory (with units chosen for convenience) was obtained for the limiting temperature rise $\Delta T_{\lim}$, namely.

$$\Delta T_{\lim} = W/4d_6, \tag{13}$$

where W is the total acoustic power in milliwatts impinging on the bone and d_6 is the -6 dB beam width in millimeters. Thus if the power is 60 mW and the beam width is 2.75 mm, the estimated limiting temperature rise is 5.4°C.

2.2. *Acoustic pressure distributions: Three dimensions*

2.2.1. *Piston in a baffle*

In the preceding equations and text, the emphasis has been on topics which can be treated by considering the ultrasound field to be a plane traveling wave propagating according to the assumptions of linear acoustics, and the temperature field to be one-dimensional. While important insight is gained in using the one-dimensional model, most applications require more general treatment. A more realistic representation of an ultrasound field is offered by a "piston-in-a-baffle" model, developed by Rayleigh (1945), which is often used and is suggested in Fig. 1. Ultrasound is produced in a homogeneous liquid by vibrations of a "piston" with surface of radius a; at rest, the surface lies in the plane $x = 0$ with axis of symmetry along the x axis. Surrounded by a motionless "baffle" in the same plane, the piston vibrates with frequency f and with velocity amplitude u_o which is uniform over the piston area. In calculating the resulting ultrasound field, the latter can be considered to be a sum of wavelets emanating from infinitesimal sources distributed over the face of the piston. The incremental contribution dp to the acoustic pressure at a point P that is at a distance r from any such infinitesimal source was given by Raleigh (1945), for an attenuation-free medium, by

$$dp = -\rho f u_o \, dS \, r^{-1} \sin(\omega t - kr), \tag{14}$$

where ρ is the liquid density and dS is the area of the elementary source; for applications to attenuating media such as soft tissues (where $\alpha^* \ll k$) the right hand side of Eq. (14) is multiplied by the factor $e^{-\alpha^* r}$ to obtain a useful approximation for soft tissues (Swindell *et al.*, 1982; Nyborg and Steele 1985). The total acoustic pressure at P is the sum of such contributions obtained by an integration over the entire area of the piston. Carrying out this integration is, in general, best done with the aid of a computer (as in examples seen later in Fig. 4), but there are important special cases where the analysis simplifies.

2.2.2. *Small source*

If the radius a of the piston is very small, the pressure amplitude p_o at the center is found to be

$$p_o = \rho c k a u_o. \tag{15}$$

Recalling Eqs. (1) and (2), we see that here the pressure amplitude is just ka times the value it has in a traveling plane wave. The nondimensional quantity ka is the ratio of the piston circumference $2\pi a$ to the wavelength λ. A condition for validity of Eq. (15) is that ka be much less than 1. A reasonable application of this approximation would be to the tip of a probe oscillating in water or tissue at a low ultrasonic frequency, the tip diameter being of the order of a few millimeters. It has been shown (Siegel,

1996; Siegel *et al.*, 1996; Tachibana and Tachibana, 1997) that this condition is commonly met by wire probes used in catheter-delivered ultrasound angioplasty; a tabulation of such probes shows tip diameters ranging from 0.8 to 2 mm and frequencies from 20 to 26 kHz. Supposing, that the radius a is 1 mm and f is 20 kHz, then λ is 7.5 cm and ka is 0.084. If the displacement amplitude ξ_o is 10 μm, the velocity amplitude $2\pi f\xi_o$ is 1.26 m/s, the pressure amplitude p_o in a traveling plane wave would be 1.9 MPa and, multiplying by 0.084, the calculated pressure amplitude at the center of the tip is found to be 0.16 MPa. The velocity amplitude is an important quantity in estimating the stresses exerted by microstreaming at the tip (see Sec. 4.2) and the pressure amplitude is important in determining the extent to which cavitation will occur during an application (see Secs. 5 and 6).

Equation (14) can also be used to estimate the acoustic power radiated into free space by a small source. At distances r, large compared to the wavelength, the relationships in Eq. (3b) apply locally, as in a plane traveling wave. Taking the area dS to be πa^2, assuming effects of attenuation can be neglected so that the pressure amplitude p_o is $\pi a^2 \rho f u_o r^{-1}$, and multiplying the intensity $p_o^2/2\rho c$ by the hemispherical area $2\pi r^2$, one obtains

$$W = \pi^3 a^4 \rho f^2 u_o^2/c. \tag{16}$$

Substituting previously assumed values for a, ρ, f and u_o, one obtains 13.1 mW for W.

2.2.3. *Acoustic field on the axis of a piston source*

In another special case, the analysis simplifies for points on the axis of a continuous piston source. It has been shown to follow from Eq. (14), modified for an attenuating media as indicated, that the acoustic pressure at a point P on the axis at any distance x from the piston is given approximately by

$$p = \rho c u_o[\cos(\omega t - kx)e^{-\alpha^* x} - \cos(\omega t - kx^*)e^{-\alpha^* x^*}], \tag{17}$$

where x^* is $(x^2 + a^2)^{0.5}$, *i.e.*, the distance from the point P to the edge of the disc. In Eq. (17), we see a rather surprising result: the acoustic pressure at any point on the axis is just the difference between contributions from two plane traveling waves, one coming from the center of the piston source, and the other (the "edge wave") from its edge. This means that

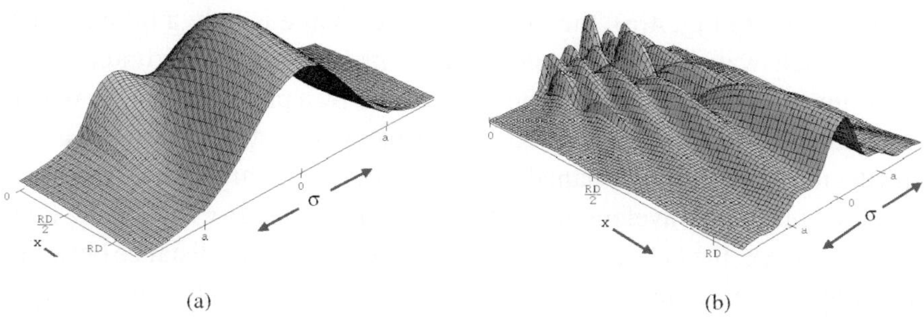

Fig. 4. Calculated spatial distribution of p_o^2 in waterlike medium produced by vibrating piston. (a) Radius $a = 0.8$ mm; $f = 1$ MHz; $\lambda = 1.5$ mm; $ka = 3.3$. (b) Radius $a = 4.0$ mm; $f = 1$ MHz; $\lambda = 1.5$ mm; $ka = 16.7$. RD = Rayleigh distance (see text).

a plot of pressure amplitude along the axis will show a series of minima corresponding (approximately) to points where the distances x and x^* differ by an even number of half wavelengths, and alternating with these, a series of maxima where the distance in half-wavelengths is approximately an odd number (when the attenuation is small there is little error in the approximation). It can be seen that if the disc radius a is very large compared to x, Eq. (17) reduces to Eq. (2), since the edge wave is highly attenuated. In another special case, if the waves are generated as very short pulses widely separated in time, the field on the axis near the source will consist partly of pulsed waves from the center and partly of edge-wave pulses, arriving separately because of the difference in path.

2.2.4. *Other situations*

When considering acoustic fields to which cells or tissues are exposed in therapeutic applications, it would of course be desireable to know the relevant acoustic parameters at all points in the region exposed. Unfortunately, the field is, by far, usually more complex than in the examples considered. The field of a sinusoidally vibrating circular "piston" source (Fig. 1) provides a very useful model of a CW field for many purposes, but it is necessary to recognize its various features. In general, the pressure distribution in such a field is not uniform, especially near the source.

Plots are shown in Fig. 4 of p_o^2, the square of the pressure amplitude, *vs* the distance x from the source and the radial distance σ from the axis of symmetry. In Fig. 4(a), the radius a of the source is only a little greater than the half-wavelength $\lambda/2$ and there is only one major maximum.

Figure 4(b) is typical of the field generated by a piston source for which the radius/wavelength ratio is larger. Here, a/λ is somewhat greater than 2.5 and the three peaks (ring-shaped because of the symmetry about the x axis) are about one half-wavelength apart in the source plane at $x = 0$. In the field near the source, the field quantity p_o^2 also varies with x, the distance between peaks at a given radial distance σ being also about one half-wavelength in this "near-field" region. However, as distance x increases, the spacing between peaks increases, the peaks decrease in magnitude and a simpler "far-field" distribution is approached. In the far-field (not shown in the Fig. 4), the pressure amplitude p_o at points on the axis falls off inversely with distance x and the relations in Eq. (3b) hold, as in a traveling plane wave. If the ratio a/λ is large, the transition between near-field and far-field occurs at a distance x approximately equal to the "Rayleigh distance" (RD), equal to a^2/λ, which is shown in Figs. 4(a) and 4(b).

In the near-field, the components of velocity are related to those of the pressure gradient according to the laws of motion, but the pressure-velocity relations are not the simple ones which apply in traveling plane continuous waves [Eqs. (1) and (2)]. As a consequence, the acoustic intensity varies through the field in a complex way, especially near the source. However, another special situation applies in the immediate vicinity of a piston source whose radius a is very large compared to the wavelength λ. Under these conditions, it has been shown (Morse 1981; Pierce 1994) that, in spite of the nonuniformity of the pressure, the total acoustic power W_o radiated by the piston is given approximately by Eq. (4) with the intensity given by $0.5\,\rho c u_o^2$. In practice, the spatial-average temporal-average intensity I_{SATA} at the surface of a piston-type ultrasound transducer is often obtained experimentally by first determining the output power W (*e.g.*, by using a radiation force technique; see Sec. 3.2), then dividing W by the area πa^2.

The quantity p_o^2 plotted in Fig. 4 is important to therapy applications, not only because cavitation (discussed later) depends on the acoustic pressure, but because of its relevance to heat production. While Eq. (4) provides a convenient means for determining the heat production in tissues or other media during exposure to ultrasound, it is strictly valid only for fields similar to traveling waves. In more complex fields, as in the near-field of a piston source, the intensity is not readily measurable and Eq. (5) is not applicable.

Instead, it was shown by Nyborg (1981) and also by Cavicchi and O'Brien (1984) that under a wide range of conditions, the rate q_v per unit volume at which heat is generated in a given locality, is determined by the pressure amplitude there; specifically, the expression

$$q_v = \alpha p_o^2 / \rho c \qquad (18)$$

is valid in homogeneous media where shear viscosity does not contribute appreciably to the absorption coefficient α. Situations where these conditions apply, as well as others where shear viscosity contributes to the absorption, are discussed by Nyborg (1986). Thus, for many conditions, the plots in Fig. 4 are plots of a quantity proportional to q_v.

Systems described in Chaps. III, IV, VI and VII for generating ultrasound can be represented, some accurately, others less so, by the "piston" model of Fig. 1. The effective a/λ ratios vary from less than 0.1 (as in catheter devices used for angioplasty; see Chap. IV) to values greater than 10 used for *in vitro* applications (see Chaps. III and VI), with intermediate values, as used in procedures for low-frequency transdermal drug delivery (Chap. VII). Space does not permit detailed discussion of the systems used in producing focused ultrasound, discussed especially in Chaps. V and VIII. These are not represented by Fig.1, of course. For them, the source is not "piston-like"; instead, the vibration varies in phase and amplitude according to a pattern designed to produce the focusing action desired. A wealth of information on the design and functioning of such systems is contained in the references provided in Chaps. V and VIII.

2.3. *Biological effects of heat: Reaction kinetics*

It has been shown that the changes produced in a tissue by increasing its temperature can often be explained in terms of reaction kinetics. Thus, Carstensen *et al.* (1974) followed Henriques (1947) in assuming accumulated tissue damage from exposure to temperature elevation for time t_e to be proportional to a **damage factor** Ω given by the integral from zero to t_e of $(t_o^{-1} e^{G(t)} dt)$, where

$$G(t) = (ER^{-1})(T_o^{-1} - T(t)^{-1}); \qquad (19)$$

$T(t)$ is the temperature at any given time t, T_o a reference temperature, R the gas constant (8.3 J/mol-deg C) and E the activation energy for the biochemical reaction which is assumed to cause the damage. Applying this reasoning to the prediction of thresholds for lesion production by focused ultrasound in mammalian brain, Carstensen *et al.* (1974) reported excellent agreement with experiments when E was chosen to be $560\,\mathrm{kJ\,mol^{-1}}$ and Ω to be 1.00. Lizzi and Ostromogilsky (1987) describe similar success in predicting thresholds for lesions in the eye.

A very useful result for comparing conditions required to produce a given amount of thermal damage is obtained by considering a special case in which the temperature is elevated by only a small amount above a reference value T_o, and is constant throughout a time interval. It is found that if the temperature elevation $(T - T_o)$ leads to an observable bioeffect in time t, the same effect will result from any other (small) temperature elevation $(T_1 - T_o)$ maintained for time t_1 given by

$$t_1 = tA^{\Delta T}, \tag{20}$$

where ΔT is the temperature difference $(T_1 - T)$ and where A is a constant involving the activation energy. Sapareto and Dewey (1984) showed that this relationship could be used in expressing conditions for treatment of cancer with hyperthermia. For exposing cells to temperatures less than $43°C$, they proposed 0.25 for the constant A, corresponding to a value of about $265\,\mathrm{kcal\,mol^{-1}\,°C^{-1}}$ for the activation energy E. With this choice, Eq. (20) expresses the simple rule that each increase (ΔT) of exposure temperature by $1°C$, leads to a decrease by a factor of four in the time required for the biological effect to occur. Miller and Ziskin (1989) found the same rule to be useful in representing conditions under which fetal damage occurred in experiments where pregnant mammals were exposed to elevated temperatures. [See also NCRP (1992).]

3. Acoustic Radiation Force and Related Topics

When the pressure amplitudes in an acoustic field are relatively low, the acoustic pressure p and particle velocity u may then vary nearly sinusoidally with time, as in Eqs. (1) and (2). If an ultrasound field impinges on an object under these conditions, any movement or deformation produced during the positive part of a cycle will be essentially reversed during the negative part, so that there is little or no net effect. At higher amplitudes, the field is altered by nonlinearity, and as a consequence, exposure of an object to ultrasound may cause irreversible changes. Solutions of the basic nonlinear equations are often expressed in series form. For example, the total pressure P may be written as

$$P = P_o + p_1 + p_2 + \cdots . \tag{21}$$

where P_o is the static pressure in the absence of sound, while $p_1, p_2, \ldots$ are functions of 1st order, 2nd order, *etc.* Similar expressions may be written for the components of the vector particle velocity $\boldsymbol{u}$, though there would usually be no term of zero order. The first-order functions are often sinusoidal functions of time; the second-order function then consist partly of a time-independent function and partly of a second-harmonic function, *i.e.*, a time-varying function with frequency twice of that of the first-order functions.

3.1. *Intensity and power*

Several quantities that are important in discussing physical, chemical or biological effects of interest are of "second-order" in that they are proportional to the product of two first-order quantities or to the square of a single first-order quantity. The acoustic intensity I, discussed in Sec. 1.2, is an example of such a second-order quantity; Eq. (3) show the proportionality of I to the combinations p_o^2, $p_o u_o$ or u_o^2. In Eq. (5), it is seen how I is related to q_v, an important quantity in connection with thermally produced biological effects. In Eq. (4), the relationship of I to the total power W is shown for a simple example.

3.2. *Radiation force and radiation pressure*

The power W is important for its relationship to another second-order quantity, the acoustic **radiation force** (F_{rad}), a time-independent quantity with the units of force. When a beam of ultrasound passes through a fluid in which the speed of sound is c and impinges on an absorbing (nonreflecting) object in an open vessel, the object responds as if a steady force were acting on it; this "effective force" is called the **radiation force**; it is given simply by

$$F_{\mathrm{rad}} = W/c, \tag{22}$$

where W is the total power absorbed by the object. If the surface of the absorbing object is a plane surface on which a beam of area S impinges normally, the **radiation pressure** averaged over S is W/cS. If, instead of being an absorber, the object acts as a perfect reflector on which the wave is normally incident, the expressions for F_{rad} and p_{rad} should each be multiplied by a factor of two, with W representing the total incident power.

Wang and Lee (1998) provided a recent discussion of the basic theory for radiation pressure and power. Beissner (1993) and Wu (1995) provided information to be considered when using radiation force techniques to measure the power output of ultrasonic devices. Carson *et al.* (1978) published data, obtained by the use of Eq. (22), on the acoustic power output of many commercial diagnostic ultrasound devices which became the basis for standards in the USA.

A number of publications report studies in which pulsed ultrasound becomes audible to humans when the ultrasound directed to sensory organs, apparently because of acoustic radiation force applied during each pulse. For example, Fig. 5 shows results of experiments by Tsirulnikov *et al.* (1988), in which 2.5 MHz focused ultrasound was delivered to the human

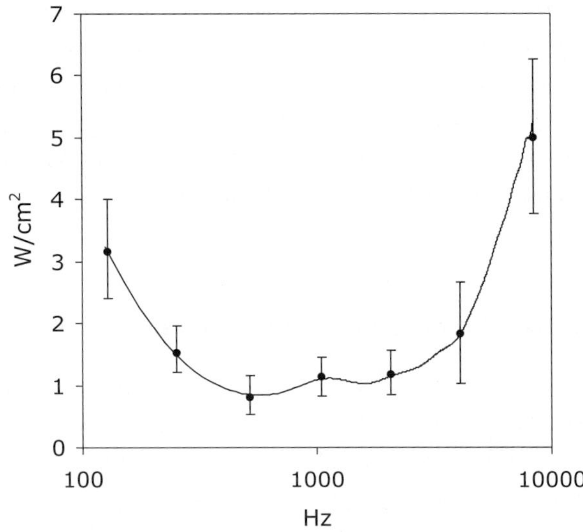

Fig. 5. Intensity threshold for hearing of sinusoidally modulated 2.5 MHz ultrasound applied to the middle ear *vs* modulation frequency. The mechanism is believed to be acoustic radiation force. See text (from Tsirulnikov *et al.*, 1988, with permission).

ear labyrinth in pulses of 50–100 μs in duration. The plot shows the intensities (in $W\,cm^{-2}$) found to be required for making these pulses audible, for pulse repetition frequencies varying from 125 Hz to 8000 Hz. The frequencies of greatest sensitivity were in the vicinity of 500 Hz, for which the required intensity was about $1\,W\,cm^{-2}$. The authors estimate the focal area of the ultrasound beam to have been about $1.75\,mm^{-2}$; hence, according to Eq. (22), the radiation force F_{rad} corresponding to $1\,W\,cm^{-2}$ at the focus is $12\,\mu N$ and the radiation pressure p_{rad} is 6.7 Pa.

In other studies, Dalecki *et al.* (1995) applied pulsed unfocused 2.2 MHz ultrasound to selected sites on the right index finger or right forearm of human volunteers and observed responses under various conditions. As the intention was to study the role of radiation force in producing the responses, the sites of interest were covered with small discs which totally reflected the incident acoustic power, and also prevented heat generation in the tissue. The radiation force F_{rad} was then calculated by using a modified Eq. (22) in which W was replaced by $2\,W$. When exposures were made with square-wave modulation at pulse repetition frequencies of 50, 100, 200, 500 and 1000 Hz, it was found that the maximum tactile sensitivity was at 200 Hz, for which the threshold value of F_{rad} was about 0.4 mN.

Further evidence that radiation force can sometimes be a primary mechanism for producing biological change with ultrasound was obtained by Mihran *et al.* (1990), during *in vitro* investigations of myelinated frog sciatic nerve. It was found that 500 μs pulses of 2, 4 or 7 MHz ultrasound focused on a small area of nerve trunk caused reproducible changes in the action potentials generated by electric stimuli. It was concluded that the temperature increases caused by the ultrasound were too small to be responsible for the effects, instead, the effects were mechanical in origin, resulting from the stretching of the nerve membranes by acoustic radiation force. Theoretical estimates of the force F_{rad} yielded 0.21 μN, 0.41 μN and 0.72 μN for the 2 MHz, 4 MHz and 7 MHz pulses respectively. Support for this conclusion came from experiments in which similar results were obtained when the ultrasound pulses were replaced by equivalent mechanical pulses from a transducer-driven glass rod whose tip (3 mm diameter) was pressed against the nerve trunk.

Since medical procedures often involve exposure of the fetal or adult heart to ultrasound, it is obviously important to understand as well as possible the conditions under which the cardiac function may be affected by exposure to ultrasound. Dalecki *et al.* (1997) carried out experiments on frog heart with 5 ms pulses of 1.2 MHz focused ultrasound, with the purpose of learning mechanisms and thus gaining understanding of ways in which ultrasound can affect heart performance. It was found that when the heart was exposed to these pulses, the results depended on when the exposure occured. If the pulses were applied during diastole (the expansion phase), premature ventricular contractions (PVCs) might occur; if applied during systole (contraction phase), the blood pressure in the aorta might decrease. To determine whether acoustic radiation force might be involved in producing these effects, the experiments were repeated while a thin acoustic reflector covered the frog; this allowed the radiation force to be transmitted while eliminating direct interaction of ultrasound with the tissue, and thus prevented heating. (Cavitation, discussed in Sec. 5, was also prevented.) It was found that with the reflector in place, the PVCs no longer occurred during diastole, but the decrease in aortic pressure still occurred during systole. However, the reduction of the latter was less with the reflector in place, apparently because the force was distributed differently. It was concluded that the mechanism for the aortic pressure decrease was indeed acoustic radiation force and it was estimated from theory that the minimum value of F_{rad} for producing these changes with 5 ms pulses was about 1 mN. (The mechanism for the PVCs was sought in other experiments, discussed in Sec. 5.)

In exploring applications of ultrasound to the eye, where 0.1 s pulses of 9.8 MHz ultrasound were focused on the choroid of rabbit eye, Lizzi *et al.* (1981) observed that blood flow was interrupted in the focal area where the intensity was about 100 W/cm^2. It was concluded that radiation force exerted on the local blood vessels was the cause.

3.3. *Radiation force on small particles*

Ultrasound produces effects of another kind by means of time-averaged forces which are exerted on biological cells or on other particles suspended in liquids. The basis for such forces was expressed by Gor'kov (1962) in an equation for the acoustic radiation force on a spherical particle of volume v in a medium where the time averaged densities of the kinetic energy density $\langle E_k \rangle$ and potential energy $\langle E_p \rangle$ are known. Letting β be the ratio of the compressibility ρ_s of the particle to that ρ_o of the surrounding medium, Gor'kov's equation, applied to the x component F_x of the force, is

$$F_x = vD^*d\Phi/dx, \qquad (23a)$$

where

$$D^* = 3(\rho_s - \rho_o)/(2\rho_s + \rho_o); \quad \Phi = \langle E_k \rangle - (1 - \beta)\langle E_p \rangle. \qquad (23b)$$

Many experiments to which this theory applies have been done by generating ultrasound in arrangements where reflections occur and standing waves are established. A perfect standing wave can be formed in a non-attenuating liquid, if a wave such as the one represented by Eq. (1) (but with $\alpha^* = 0$) is superposed on another which is the same except that it travels in the "$-x$" direction (represented in the equations by replacing the argument "$\omega t - kx$" with "$\omega t + kx$"), obtaining

$$u(x, t) = 2u_o \cos kx \cos \omega t. \qquad (24)$$

The time-averaged kinetic energy $\langle E_k \rangle$ is proportional to the square of the particle velocity amplitude; since the velocity amplitude is just $2\, u_o \cos kx$ in the standing wave field, maxima of $\langle E_k \rangle$ occur one-half wavelength apart, *i.e.*, when $\cos kx$ is equal to ± 1. Since the net energy transported in a perfect standing wave is zero, it follows that d $\langle E_p \rangle/dx$ is equal and opposite to $d\langle E_k \rangle/dx$. Most biological cells in saline solution or in body fluids are more dense and less compressible than the surrounding fluid; for these, $D^* > 1$ and $\beta < 1$. Hence, F_x is in the direction of increasing $\langle E_k \rangle$. Thus, theory predicts that when a plane standing wave of ultrasound is established in a cell suspension, the cells will migrate toward planes where $\langle E_k \rangle$ is maximum, *i.e.*, toward planes separated by a distance of $\lambda/2$ (one-half wavelength).

Many investigators have found the above prediction to be confirmed. When cell suspensions are exposed to ultrasound under conditions where the field resembles a one-dimensional standing wave, the cells tend to gather into equally spaced layers with $\lambda/2$ as the inter-layer distance. The speed at which the layers form depends on the size, density and compressibility of the cell, a fact which has been utilized in techniques for cell separation. (Allman and Coakley, 1994; Benes *et al.*, 1993; Hawkes and Coakley, 1996; Weiser and Apfel, 1982; Whitworth and Coakley, 1992).

It was discovered by Dyson *et al.* (1971, 1974) that similar behavior of cells can occur *in vivo*. They used an arrangement suitable for viewing blood flow in vessels during exposure to ultrasound. In this arrangement, chick embryos, dissected from the yolk, were transferred to an irradiation chamber on a microscope stage; ultrasound of frequency 1, 3 or 5 MHz from a transducer at one end of the chamber was projected across the stage and reflected from the wall at the opposite end. Applying continuous ultrasound at an acoustic pressure level of about 0.2 MPa (corresponding to a plane wave intensity of about $1\,\mathrm{W\,cm^{-2}}$) for a few tenths of a second, the normal blood flow ceased and a series of parallel red stripes or bands formed across the embryo. It was observed that this was generally a reversible effect; the bands disappeared soon after the irradiation ceased. Sometimes, however, small vessels seemed to be permanently blocked. Similar results were obtained in further experiments by ter Haar and Wyard (1978); see Fig. 6.

The latter authors also measured the rate at which bands were formed under various conditions and compared measured results with expectations from computations, based on the assumption that the motion was governed

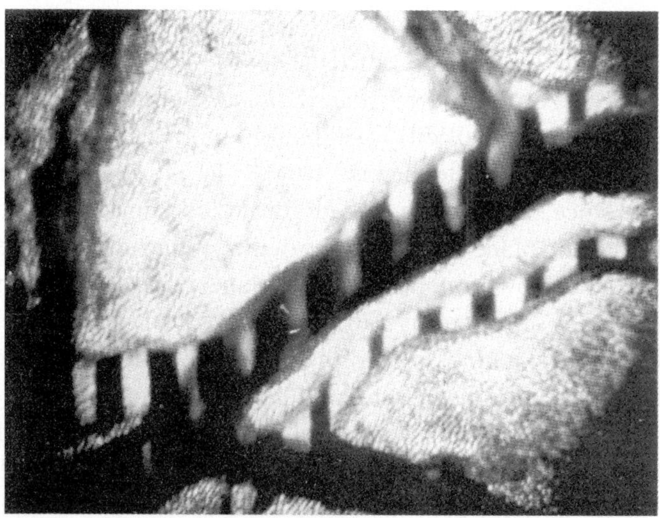

Fig. 6. Bands of red blood cells in blood vessels of chick embryos, formed by radiation force in 3 MHz ultrasound standing waves. See text. [From ter Haar and Wyard (1978) with permission.]

by Eq. (23). If a particle of effective radius, r_{eff}, is driven through a viscous fluid by a radiation force given by Eq. (23), proportional to $(r_{\text{eff}})^3$, and is subject to a drag force given by Stoke's Law, proportional to r_{eff}, the speed expected is proportional to $(r_{\text{eff}})^2$. Comparing theory of this kind with measured speeds, ter Haar and Wyard concluded that the bands formed more quickly than they would have, if the particles forming them were no larger than red cells. They proposed that the ultrasound caused cells to combine and that the aggregates so formed traveled to the maxima of $\langle E_k \rangle$ to form the bands. The proposal that the cells combined to form aggregates is consistent with the theory for another kind of acoustic radiation force, namely, the force between two small spheres in a sound field (Nyborg and Gershoy, 1973). According to this theory, the force is repulsive if the axis connecting the two spheres is parallel to the direction of oscillatory motion in the sound field, and is attractive if the axis is perpendicular to the oscillatory motion. The consequence is that cells in a suspension exposed to an ultrasound field tend to form linear aggregates perpendicular to the direction of oscillatory motion. The fact that linear aggregates are indeed formed is shown by an example in Fig. 7 from Miller (1976). These aggregates are strikingly similar to the "pearl chains", shown by Herrick (1958) to form when cells are exposed to microwave radiation A theoretical criterion for

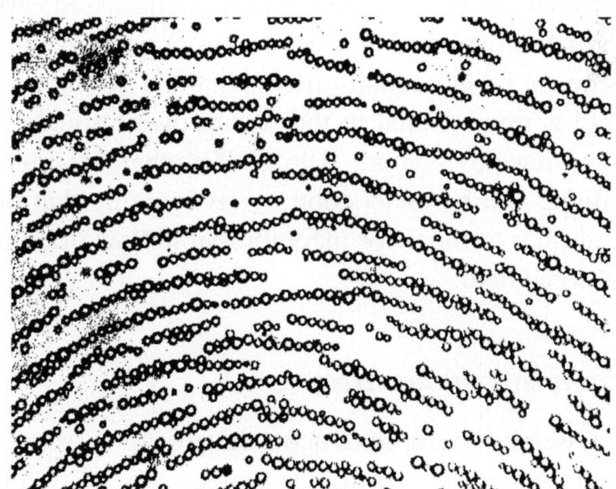

Fig. 7. Linear aggregates ("pearl chains") of sphered erythrocytes formed in a 1 MHz ultrasound field. See text (From Miller, 1976).

the formation of such aggregates in an ultrasound field was derived by Nyborg (1989), following procedures developed by Schwan (1982) for the analogous process of "pearl chain" formation by electromagnetic radiation. The pressure amplitudes used by ter Haar and Wyard (1978) are found to be fully adequate in satisfying the above criterion.

A novel application of Eq. (23) is to a manipulative technique ("acoustic tweezers") for trapping and positioning a small biological object of interest (Wu, 1991). This technique utilizes two ultrasound beams, opposing each other so that their focal regions are superposed and form the desired trap. Hu (2004) cites later developments of ultrasonic methods based on radiation force, for manipulating cells and the other small objects. In particular, he describes working details of a new technique based on the tweezers concept.

4. Acoustic Streaming and Acoustic Radiation Torque

When a sound field is produced in a liquid or gaseous medium by a source operating continuously at a fixed frequency, the motion in the medium consists not only of an oscillatory part [as exemplified in Eq. (1)] but also includes a steady (*i.e.*, time-independent) flow called **acoustic streaming**, or if it is of a small scale, **acoustic microstreaming**. Like other acoustical quantities (intensity, power, radiation force) discussed earlier, acoustic streaming is commonly treated as a second-order quantity mathematically. One consequence of being second-order is that the flow speed at any point in a sound field is proportional to the square of the source amplitude. It was shown in reviews by Nyborg (1965, 1998) that important features of acoustic streaming can be understood by recognizing that the governing equations are similar to those for incompressible flow of a fluid produced by an external force field.

4.1. *Quartz-wind streaming*

A commonly observed example of acoustic streaming, sometimes known as "quartz wind", occurs when a source projects a beam of ultrasound into a tube containing an absorbing fluid. The theory for this situation was first derived by Eckart (1948). In a simplified treatment, the ultrasound field can be considered to be a traveling wave, confined to the central region of the tube, which propagates without reflection; within the beam the acoustic pressure, particle velocity and intensity are as given in Eqs. (1)–(3). According to Eq. (5), the rate (q_v) at which energy is lost from the beam per unit volume is $2\alpha I$. Hence, extending the idea expressed in Eq. (22), the radiation force in the propagation direction exerted on the unit volume of the liquid at each point in the beam is $2\alpha I/c$, and the total force would be obtained by an integration over the entire beam. As might be expected, the force produces flow along the axis in the direction of propagation, with return flow in the outer region. The expression obtained by Eckart (1948) for the velocity, U_o, along the axis can be written as

$$U_o = \alpha W\Phi/\pi\eta c, \tag{25}$$

where W is the total power in the beam, η is the coefficient of shear viscosity for the liquid, and Φ is a function of the beam and the tube diameters. It is seen that for given values of the power W and the function Φ, the velocity U_o is proportional to the ratio α/η. It has been noted (NCRP, 2002) that this ratio is about 30 times greater in blood than in water or in fluids such as urine or amniotic fluid that are acoustically similar to water. Even in the latter fluids, the ratio α/η can become very high under conditions of nonlinear propagation. "Quartz-wind" type acoustic streaming can occur when a beam of ultrasound passes through the bladder or any other part of a patient's body where a sizeable pool of fluid exists. Stavros and Dennis (1993) reported that benign breast cysts can be distinguished from others by observation of the flow produced within the cyst by ultrasound. Later, Nightingale *et al.* (1999) carried out a more extended clinical study confirming this possibility and determining the conditions for most effective use.

Under some circumstances, the convection associated with quartz-wind streaming can affect rate processes such as heat transport or chemical reactions. It was shown by Wu *et al.* (1994) in *in vitro* experiments that the temperature produced when an ultrasound beam impinges on bone in an arrangement which allows acoustic streaming to convect heat away, was much lower than in arrangements where the convection was prevented.

4.2. *Near-boundary streaming*

In Eckart's theory for acoustic streaming, it is assumed, for simplicity, that the ultrasound is generated in a homogeneous fluid and is strictly confined

                    W. L. Nyborg

to a cylindrical space projected forward from the source which does not intersect the wall of the tube. In this situation, the radiation force which causes the streaming is confined to the same cylindrical space. Under other conditions, the ultrasound field of interest is in the vicinity of boundaries which affect both the oscillatory motion and the steady flow. A streaming situation of this kind, which has probably received more attention than any others, is that of the infinite solid cylinder, vibrating transversely in a viscous liquid (Fig. 8). Theory has been given for this by Holtzmark *et al.* (1954) and by Raney *et al.* (1954). The cylinder vibration sets up an oscillatory motion in the liquid which is typically subject to steep gradients near the cylindrical surface because of the non-slip condition which typically applies there. A boundary layer is established at that point with characteristic thickness δ given by

$$\delta = (\eta/\pi\rho f)^{0.5} \tag{26}$$

where η is the coefficient of shear viscosity, ρ is the density and f the frequency. At a frequency of 1 MHz in water, the boundary layer thickness δ is 0.56 μm. Due to time-averaged forces established in the boundary layer,

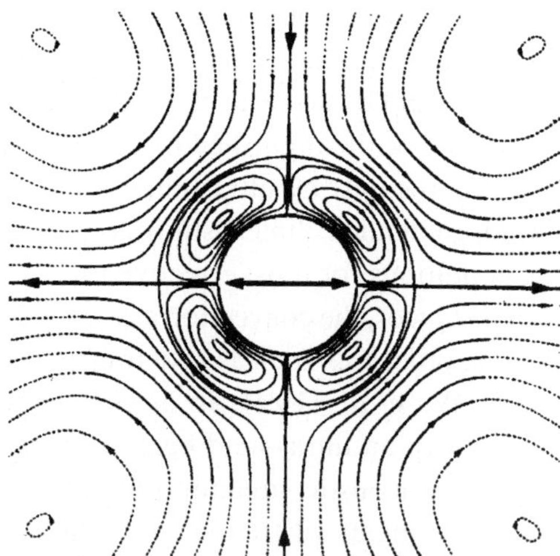

Fig. 8. Acoustic streaming near a vibrating cylinder. Double-headed arrow at center shows direction of cylinder oscillation. Other arrows show direction of steady fluid flow. See text (Adapted from Holtzmark *et al.*, 1954, with permission). The flow relative to the cylinder is similar to that for a fixed cylinder in an oscillating fluid.

a pattern of streaming is established as shown in the figure. It was shown by Westervelt (1953, 1955) that, to the usual second-order approximation, the streaming is the same (relative to the cylinder) for a cylinder oscillating in a quiescent fluid, as for a cylinder fixed in an oscillating fluid. Wang (1982) developed analogous theory for the streaming near a rigid sphere which vibrates relative to the surrounding fluid. The topic has been reviewed by Nyborg (1965, 1998).

Streaming occurs in four symmetrical counter-rotating circulations as shown in Fig. 8. The "Schlichting approximation" gives the simplest analysis; this holds when the amplitude of the oscillation and the boundary layer thickness δ [see Eq. (26)] are each small, compared with the cylinder radius a_c. Using this approximation, an expression is obtained for the maximum velocity gradient at the surface of the cylinder; from the product of this with η, the coefficient of shear viscosity, the maximum viscous stress $S_{\max}$ at the boundary is found to be

$$S_{\max} = \eta u_o^2 / \omega a_c \delta, \tag{27}$$

where u_o is the velocity amplitude of the cylinder vibration and $\omega = 2\pi f$. Small-scale acoustic streaming, of this kind, often named **microstreaming** or **boundary-layer streaming**, which occurs near a small vibrating cylinder or sphere, and in other related situations, has been found capable of producing biological effects in a variety of *in vitro* experiments which have been reviewed by Williams (1983). In an experiment by Williams *et al.* (1970), a tungsten wire of 0.025 cm in diameter was set into transverse vibration at a frequency of 20 kHz, while immersed in a suspension of human or canine erythrocytes in a saline-dextran solution with shear viscosity coefficient (30 times that of water) of 0.3 poise (0.03 Pa s). From Eq. (26), the boundary layer thickness δ for these conditions was 22 μm. Five minute exposures led to detectable hemolysis when the vibration amplitude exceeded a threshold value of about 20 μm, corresponding to a velocity amplitude u_o of 2.5 m/s. According to Eq. (27), the threshold value of the stress $S_{\max}$ was 560 Pa. The hemolysis increased rapidly as the amplitude was increased, *i.e.*, >90% when an amplitude of 30 μm was used.

In other *in vitro* experiments reviewed by Williams (1983), it is shown that microstreaming generated with vibrating wires, needles and specially constructed probes, operating at frequencies from 20 kHz to 1 MHz, can

produce effects such as reduction of protozoan motility, release of sero-
tonin from human platelets, and deformation of nuclei within eggs of marine
invertebrates. Crowell *et al.* (1977) carried out a 5-minute 20 kHz vibrating-
wire experiments with suspensions containing white blood cells and bacteria, and in calculations based on these, calculated the stress threshold for
microstreaming-produced lysis of the white cells to be 50 Pa. Also, functional effects occurred for which the threshold was much less; for example,
the antibacterial index for the white cells was reduced by an amount that
increased approximately linearly with vibration amplitude ξ_o, and thus the
threshold for the effect was not significantly different from zero. In addition,
it was found for amplitudes ξ_o below the threshold for lysis that bacteria
tended to collect on the surfaces of the white cells, as if the latter had been
made "sticky".

Directly relevant to the topics of this book is the demonstration of
reparable sonoporation produced in Jurkat lymphocytes *via* microstreaming
near a small vibrating horn tip at 21 kHz (Wu *et al.*, 2002), using a range of
amplitudes and exposure times; from calculations, it was estimated that the
change in permeability was produced when the lymphocytes were subjected
to a viscous stress of 12 Pa or more for 7 minutes.

In vivo experiments have included production of eddies and consequent
formation of platelet thrombi within blood vessels, by pressing the tip of a
vibrating probe against the vessels (Williams, 1983). In general, the opac-
ity of most mammalian tissue makes it difficult to observe microstreaming which may be produced in such tissues by ultrasound. However, it is
expected to occur wherever there is fluid, especially if the ultrasound field
is non-uniform. For example, ultrasound would be expected to produce
eddying in the blood near sharp edges of fractured bone, and thus might be
involved in procedures where low intensity ultrasound is used to enhance
the healing of bone fractures (NCRP, 2002).

5. Activation of Gas Bodies; Cavitation; Bubbles

In the early experiments with physical, chemical and biological effects of
ultrasound in liquid media during the 1920s and 1930s, it was discovered
that many of these were caused by **cavitation**, an activity which depends
on the presence of small bubbles, *i.e.*, cavities filled with gas or vapor.

The cavitation could be destructive by eroding solid surfaces or could be beneficial by killing bacteria on surgical instruments. The bubbles which caused the effects became visible by growth from microscopic or submicroscopic ones, called "cavitation nuclei", which are usually present in cracks or other irregularities on container walls, or on small impurity particles. In time, methods were developed to control the production and distribution of bubbles. The last decade has seen the industrial production of specially coated gas bodies of controlled size small enough for insertion into blood vessels; these serve as ultrasound contrast agents (*UCAs*) in the applications of diagnostic ultrasound. The UCAs are also promising in techniques for modifying cells in medical applications.

Mathematical theory for the behavior of small gas-filled cavities has been developed, starting from basic equations of motion. It is useful to distinguish between two categories of cavity activation in a sound field. In **inertial cavitation**, produced when the pressure amplitude is above a threshold level, a cavity may implode violently; if its contents are gases of low molecular weight, very high temperatures may result during implosions and highly reactive free radicals may be generated. For some biological effects, inertial cavitation seems to be required. However, it has been found that under other conditions, biological effects of interest can be produced by means of a less violent **non-inertial** activity of bubbles in which implosions are avoided. In discussing the manifold aspects of bubble activity which can be produced by ultrasound, attention is now first given to relationships which apply when the acoustic pressure is of moderate level. Under these conditions, the relevant theory can be obtained from approximations of first-order and second-order to the basic equations of motion. For dealing with effects which occur at higher levels, it is necessary to obtain and use more exact solutions by computational techniques.

5.1. *Bubble dynamics; moderate amplitudes*

Consider a small bubble in a body of liquid where a continuous ultrasound field is present in which the acoustic pressure is given by $p_o \cos(2\pi ft)$. If the pressure amplitude p_o is not too high, the bubble volume will vary approximately sinusoidally in time with the same frequency. The linear response of an air bubble in water was first analyzed by Minnaert (1933);

biophysical implications are discussed by Coakley and Nyborg (1978) and there is a recent thorough discussion of the topic by Leighton (1994). Letting $R(t)$ be the radius of the bubble at any time t when the sound is present, and R_o its radius in the absence of sound, the displacement $\xi(t)$ at any time t is $R(t) - R_o$, and can be written as

$$\xi(t) = \xi_o \cos(\omega t - \alpha), \tag{28}$$

where ξ_o is the displacement amplitude and α is a phase constant. It is found that the dimensionless quantities ξ_o/R_o and $(p_o/3\gamma P_o)$ are proportional to each other according to the relationship

$$\xi_o/R_o = (p_o/3\gamma P_o)\chi(\Omega, \delta), \tag{29a}$$

where γ is the ratio of specific heats for the gas in the bubble, P_o is the static pressure in the absence of sound, and

$$\chi(\Omega, \delta) = [(1 - \Omega^2)^2 + \Omega^2\delta^2]^{-0.5}; \tag{29b}$$

Ω is the ratio f/f_o, where f_o is the **resonance frequency** of the bubble and δ its **damping constant**.

Figure 9 shows χ plotted against Ω for several values of δ; at resonance, Ω reduces to unity and $\chi(\Omega, \delta)$ to δ^{-1}. The resonance frequency depends on properties of the gas, the liquid and the gas/liquid interface as seen in the equation:

$$f_o = (1/2\pi)(k_s/m)^{0.5}, \tag{30}$$

where k_s is the "stiffness" and "m" the "mass", by analogy to the mass–spring combination whose resonance characteristics are a traditional topic in physics courses. The mass m is determined by the density ρ_o of the liquid outside the bubble and is given specifically by $4\pi R_o^3\rho_o$; thus, m is equal to just three times the mass of water which could fill the bubble when it is not vibrating. The stiffness k_s depends on the nature of the interface at the bubble surface. If there is a thin film or shell at this surface, as there is for a typical UCA, properties of the surface material must be taken into account. If the surface is free, and is simply an interface between the gas in the bubble and the liquid outside, the surface tension σ at the surface may be important. However, if the radius R_o is much larger than $2\sigma/P_o$, the

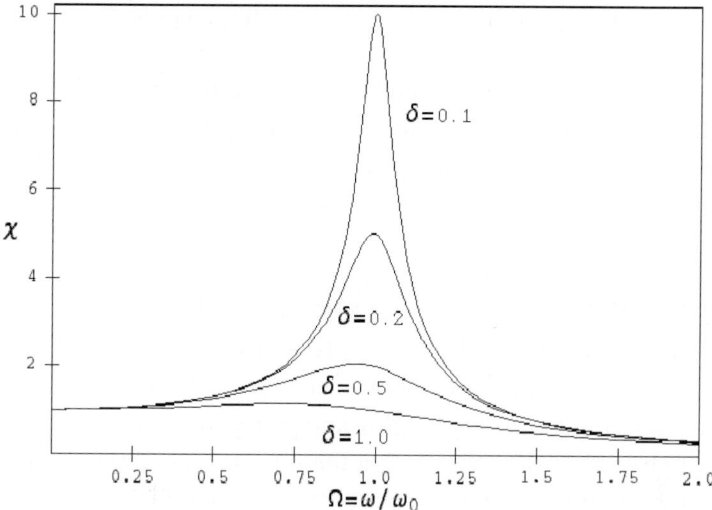

Fig. 9. Nondimensional vibration amplitude (χ) of gas-filled sphere *vs* nondimensional frequency (f/f_o) for several values of the damping constant (δ). See Eq. (29).

effect of surface tension is negligible and the stiffness is given by

$$k_s = 12\pi\gamma R_o P_o,\tag{31}$$

where γ is the polytropic index for the gas. For air or other diatomic gases, this index varies from 1.4 (if volume changes occur adiabatically) to 1.0 (if they occur isothermally). It has been shown by de Jong (1992) that for a UCA which is encapsulated by a thin shell at its surface, the expression for k_s should be modified by adding to P_o a term that depends on the elastic properties of the shell. For a free air-filled bubble in water whose radius R_o is large enough to satisfy the above criterion for validity of Eq. (29), the resonant frequency is given by the simple formula

$$f_o = 3.28/R_o;\tag{32}$$

here f_o is in kHz when R_o is in mm; it is assumed that $\gamma = 1.4$. For a free bubble or UCA resonant in the megahertz range it is necessary to take surface tension into account and the relationship is modified from that in Eq. (32). In a review of the topic (Table A.1, Chap. VI), the radii for resonance at 1 MHz and 3 MHz are given as 3.2 μm and 1.2 μm respectively for a free air bubble in water, and as 6.5 μm and 3 μm for a contrast agent with shell encapsulation.

As seen in Fig. 9, in plots of displacement amplitude ξ_o *vs* frequency, the heights of the maxima decrease and the breadths increase with increasing values of the damping constant δ. The latter quantity depends on the size of the bubble, and also for UCAs, on the properties of the encapsulating layer. The topic has been reviewed by Coakley and Nyborg (1978) and by de Jong (1992). Representative values of δ at resonance have been given (NCRP, 2002, Table 4.1) for frequencies of 1 MHz and 3 MHz respectively as 0.13 and 0.19 for free bubbles, and as 0.25 and 0.85 for shell-encapsulated UCAs.

As the bubble vibrates, it removes energy from the local sound field, partly by scattering it out of the region and partly by converting the acoustic energy into heat. It can be shown that the time-averaged rate W at which a single resonant bubble removes energy from the field is

$$W = R_o p_o^2 / \rho \delta f_o, \tag{33}$$

where p_o is the local pressure amplitude. For comparison, in Eq. (18), the rate q_v per unit volume at which absorption processes remove energy from a plane wave traveling through a homogeneous medium is given as $\alpha p_o^2 / \rho c$, where α is the absorption coefficient for the medium. Thus, n identical resonant bubbles per unit volume would remove energy from a traveling wave at the same rate as the absorption mechanisms in a homogeneous medium with absorption coefficient α if

$$n = \alpha \delta f_o / c R_o. \tag{34}$$

Here, f_o and R_o are related as required for resonance. Suppose f_o is 2 MHz, then from theory for resonance of a free bubble, taking surface tension into account (NCRP, 2002), one obtains 1.9 μm for R_o. Supposing α is 10 Np/m (0.87 dB cm^{-1}), which is typical at a frequency of 2 MHz for soft tissues such as liver; then if δ is 0.2 and c is 1700 m/s, one obtains from Eq. (34), the value 1.4×10^9 m^{-3} (1400 ml^{-1}) for the bubble number density n.

While experimental data are not available on absorption coefficients α for suspensions of identical free bubbles in liquids with number densities this large, Marsh *et al.* (1997) have measured α at a range of frequencies for suspensions of the UCA Albunex$^{\circledR}$ with values of n up to 1.9×10^6 ml^{-1}. For the latter value of n, the maximum value of α was found to be 75 dB cm^{-1}

$(8.6\,\mathrm{Np\,cm^{-1}})$ and occurred at an ultrasound frequency of 2 MHz. This is an extremely high value for the absorption coefficient, higher than reported for any normal mammalian tissue. In applications of UCAs to ultrasound imaging, even higher values of the number density n are common, and the high absorption is recognized. In comparing the values of α for the Albunex® suspensions measured by Marsh *et al.* with those expected from Eq. (34) for a hypothetical suspension of identical free bubbles with the same number density, we find that the predicted absorption for the hypothetical suspensions would be even greater. The difference comes partly from the shells which envelop the UCAs, causing the damping coefficient δ to be greater so that the vibration amplitude (and the energy extracted from the ultrasound field) is smaller than it would be for a resonant free bubble. However, most of the difference probably comes from the fact that the measured number density n of the UCAs includes a large proportion of bubbles that are smaller than resonance size and contribute little to the absorption.

5.2. *Heating*

As UCAs are effective absorbers, one would expect that heat production would be increased in a region where UCAs of high number density are present. Wu (1998) estimated the temperature rise to be $\sim$2°C if a 2 MHz beam of ultrasound of diameter 4.2 mm and intensity 0.3 W cm^{-2} impinges for 10 s, normally on the boundary of an Albunex® suspension of number density $2.6\,\times\,10^7\,\mathrm{cm^{-3}}$. For comparison, one obtains from Eq. (6) that a wide beam of the same frequency and intensity traveling through soft tissue ($\alpha = 0.1\,\mathrm{Np\,cm^{-1}}$) would produce a temperature rise of 0.14°C at the same time.

5.3. *Bubble growth*

Effects produced by cavitation when a biological cell suspension is exposed to ultrasound do not come from pre-existing free bubbles. A small free bubble would quickly dissolve because of the excess internal pressure caused by surface tension. This excess pressure is $2\sigma/R_o$; for an air bubble in water, σ is about 0.072 N/m, so the excess pressure in an air bubble of 1 μm radius would be 0.24 MPa, and the bubble would dissolve in a few milliseconds

38   *W. L. Nyborg*

(Epstein and Plesset, 1950). If UCAs or other gas bodies are not deliberately provided, the cavitation activity comes from bubbles which were caused to grow from minute pre-existing gas bodies stabilized in recesses provided on rough surfaces of vessel walls or microscopic impurity particles. The ultrasound causes growth of free bubbles from these "cavitation nuclei" by a combination of processes. One of these is "rectified diffusion", a phenomenon which depends on the influx of gas during the expansion of a bubble exceeding the efflux during contraction. The theory for this interesting topic has attracted the attention of numerous investigators. Leighton (1994) and the NCRP (2002) have provided recent reviews. The other process for bubble growth involves coalescence of existing bubbles through radiation force and is discussed below.

Experimental evidence for ultrasonically induced growth of bubbles in mammalian tissue was reported by ter Harr and Daniels (1981) and discussed further by Daniels and ter Haar (1992); they observed the growth of gas bubbles in animal tissue produced by 0.75 MHz CW ultrasound at spatial average intensities up to $1\,\mathrm{W\,cm^{-2}}$. It was shown in theoretical analysis by Crum *et al.* (1987) that the growth may have been a consequence of rectified diffusion.

5.4. *Radiation force on a small gas body in a plane traveling wave*

According to Eq. (22), a plane traveling wave of ultrasound will act on an absorbing body with a steady radiation force, F_{rad}, equal to W/c, where c is the speed of sound and W is the rate at which the body removes energy from the wave. For a free bubble, W is given by Eq. (33) and we obtain for the force, F_{bub}, the expression

$$F_{\mathrm{bub}} = R_o p_o^2/(\rho c \delta f_o) = 2IR_o/\delta f_o; \tag{35}$$

here, an expression from Eq. (3b) is used for the intensity I.

Miller *et al.* (1991) used equations equivalent to Eq. (35) to estimate the effects of radiation force produced by a 1.6 MHz traveling wave of intensity $0.3\,\mathrm{W\,cm^{-2}}$ on a free resonant bubble of radius $2\,\mu\mathrm{m}$ in a water-like liquid. (They recognized, though, that since Eq. (35) is based on a second-order approximation, it may not be highly accurate under these conditions.) Further, they applied a modified Stokes formula to calculate the speed that this radiation force would produce, and found it to be of the order of 10 m/s, in agreement with observations. Consideration of the viscous stress produced at the boundary of such a speeding bubble led to the conclusion that if this motion occurred in a cell suspension, the stress would be sufficient to lyse or otherwise alter some of the biological cells lying in the bubble path.

Dayton *et al.* (1997) investigated the paths followed by UCAs in a 200 μm diameter cellulose vessel, when displacements produced by radiation force along the axis of a pulsed ultrasound beam are superposed on the flow from a syringe pump. Using frequencies from 2 to 38 MHz and pressure amplitudes from 60 to 800 kPa, they measured displacements under varying conditions and found reasonable agreement with expectations from theory [such as Eq. (35)] for radiation force. This work was followed by Dayton *et al.* (1999) with an emphasis on directing the force oward the vessel wall. This was done both *in vitro* by using the cellulose vessel and *in vivo* by using a 50 μm diameter blood vessel in the mouse cremaster muscle. The authors found that by manipulating the source transducer, and thus its axially directed radiation force, the UCAs could be brought into contact with cells at the wall of the blood vessel. The ultrasound also causes the UCAs to form aggregates, a process which comes about through inter-particle radiation forces discussed below.

That the radiation force on UCAs can be important in therapeutic applications is seen in the results of *in vivo* experiments by Hwang *et al.* (2005), who exposed rabbit carotid artery to focused 1.13 MHz ultrasound of high pressure amplitude (above 3 MPa). They found that when Optison® UCAs were present in the artery, endothelial cells on its distal side were destroyed by the ultrasound, while those on its proximal side were not significantly affected.

The theory on which Eq. (35) is based, has also been found useful in explaining a phenomenon discovered by Clarke and Hill (1969) during experiments in which 1 MHz CW ultrasound was applied to suspensions of mammalian cells, and information was obtained on the conditions under which the cells were destroyed. In their arrangement shown schematically in Fig. 10, the ultrasound beam was directed at a polystyrene tube containing a suspension of interest which could be rotated slowly about its axis. They discovered, very surprisingly, that the number of cells destroyed

                    W. L. Nyborg

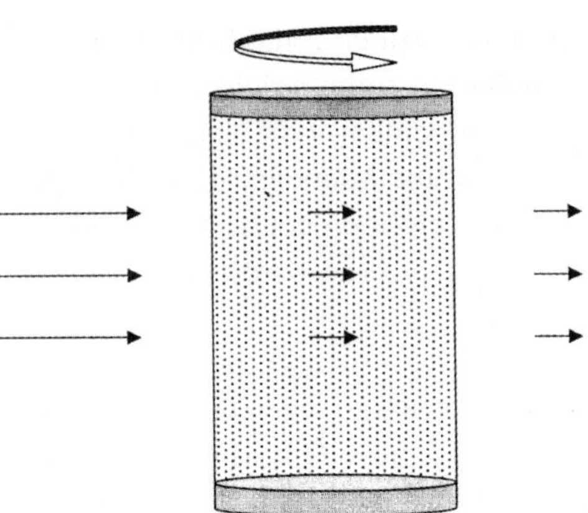

Fig. 10. Schematic of arrangement for employing "rotation effect". Beam of ultrasound passes through cell suspension in thin-walled tube which is rotated (continuously or periodically) about its axis. See text.

was reduced "by a factor of at least 100" when the tube was not rotated. When this "rotation effect" became widely known, it had considerable influence on subsequent practice; rotating the exposure vessel became a normal procedure in subsequent *in vitro* experiments. In explaining the phenomenon, the authors hypothesized that cell disruption requires close interaction between the cells and active bubbles. They suggested that in the absence of rotation, the radiation force along the beam direction forces bubbles to the far side of the vessel where they have little interaction with cells. This was confirmed by Miller and Williams (1989) who obtained evidence that vessel rotation had the effect of bringing these bubbles to the location where the beam enters the vessel, so that they would again be forced to the far region and would destroy cells along the path. In a novel demonstration, they showed that even if the vessel rotation continued, the cell destruction activity would be greatly reduced if the ultrasound was present only during alternate half-periods of the rotation cycle, during which the entry region was devoid of bubbles. Carstensen *et al.* (1993) went further and showed that continuous rotation of the vessel is not necessary for maintaining the cell-destruction activity; instead, they obtained equivalent results by manually turning the vessel through 180° quickly at regular intervals during the exposure.

5.5. *Radiation force on a small gas body in a plane standing wave*

When CW ultrasound is applied to cell suspensions *in vitro*, precautions are often taken to avoid reflections at container walls or at gas-liquid interfaces. Otherwise standing waves are likely which will perturb the exposure conditions. In applications to mammalian tissues, standing waves are possible at interfaces with bone or lung. If UCAs or other gas bodies are present in liquids where standing waves exist, they will be acted on by radiation forces of a special nature. An expression for the acoustic pressure in a perfect standing wave can be formed by superposing the expression for a traveling wave in Eq. (2) (letting α^* be zero) on another that is the same, except that "$\omega t - kx$" is replaced by "$kx - \omega t$"; one obtains

$$p(x, t) = 2p_o \cos kx \cos \omega t. \tag{36}$$

(This can be compared with the corresponding expression in Eq. (24) for the particle velocity $u(x, t)$ in the standing wave.) From Eq. (36), the pressure at any point in this field varies sinusoidally with time, with pressure amplitude $2p_o \cos kx$. The pressure amplitude is maximum ($2p_o$) on a series of equally spaced planes at $x = n\lambda/2$, where n is any integer or zero. The pressure amplitude is zero on the intermediate planes $x = \lambda/4 + n\lambda/2$.

From theory (Coakley and Nyborg, 1978; Leighton, 1994), it has been shown that the radiation force on a small gas body of radius R (resonant radius R_o) in a plane standing-wave field is such that the following rules hold:

(1) The force is zero if $R = R_o$
(2) The force is toward a plane where the pressure amplitude is maximum ($2\,p_o$) if $R < R_o$
(3) The force is toward a plane where the pressure amplitude is minimum (0) if $R > R_o$

Thus, small bubbles or UCAs will tend to collect at pressure maxima and become active there, while large ones will collect at pressure minima and become quiescent. This suggests that under some circumstances, the presence of standing waves in an *in vitro* exposure of a cell suspension will reduce the interaction between these gas bodies and biological cells, since according to the discussion of Eq. (23), radiation force will then cause most cells to migrate to pressure minima. These possibilities are discussed by Church *et al.* (1982).

5.6. *Radiation force between two small gas bodies in a sound field*

Suppose A and B are two neighboring bubbles or UCAs in a liquid and are set into vibration in a sound field, named the *incident* field; both of these vibrating gas bodies will then generate additional sound fields of the same frequency. Both A and B will then be acted on by two sound fields: the incident field and the field from the other gas body. As a result, they will also both be acted on by a radiation force, derived from the two superposed sound fields, whose nature depends on the characteristics of A and B, on the frequency of the incident field, and on the distance between A and B. Of the various possibilities, one is of special interest, since it relates to a mechanism for bubble growth. If the resonance frequencies for A and B are each higher than the frequency of the incident field, then it can be shown that for each of them, the pressure amplitude in the immediately surrounding field decreases monotonically with distance. As a result of this, the force on each is toward the other, *i.e.*, the radiation force between the two is attractive. They will move toward each other and may combine to form a single gas body of larger size. This and other possibilities are discussed further by Leighton (1994) and by Coakley and Nyborg (1978).

5.7. *Radiation force on a particle near a small gas body*

Cells and other suspended particles with comparable density and compressibility tend to collect at vibrating bubbles and UCAs. For example, it was found (Nyborg and Miller, 1982; Miller, 1988) that when 2 MHz ultrasound of modest pressure amplitude was applied to a suspension of human erythrocytes in the presence of a membrane containing small gas-filled pores (see Sec. 5.8), the cells quickly moved toward the pores and became concentrated there. This response of the cells can be understood by referring to Eq. (23) and assuming that the gas-filled pore is, for this purpose, equivalent to a small bubble. These equations can be used to determine the radiation force on a small particle at a short distance r from the center of a small spherical gas body of radius R_o, which has been set into vibration at a frequency near resonance by an incident sound field. For this situation, the term in Eq. (23) involving the time-average of the potential energy density E_p can be neglected, since the kinetic energy density E_k is greatly elevated in the liquid near the vibrating surface of the gas body. Just outside the vibrating surface, the oscillatory flow is essentially incompressible and the velocity amplitude u_o is inversely proportional to the square of the distance r; it can be written as $U_o R_o^2 r^{-2}$, where U_o is the velocity amplitude of the vibrating surface at $r = R_o$. Since the time-averaged kinetic energy density $\langle E_k \rangle$ is 0.25 ρu_o^2, one obtains for the radiation force, F_{rad}, from Eq. (23),

$$F_{\text{rad}} = 0.25 \rho v D^* U_o^2 R_o^4 r^{-5}. \tag{37}$$

It is this force that drives particles toward the bubble. By invoking the Stokes relationship, Nyborg and Miller (1982) estimated that particles in the vicinity of a vigorously vibrating bubble would approach it with speeds comparable to those which would apply if the same particles were in the chamber of a high speed centrifuge.

Influence of the same force was recognized in explaining results of *in vitro* experiments, in which ultrasound was applied to cell suspensions and lysis was caused by cavitation. In these experiments, the percentage of cells lysed in a given exposure was shown to decrease as the number density of the cells was increased. Brayman and Miller (1993) carried out experiments on erythrocyte suspensions of varying density and concluded that much of the effect comes about because radiation forces bring cells to the surface of active bubbles and, as the number accumulated on a given bubble increases, the lytic effectiveness decreases. Thus, the number of cells that can be lysed by each bubble is limited.

5.8. *Role of gas bodies in acoustic streaming and microstreaming*

In Sec. 4, the flow produced in a tube by a beam of ultrasound is discussed, and in Eq. (25), the axial flow speed U is shown to be proportional to the ratio α/η, where α is the attenuation coefficient and η is the coefficient of shear viscosity. In Sec. 5.1, results are discussed of experiments in which measurements of α were made in UCA suspensions. It was found in agreement with expectations from the theory that α can be very great in suspensions where the number density of UCAs is comparable to the (high) values commonly used in clinical practice with diagnostic ultrasound. Since the viscosity of a suspension of UCAs in a water-like liquid is probably not very different from water, it is to be expected that relatively vigorous acoustic streaming will be produced when an ultrasound beam passes through a suspension of UCAs.

In Sec. 4, examples were discussed of near-boundary streaming, a class of acoustic streaming which is generated when a sound field exists near a boundary that perturbs the oscillatory flow within a boundary layer. Figure 8 shows the kind of streaming known as "microstreaming" if it is of small scale, which is of special interest here. In the thin boundary layer which is formed in the microstreaming near a wire vibrating transversely at a frequency of 20 kHz, the time-independent viscous stress can be high enough to lyse or otherwise affect biological cells, as discussed in Sec. 4. It was found by Elder (1959) that an analogous kind of microstreaming occurs when a small bubble vibrates at a frequency of 10 kHz, while resting on a solid boundary (Fig. 11). Marmottant and Hilgenfeldt (2003) have recently made experimental and theoretical studies of near-boundary bubble-associated streaming at 185 kHz.

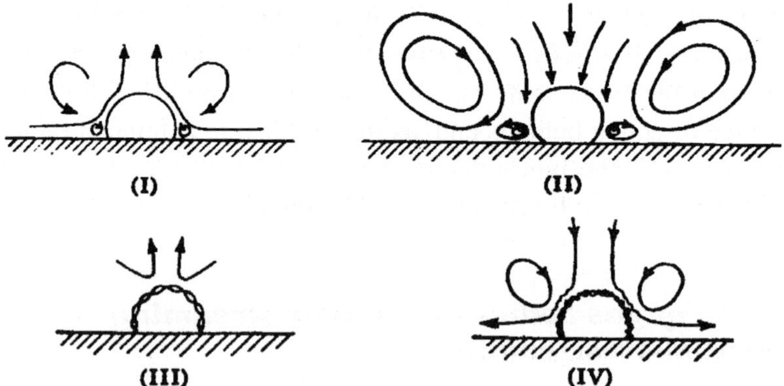

Fig. 11.   Streaming patterns near a vibrating bubble situated on a solid boundary, observed by Elder (1959).

Elder's findings led to further investigations (Hughes and Nyborg, 1962) motivated by possibilities of developing improved ultrasonic methods for disrupting bacteria and other microorganisms, without generating unwanted free radicals. An arrangement was devised for producing 20 kHz ultrasound in a liquid or suspension of interest at amplitudes which could be varied, in the presence of an array of air bubbles approximately of resonance size. In water, it was found that cavitation streamers appeared on the surface of the source when the amplitude exceeded a critical level (L). In the tests for free radical production, iodine was produced from potassium iodide in the presence of carbon tetrachloride if the amplitude was greater than "L", but not otherwise. However, disruption of E.Coli bacteria occurred at amplitudes well below "L" and increased monotonically with amplitude. These and other tests led to the conclusion that such structural effects as bacterial disruption can be produced by bubble action *via* mechanical stresses associated with microstreaming, which occur at lower amplitudes than those required for the production of free radicals. The latter may be generated if the activity is of a violent kind now referred to as *inertial cavitation*, a topic discussed in Sec. 6.

The above findings by Hughes and Nyborg showed that an array of approximately 50 stable vibrating bubbles could produce mechanical stresses sufficient to disrupt biological cells; the question then arose as to whether similar results could be obtained with a single bubble. Rooney (1970) found this to be possible, indeed, by using a special arrangement in which 20 kHz ultrasound was produced in a saline suspension of human erythrocytes in the presence of a single hemispherical bubble. The latter, of radius R_o equal to 130 μm, was formed at the end of a length of stainless-steel tubing which was connected to a gas reservoir through a capillary of very small bore so that the pressure could be carefully controlled. The suspension was contained in a small plastic vessel which allowed measuring the bubble vibration and viewing accompanying fluid motion through a microscope. Dextran was added to the saline, thus increasing its viscosity by about a factor of 30, in order to prevent surface-wave instabilities from occurring. The bubble then executed simple volume oscillations for which the amplitude was proportional to the amplitude of the voltage applied to the source transducer. Along with the oscillations, a pattern of acoustic microstreaming appeared which was similar to Pattern II reported by Elder

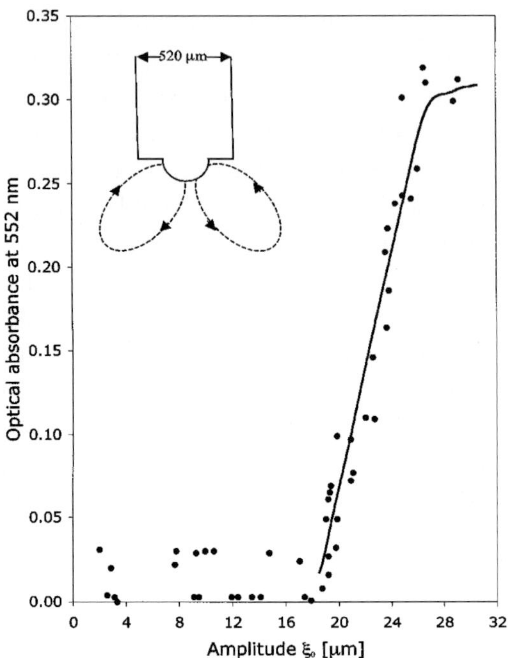

Fig. 12.   Hemolysis of canine red cells in the microstreaming field near a single air bubble set into stable volume oscillation at a frequency of 20 kHz. The Hb release was detectable when the displacement amplitude ξ_o exceeded about 14% of the initial bubble radius R_o. [From Rooney (1970) with permission.]

(1959), see Fig. 11. Hemoglobin release, determined by measurements of optical absorption, was observed after 5-minute exposures when the bubble oscillation amplitude exceeded a threshold of 18 μm, *i.e.*, about 0.14 R_o. Results are shown in Fig. 12. Since the oscillation amplitudes were modest, it is clear that inertial cavitation was not involved in producing the hemolysis. Instead, the cause was evidently the stress exerted by microstreaming in the boundary layer near the rigid boundary surrounding the bubble. Calculations based on approximate theory gave 450 Pa for the stress under threshold conditions. The theory employed is similar to that for the vibrating cylinder in Eq. (27) (see also Eq. (3) in Chap. VI). This compares favorably with the value of 560 Pa obtained by Williams *et al.* (1970) for the minimum stress required for detectable hemolysis after 5-minute exposure to analogous microstreaming produced near a vibrating wire.

The methods used at frequencies in the 10–20 kHz range have not proved feasible for studying the response of single or designed arrays of small gas bodies to ultrasound in the megahertz range, since in this range, the resonance dimensions are typically smaller by a factor of 100 or more. However, commercially available Nuclepore® filters (Nuclepore Corporation, Pleasanton, California) include membranes that have proved very useful for ultrasound studies. In experiments with these, it was found that when their hydrophobic membranes with cylindrical pores several micrometers in diameter are immersed in water, most of the pores retain their air and thus provide a source of stabilized gas bodies for use in experiments. In a review of literature, Miller (1987) includes discussions of many investigations that had been carried out in which these membranes were used to study effects of megahertz frequency ultrasound on biological cells when gas bodies of near-resonance size are present. For example, when suspensions of erythrocytes, platelets and other cells were exposed to low intensity ultrasound of frequency in the range 2–4 MHz, it was found that cells tended to gather near the gas-filled pores and to follow the microstreaming flow which occurred there. Sometimes, the flow would cease as the gathered cells blocked the pore entrance. In some experiments with platelet-rich plasma, the platelets formed permanent aggregates after a short exposure. In the other experiments with Nuclepore® membranes, measurements were made of ATP released from erythrocytes, platelets and white cells during exposure to 2 MHz ultrasound of low intensity.

In the late 1900s, the clinical importance was increasingly recognized of understanding the consequences of exposing cells and tissues to megahertz-frequency ultrasound in the presence of small stabilized gas bodies. During this time, the ultrasound contrast agents (UCAs) mentioned earlier in this chapter (and discussed in the other chapters in this book) came into common use and became available commercially. Much has been learned from research in which these agents are used. For example, numerical calculations indicate that if a UCA is set into vibration by 1 MHz or 2 MHz ultrasound with a pressure amplitude of about 0.1 MPa, the shear stress caused by microstreaming will be sufficient for causing reparable sonoporation of cells in its immediate vicinity (Wu, 2002). Later, Miller and Dou (2004a, b) reported that in experiments where arrangements were used to bring UCAs into contact with mouse macrophage-like cells while ultrasound in the frequency range of 1 to 10 MHz was applied, pressure amplitudes lower than those required for inertial cavitation caused damage to the cell membranes. Results of investigations at higher acoustic pressures where inertial cavitation is involved, are discussed in Sec. 6 and in the other chapters in this book.

6. Nonlinearity

In Secs. 1–5, phenomena were discussed for which the relevant theory is dealt with by using approximations of first-order and second-order to solutions of the basic equations. These approximations are sufficiently accurate for sound fields in which the pressure amplitude is relatively small, and considerable useful information is obtained from their use. However, medical applications often require the use of conditions where the approximations are inadequate. Computational techniques are then usually required for obtaining the desired information.

6.1. *Nonlinear propagation and some of its implications*

When a traveling wave is generated in which the total acoustic pressure $p(x, t)$ is not small compared with the hydrostatic pressure P_o, the pressure $p(x, t)$ in the wave does not have the simplified form of Eq. (2). Instead, although a wave of this form exists, its frequency f, being now the **fundamental** frequency, is accompanied by other waves whose frequencies are **harmonically** related to the fundamental; *i.e.*, their frequencies have the values $2f$, $3f$, etc. Plots of the **waveform** (*i.e.*, plots of total acoustic pressure $p(x, t)$ in the wave *vs* time) at various distances x show that under nonlinear conditions, the waveform becomes distorted as the wave travels; the positive portion of the wave tends to move forward and the negative part lags. If the amplitude is high, the distortion may increase with distance until a shock wave is formed.

The formation of harmonics increases the potential for a beam of ultrasound to cause biological effects. Since the absorption coefficient increases with frequency, the presence of harmonics increases the heat produced per unit volume. Also, the increased rate of energy loss in an absorbing object leads to increased radiation force along the axis of a beam, as might be inferred from Eq. (22). As an ultrasound beam passes through an absorbing fluid, the fluid itself is acted on by increased force, as shown by Starritt *et al.* (1989, 1991) in measurements of the acoustic streaming speeds produced by ultrasound beams in water. These investigators found that, in accordance with Eq. (25), the large increase in attenuation resulting from harmonic generation, caused a greatly increased speed of the flow. Other implications of nonlinear propagation, relevant to biomedical applications, are discussed in NCRP (1992, 2002) and by Carstensen and Bacon (1998).

6.2. *Nonlinear activation of gas bodies; inertial cavitation*

In Sec. 5, the discussion of activities in sound fields when gas-filled cavities are present, *i.e.*, of cavitation, was restricted to those which occur when the incident pressure $p(t)$ (*i.e.*, the acoustic pressure in the immediately surrounding liquid) is fairly low. Under these conditions, the radius $R(t)$ of a spherical gas body varies linearly with $p(t)$. Specifically, if the incident pressure is $p_o \cos(2\pi ft)$, where p_o is small, the radial displacement $\xi(t)$ (after an initial transient) will be sinusoidal with the same frequency f, as in Eqs. (28) and (29). The acoustic pressure $p_r(t)$ in the spherical wave radiated by the vibrating sphere will also vary sinusoidally in time with the same frequency f. However, at higher levels of p_o, the linearized equations of motion are no longer valid and the time dependence of $\xi(t)$ and of the radiated pressure $p_r(t)$ are more complex. The functions $\xi(t)$ and $p_r(t)$ then include not only fundamental components of frequency f, but also harmonics of frequency $2f$, $3f$, *etc.*, whose amplitudes, relative to that of the fundamental, increase with increasing amplitude of the incident pressure $p(t)$. In addition, subharmonics with frequencies $f/2$, $f/3$, etc., as well as other components, become increasingly evident, and disturbances appear on the bubble surface.

If the incident pressure amplitude is increased until it exceeds a critical value, a more dramatic form of cavitation occurs, in which the gas-filled spherical cavity expands during part of a cycle, then contracts very rapidly in a "collapse" phase which is aided by inertia of the in-rushing mass of liquid. Noltingk and Neppiras (1950) were among the first to form the nonlinear equations required for analyzing this acoustically produced phenomenon.

Using an early form of a computer, they made calculations which revealed the possibilities now known for the occurrence of very high pressures and velocities during the collapse of a gas-filled cavity. Flynn (1964) greatly extended the analysis of collapse behavior, now known as **inertial cavitation**. In plots of radius R vs time t, it was found that for a spherical bubble in water with a resting radius of 1 μm, its response to a sound field in which p_o is 0.45 MPa, would include a "collapse" portion during which it would rapidly collapse to one-third of it original radius. Thus, its volume would decrease by a factor of 27 and the pressure would increase accordingly. The contraction would occur almost adiabatically and, for a bubble containing air or other gas of low atomic number, the temperature would rise momentarily to a very high value. That such high temperatures occur has been confirmed by many investigators who have investigated the chemical reactions involved; these often include the production of free radicals and are accompanied by the production of visible light, $i.e.$, **sonoluminescence** (see, Suslick, 1989; Young, 1989, 2005; Leighton, 1994; NCRP, 2002). Much detailed information about the sonoluminescence has been obtained since the discovery that, under suitable conditions, a single bubble can be caused to contract periodically in a stable manner and emit a very short flash of light during each contraction (Gaitan and Crum, 1990; Gaitan $et\ al.$, 1992). If the gas in the contracting bubble is of very high atomic number, as is common in present-day UCAs, the expected temperature rise during contraction is much less; hence, free radical production is unlikely to result from inertial cavitation involving UCAs containing such gases (Suslick and Kemper, 1993).

In a study of R vs t curves for a range of conditions, Flynn (1964) arrived at a simple approximate generalization, namely, that inertial cavitation occurs if the largest value of the radius R during a cycle exceeds twice the resting value R_o. More detailed information on the thresholds for pulsed ultrasound came from later computations by Flynn and Church (1988). In an approximate analytical approach, Apfel and Holland (1991) arrived at a convenient (though less generally accurate) alternative criterion based on the pressure amplitude p_o and frequency f of the incident field, namely, that inertial cavitation may occur in a waterlike liquid, if the quantity $p_o/f^{-0.5}$ exceeds a critical value, where p_o and f have the units MPa and MHz respectively. It is an estimate of this quantity known as the **mechanical index** or the "MI", which is sometimes displayed on the screen of diagnostic ultrasound equipment as an indication of the likelihood that inertial cavitation might be produced in the region being examined. In the USA, the MI must not exceed 1.9 for megahertz-frequency commercial medical diagnostic equipment. At lower ultrasound frequencies, *e.g.*, 20 kHz, the threshold value of p_o for inertial cavitation is typically in the vicinity of standard atmospheric pressure, *i.e.*, 0.1 MPa (Flynn, 1964).

The above analysis is for "symmetrical collapse" of a cavity in a region well removed from boundaries that would influence its motion. Plesset and Chapman (1971) used numerical methods to obtain an approximate description for "asymmetrical collapse" of a cavity near a solid wall. In this situation, liquid above the cavity flows toward the wall and forms a jet which impinges on the wall (see Fig. 13).

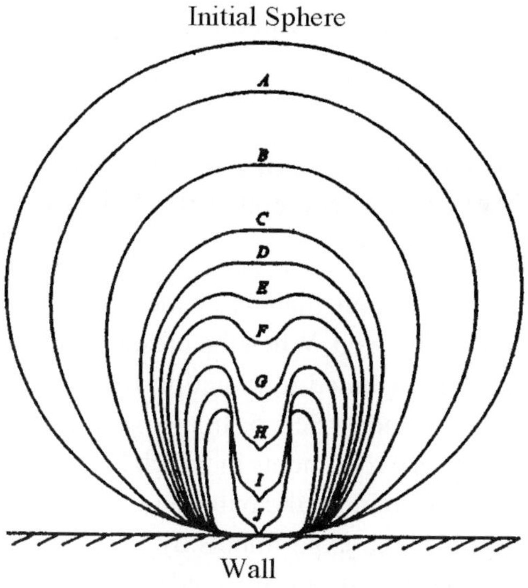

Fig. 13. Computed plots of the surface of a small gas-filled cavity at a series of times (in μs) after the onset of asymmetric collapse. A, 0.63; B, 0.89; C, 0.99; D, 1.01; E, 1.03; F, 1.05; G, 1.07; H, 1.08; I, 1.10; J, 1.12. [From Plesset and Chapman (1971) with permission.]

6.3. *Techniques for detection of small gas-filled cavities and monitoring of cavitation activity*

Since cavitation can cause biological effects on cells and tissues, techniques have been developed for detecting small gas bodies and monitoring their activity during ultrasound exposures. A Technical Report (ANSI, 2002) includes descriptions of 25 techniques that have been used for these purposes. Those which have been used with *in vitro* experiments, in which biological suspensions or tissues are exposed to ultrasound, include detection of harmonics, subharmonics and noise generated during the exposure, observation of backscatter synchronized with ultrasonic pulses, detection of light production, detection of free radicals, and studies of biological effects.

The above methods, except for those requiring observation of light, have also been used for detecting gaseous cavities and/or cavitation activity during *in vivo* experiments in which ultrasound is applied to living subjects. In addition, for *in vivo* experiments, ultrasonic imaging and Doppler techniques have been used, as well as methods in which effects of ultrasound exposure are observed with and without applying increased hydrostatic pressure to the subject.

6.4. *Bioeffects resulting from activation of gas bodies, including inertial cavitation*

In applications where ultrasound produces effects by activation of gas-filled cavities, *i.e.*, by cavitation, there is a wide range of possibilities for the detailed mechanism(s) involved. When the pressure amplitude is fairly low, bioeffects can often be attributed to radiation force or acoustic streaming as in the examples discussed in Sec. 5. In this section, we discuss more of such examples, as well as experiments in which higher amplitudes are used and results are attributed to inertial cavitation.

In Chap. VI of this book, experiments by Ward *et al.* (1999, 2000) are discussed. In these experiments, it was found that cervical cancer cells were temporarily made permeable to dextran molecules, after exposure to 2 MHz ultrasound of pressure amplitude 0.2 MPa for 5 minutes in the presence of Optison® UCAs. According to calculations by Wu (2002), the vibration amplitude ξ_o of a typical intact UCA under these conditions would only be a small fraction of its original radius R_o; hence, linear theory is adequate for analyzing the vibration. Since it had been shown that vibrating UCAs can produce microstreaming (Gormley and Wu, 1998), it was considered possible that the cellular changes might have been caused by such microstreaming, and Eq. (3) in Chap. VI was used to estimate the stress applied to the cells. In this manner, the stress was determined to be approximately in the range of 18 to 92 Pa, where the specific value depended on the UCA resting radius R_o. This range is comparable in magnitude to the values calculated by Wu *et al.* (2002) for stresses applied in producing reparable sonoporation by microstreaming near a horn tip vibrating at a frequency of 21 kHz. It is also comparable to thresholds for lysis of white blood cells (polymorphonuclear neutrophiles) as determined by Crowell *et al.* (1977). In contrast, the microstreaming-produced stresses required for lysis of red blood cells are much higher, being determined as 560 Pa and 450 Pa respectively, in the experiments of Williams *et al.* (1970) and Rooney (1970), which are discussed in Secs. 4 and 5.

Thus, bioeffects of interest can be produced by exposing cells to ultrasound of relatively low pressure amplitude in the presence of UCAs. Microstreaming-produced stresses appear to be involved, but further development of understanding for specific situations will be useful in optimizing applications. A complication in determining mechanisms is that the UCAs will be altered or destroyed by the ultrasound when the pressure amplitude and exposure time exceed limits which depend on the size and narure of the UCA. Chomas *et al.* (2001) used high-speed optical techniques to study the fragmentation of MP1950® UCAs (mfg. by Mallinckrodt, Inc) and found, *e.g.*, that a UCA of resting diameter 3 μm is destroyed by two cycles of 2.25 MHz ultrasound, if the pressure amplitude exceeds 0.3 MPa; the critical pressure increases with diameter, being 0.6 MPa when the diameter is 4 μm. Also, the critical pressure decreases as the pulse length increases. In some of the experiments of Ward *et al.* (1999) discussed in Chap. VI, in which cells were exposed to 2 MHz ultrasound at a pressure amplitude level of 0.2 MPa in the presence of Optison® UCAs, it was found that the UCAs were no longer functional after 5 minutes and had presumably fragmented. When a UCA is fragmented, the gas escapes as free bubbles. These may dissolve in the liquid fairly quickly, but will respond vigorously to the ultrasound before dissolution. According to the analysis by Wu (2002), the radius of the free bubble in an ultrasound field where the pressure amplitude is 0.1 MPa or greater, may (depending on its size) expand to a radius R

more than twice its resting value R_o during an oscillation; if so, Flynn's criteron (Flynn, 1964) for inertial cavitation will be satisfied. This possibility creates uncertainty about the mechanisms involved in procedures where cells are exposed to ultrasound in the presence of UCAs. When the pressure amplitude is fairly low, the action may be partly a result of stresses associated with microstreaming generated by intact vibrating UCAs, and partly a result of inertial cavitation involving gas bubbles released from the fragmented UCAs. Free radicals were probably not produced in the experiments of Ward *et al.* (1999, 2000), since the gas used in Optison® UCAs is octafluorocarbon, a gas of very high atomic number.

In earlier experiments, Bao *et al.* (1997) applied 2.25 MHz ultrasound to suspensions of Chinese hamster ovary cells in the presence of DNA plasmids and Albunex® UCAs in a series of 60 s exposures at a series of pressure amplitude levels. Transfection was significant at the 0.1 MPa level and increased rapidly at levels above 0.3 MPa, lysis of the cells was observed above 0.2 MPa, and H_2O_2 became evident at levels above 0.4 MPa. Albunex® UCAs are air-filled and the appearance of H_2O_2 in these experiments was evidence of free radicals resulting from inertial cavitation involving gas bubbles released from fragmented UCAs. The findings would seem consistent with an assumption that the transfection at levels around 0.1 MPa was enabled by microstreaming from intact UCAs and that lysis, together with increased rate of transfection, occurred at higher levels as fragmentation of the UCAs occurred and free gas bubbles became available.

It was shown by Lindner *et al.* (2000) that when UCAs are introduced into the bloodstream, they may become attached to activated leukocytes on the endothelium of blood vessels. Dayton *et al.* (2001) used high-speed photography with an inverted microscope to study the dynamics of UCAs, which were on the interior of leucocytes after phagcytosis had occurred. They found that the UCAs vibrated in response to an ultrasound field, but with reduced amplitude, probably because of cytoplasmic viscosity. Miller and Dou (2004a, b) used a novel method for inducing mouse macrophage-like cells to phagocytose UCAs *in vitro* in a controlled manner, so that detailed studies could be made on effects produced by exposing the UCA-linked cells to ultrasound. They found that the cell membranes were made permeable at pressure amplitude levels well below the thresholds for UCA fragmentation or for inertial cavitation. The findings are discussed much further in Chap. VI.

The investigations discussed above indicate that biological cells can be made permeable *in vitro* by low-megahertz ultrasound in the absence of inertial cavitation, if intact UCAs are present. To prevent fragmentation of the UCAs, it is necessary to limit the pressure amplitude and the duration of exposure to an extent that depends on the nature of the agent, as well as on the experimental conditions. In the absence of UCAs or other means to provide gas bodies in a controlled manner, one typically uses higher pressure amplitudes to obtain nonthermal cellular effects with ultrasound in the megahertz frequency range. With higher amplitudes inertial cavitation occurs, but in a highly variable manner, since it is dependent on the presence of **cavitation nuclei**, *i.e.,* small gas-filled cavities which may be provided *in vitro* in crevices at container walls or may be associated wth microscopic impurity particles in the medium (see review by Miller *et al.*, 1996). The pressure level must be high enough to cause the growth of the nuclei to a size required for inertial cavitation. If monatomic or diatomic gases are involved, high temperatures will be generated during collapse events and highly reactive sonochemicals will be generated. (Suslick, 1988; ANSI, 2002; Fowlkes and Crum, 1988). It was shown by Miller and Thomas (1996) that *in vitro* exposure of Chinese hamster ovary cells to 2.17 MHz ultrasound at a pressure amplitude of 0.6 MPa for 4 minutes produced inertial cavitation with consequent production of hydrogen peroxide in the solution and DNA breaks within the cell.

Everbach *et al.* (1997) describe a device, designed to provide a measure of inertial cavitation activity, which detects ultrasound emissions with frequencies lying within a narrow band centered at 20 MHz. It was employed during experiments in each of which red cells in plasma were exposed for one minute to 20 pulses of 1 MHz ultrasound with pressure amplitude ~5 MPa, varying in duration from 20 to 1000 μs. When Albunex® was present in the suspension, hemoglobin was released under all conditions in amounts which correlated well with the output of the 20 MHz emissions detector. Without Albunex®, there was no measureable hemoglobin release.

In many *in vitro* experiments, there is evidence that inertial cavitation is occurring, *e.g.*, because of acoustic emissions or sonochemicals, but it is not known whether the action involved collapse of a spherical gas body without change in shape, or if the collapse occurs asymmetrically as indicated in Fig. 13. Miller *et al.* (2000) give plausible arguments in favor of the latter, especially as applied to suspensions of high cell density, and Coleman *et al.* (1987) give evidence for its relevance to applications of extracorporeal shock wave lithotripsy (ESWL). When the shockwaves generated in lithotripsy procedures are focused on aluminum foil or other surfaces immersed in water, deep pits and cracks are produced in the surfaces, These are evidently caused by jetting action which occurs during asymmetric collapse. Kudo *et al.* (2002), using high speed microphotography, obtained photographs of a UCA during asymmetric collapse while in contact with a cell, such that a small liquid jet penetrated the cell, causing it to be deformed.

When applying focused ultrasound to experimental animals in therapy-related research, relatively high values of the pressure amplitude are often used and cavitation is sometimes observed. During investigations of focal lesions produced in the cat brain by ultrasound at frequencies of 1, 3 and 4 MHz, Fry *et al.* (1970) found that when the pressure amplitude exceeded $\sim$8 MPa, the tissue destruction was of a very different character than that observed at lower levels; the difference was attributed to (inertial) cavitation. In later studies, Frizzell (1988) determined the time (t) required for the production of lesions in the cat liver using 3.5 MHz ultrasound at various focal intensities (I). For intensities below $\sim$1000 W/cm^2 (pressure amplitude 5.6 MPa), he found the quantity $It^{0.5}$ to be consistently constant, but at higher intensities, less time was required than expected from this rule. His conclusion was that temperature elevation was the mechanism for lesion production at the lower intensities, but that cavitation was involved at the higher levels. In a review of other studies of the heating and cavitation which can occur during therapeutic applications of focused ultrasound, Holt and Roy (2001) found considerable evidence that the cavitation itself can be a significant source of heating, and proceeded to make a systematic investigation of the phenomenon using tissue-mimicking materials. That cavitation can be useful for targeted drug delivery is indicated by recent findings of Sheikov *et al.* (2004) who exposed rabbit brain to focused ultrasound and showed that this produced local openings of the blood-brain barrier. The significance of various aspects of cavitation to therapeutic applications of focused ultrasound is discussed further in Chaps. V and VIII.

When a patient is examined with diagnostic ultrasound, effective transmission of the ultrasound requires that the coupling medium between transducer and tissue have acoustic properties similar to water. An aqueous gel is commonly employed, partly because unwanted cavitation might occur if water itself were used. However, if ultrasound is being applied in an application of transdermal drug delivery, it is found that cavitation is required, and is probably of the asymmetrical inertial type to which Fig. 13 applies. The coupling medium for this purpose is an appropriate aqueous solution (Mitagotri *et al.*, 1995). The mechanisms involved in enhancing drug transmission across the skin are discussed in Chap. VII. Using 0.88 MHz ultrasound in a related technique for transmitting drugs across the cornea into rabbit eye, Zderic *et al.* (2004) found cavitaton activity to be involved, with contributions from both streaming motions and asymmetric collapse.

In their natural states (and in the absence of ultrasound contrast agents), the only organs in the mammalian body that are known to contain stable bodies of undissolved gas are the lung and the intestinal tract. In the lung, it is found that exposure to ultrasound in the lower megahertz frequency range with pressure amplitudes of the order of 1 MPa can cause hemorrhage; the detailed mechanism is yet unknown, but does not appear to be inertial cavitation. In the intestine, small areas of hemorrage occur at sites of individual bubbles; the pressure amplitude required is somewhat higher and the mechanism is probably inertial cavitation. The topic is reviewed in NCRP (2002).

7. Conclusions

It has been the purpose of this chapter to discuss physical attributes and capabilities of ultrasound which are believed to be relevant to its therapeutic applications. Of ultrasound's capabilities, the best known is undoubtedly the ability to produce heat within tissue. With unfocused ultrasound in the low MHz frequency range, the temperature of soft tissue can be raised a few degrees Celsius to depths of several centimeters with a variety of consequent beneficial physiological effects. With focused ultrasound, relatively high temperatures can be produced at selected sites in tissue, sufficiently localized so that malignant tissue can be treated without appreciable damage to the surrounding tissue. In any of these applications, it is important to be able to control the magnitude and duration of the temperature rise wherever the ultrasound is applied. Computations based on available theory for heat conduction and perfusion, together with current knowledge on acoustical properties of tissue, are very useful as a general guide and have been shown capable of predicting the temperature rise well in experiments with tissue-mimicking models. Also, prediction of the temperatures has proved sufficiently accurate for therapeutic applications in some experiments with animal models, especially in brief exposures, or in other conditions where uncertainties about perfusion are minimal. In addition, available information from reaction rate studies has proved very useful for understanding the temperature sensitivity of various tissues. In general, however, there is a need for better means of mapping the temperature fields generated in applications of ultrasound. A promising technique, based on the use of MRI, is described in Chap. V.

Another very important capability of ultrasound, unique to sonic techniques, is the ability to produce cavitation, *i.e.*, to activate small or large gas bodies which may be present in tissue or other media of interest. By this means, a wide variety of physical, chemical or biological effects can be produced. The action is strongly dependent on the pressure amplitude p_o in the ultrasound field. At the lower levels of p_o, regular oscillatory movements of the gas bodies occur, along with steady eddying (microstreaming) and translation. At the higher levels, the action includes violent collapse phenomena, symmetric or asymmetric, which are characteristic of inertial cavitation. Collapse phenomena are invoked in Chap. VII as the mechanism for producing the increase in skin permeability required for the enhancement of transdermal drug delivery. However, when cells are to be subjected to more gentle stresses, as in some applications of ultrasound to sonoporation and transfection discussed in Chaps. III, IV and VI, inertial cavitation is often not required and the gas body activity consists primarily of microstreaming and allied phenomena. The use of ultrasound contrast agents, which became widely available only within the last decade, has made it possible to control cavitation activity to a much greater extent than was formerly possible. Besides the mechanical characteristics of cavitation, there are also thermal effects; in Chap. V, it is shown that therapeutic applications of focused ultrasound can be enhanced by the heating that accompanies cavitation activity.

While good progress has been made in learning the mechanisms underlying therapeutic applications of ultrasound, challenges remain for the future. As examples among mechanisms, consideration might be given to the roles that radiation force and acoustic streaming, now utilized in novel modes of imaging, might play in therapy. As an example among therapies, the mechanisms have yet to be determined for the healing of bone fractures by low intensity ultrasound.

Acknowledgments

The author wishes to thank Professors Jun-ru Wu and Douglas Miller for their useful suggestions, and Christopher Layman for his considerable help in preparing this manuscript.

References

Allman R, Coakley WT. Ultrasound enhanced phase partition of microorganisms. *Bioseparation* (1994) **4**: 29–38.

ANSI Technical Report S1.24 TR-2002. Bubble detection and cavitation monitoring. (2002) Acoustical Society of America, Melville, New York, Standards Secretariat.

Apfel RE, Holland CK. Gauging the likelihood of cavitation from short-pulse, low duty-cycle diagnostic ultrasound. Ultrasound Beissner K. Measurement techniques, in *Ultrasonic Exposimetry*, Ziskin MC, Lewin PA (eds.) (1993) Boca Raton.

Bao S, Thrall BD, Miller DL. Transfection of a reporter plasmid into cultured cells by sonoporation *in vitro*. *Ultrasound Med Biol* (1997) **23**: 953–959.

Beissner K, Measurement techniques, in *Ultrasonic Exposimetry*, Ziskin MC, Lewin PA (eds.) (1993) Boca Raton.

Benes E, Burger W, Groschl M, Schaffner A, Trampler F, Bolek W, Gaida T, Doblhoff O, Hager F. Trapping of suspended biological particles by use of ultrasonic resonance fields, in *Ultrasonics International '93 Conference Proc* (1993) Butterworth-Heinemann Ltd.: Oxford, pp. 517–518.

Brayman AA, Miller MW. Cell density dependence of the ultrasonic degassing of fixed erythrocyte suspensions. *Ultrasound Med Biol* (1993) **19**: 243–252.

Carson PL, Fischella PR, Oughton TV. Ultrasonic power and intensities produced by diagnostic ultrasound equipment. *Ultrasound Med Biol* (1978) **3**: 341–350.

Carstensen EL, Bacon DR. Biomedical applications, in Hamilton MF, Blackstock DT (eds.) *Nonlinear Acoustics* (1998) Academic Press: San Diego, pp. 421–447.

Carstensen EL, Child SZ, Norton S, Nyborg WL. Ultrasonic heating of the skull. *J Acoust Soc Am* (1990) **87**: 1310–1317.

Carstensen EL, Miller MW, Linke CA. Biological effects of ultrasound. *J Biol Phys* (1974) **2**: 173–192.

Carstensen EL, Kelly P, Church CC, Brayman AA, Child SZ, Raeman CH, Schery L. Lysis of erythrocytes by exposure to CW ultrasound. *Ultrasound Med Biol* (1993) **19**: 147–165.

Cavicchi TJ, O'Brien WD, Jr. Heat generated by ultrasound in an absorbing medium. *J Acoust Soc Am* (1984) **76**: 1244–1245.

Chomas JE, Dayton P, May D, Ferrara K. Threshold of fragmentation for ultrasound contrast agents. *J Biomed Optics* (2001) **g**: 141–170.

Church CC, Flynn HG, Miller MW, Sacks PG. The exposure vessel as a factor in ultrasonically-induced mammalian cell lysis — II. *Ultrasound Med Biol* (1982) **8**: 299–309.

Clarke PR, Hill CR. Physical and chemical aspects of ultrasonic disruption of cells. *J Acoust Soc Am* (1969) **47**: 649–653.

Coakley WT, Nyborg WL. Cavitation; dynamics of gas bubbles; applications, in Fry FJ (ed.) *Ultrasound: Its Applications in Medicine and Biology. Vol. 3, Methods and Phenomena: Their Applications in Science and Technology* (1978) Elsevier Scientific Publishing Co.: Amsterdam, pp. 77–179.

Coleman AJ, Saunders JE, Crum LA, Dyson D. Acoustic cavitation generated by an extracorporeal shockwave lithotripter. *Ultrasound Med Biol* (1987) **13**: 69–76.

Crum LA, Daniels S, ter Haar GR, Dyson M. Ultrasonically induced gas bubble production in agar based gels: Part II, theoretical analysis. *Ultrasound Med Biol* (1987) **13**: 541–554.

Crowell JA, Kusserow BK, Nyborg WL. Functional changes in white blood cells after microsonation. *Ultrasound Med Biol* (1977) **3**: 185–190.

Dalecki D, Child Z, Raeman CH, Carstensen EL. Tactile perception of ultrasound. *J Acoust Soc Am* (1995) **97**: 3165–3170.

Dalecki D, Raeman CH, Child SZ, Carstensen EL. Effects of pulsed ultrasound on the frog heart. III. The radiation force mechanism. *Ultrasound Med Biol* (1997) **23**: 275–285.

Daniels S, ter Haar GR. Formation of bubbles in guinea-pig leg *in vivo*. *Ultrasonics* (1992) **30**: 197.

Dayton PA, Morgan KE, Klibanov AL, Brandenburger G, Nightingale KR, Ferrara KW. A preliminary evaluation of the effects of primary and secondary radiation forces on acoustic contrast agents. *IEEE Trans Ultrason Ferroelec Freq Control* (1997) **44**: 1264–1277.

Dayton P, Klibanov A, Brandenburger G, Ferrara K. Acoustic radiation force *in vivo*: A mechanism to assist targeting of microbubbles. *Ultrasound Med Biol* (1999) **25**: 1195–1201.

Dayton PA, Chomas JE, Lum AFH, Allen JS, Lindner JR, Simon SI, Ferrara KW. Optical and acoustical dynamics of microbubble contrast agents inside neutrophils. *Biophys J* (2001) **80**: 1747–1756.

de Jong N. Absorption and scatter of encapsulated gas filled microspheres: Theoretical considerations and some measurements. *Ultrasonics* (1992) **30**: 95–103.

Duck FA, Starritt HC, ter Haar GR, Lunt MJ. Surface heating of diagnostic ultrasound transducers. *Brit J Radiol* (1989) **62**: 1005–1013.

Dyson M, Woodward B, Pond JB. Flow of red blood cells. Stopped by ultrasound. *Nature* (1971) **232**: 572–573.

Dyson M, Pond JB, Woodward B, Broadbent J. The production of blood cell stasis and endothelial damage in the blood vessels of chick embryos treated with ultrasound in a stationary wave field. *Ultrasound Med Biol* (1974) **1**: 133–148.

Eckart C. Vortices and streams caused by sound waves. *Phys Rev* (1948) 73; **68**: 68–76.

Elder SA. Cavitation microstreaming. *J Acoust Soc Am* (1959) **31**: 54–64.

Epstein PS, Plesset MS. On the stability of gas bubbles in liquid-gas solutions. *J Chem Phys* (1950) **18**: 1705–1709.

Everbach EC, Makin IRS, Azadniv M, Meltzer RS. Correlation of ultrasound-induced hemolysis with cavitation detector *in vitro*. *Ultrasound Med Biol* (1997) **23**: 619–624.

Flynn HG. Physics of acoustic cavitation in liquids, in Mason WP (ed.) *Physical Acoustics: Principles and Methods, Vol. 1* (1964) Academic Press: New York, pp. 57–172.

Flynn HG, Church CC. Erratum: Transient pulsations of small gas bubbles in water. *J Acoust Soc Am* (1988) **84**: 1863–1876.

Fowlkes JB, Crum LA, Cavitation threshold measurements for microsecond pulses of ultrasound. *J Acoust Soc Am* (1998) **83**: 2190–2201.

Frizzell LA. Threshold dosages for damage to mammalian liver by high intensity focused ultrasound. *IEEE Trans Ultrason Ferroelec Freq Control* (1988) **35**: 578–581.

Fry FJ, Kossoff G, Eggleton RC, Dunn F. Threshold ultrasonic dosages for structural changes in mammalian brain. *J Acoust Soc Am* (1970) **48**: 1413–1417.

Gaitan DF, Crum LA. Observation of sonoluminescence from a single, stable cavitation bubble in a water/glycerine mixture, in Hamilton MF, Blackstock DT (eds.) *Frontiers of Nonlinear Acoustics: Proc of the 12th International Symposium of Nonlinear Acoustics* (1990) Elsevier Applied Science: New York.

Gaitan DF, Crum LA, Church CC, Roy RA. Sonoluminescence and bubble dynamics for a single, stable cavitation bubble. *J Acoust Soc Am* (1992) **91**: 3166–3183.

Gormley G, Wu J. Observation of acoustic streaming near Albunex® spheres. *J Acoust Soc Am* (1998) **104**: 3117–3118.

Gor'kov LP. On the forces acting on a small particle in an acoustic field in an ideal fluid. *Sov Phys Dokl* (1962) **6**: 773–775.

Guzmán HR, Nguyen DX, Khan S, Prausnitz MR. Ultrasound-mediated disruption of cell membranes. I. Quantification of molecular uptake and cell viability. *J Acoust Soc Am* (2001) **110**: 588–596.

ter Haar G, Daniels S. (1981). Evidence for ultrasonically induced cavitation *in vivo*. *Phys Med Biol* (1981) **26**: 1145–1149.

ter Haar G, Hopewell JW. The induction of hyperthermia by ultrasound: Its value and associated problems. I. Single, static, plane transducer. *Phys Med Biol* (1983) **28**: 889–896.

ter Haar G, Wyard SJ. Blood cell banding in ultrasonic standing wave fields: A physical analysis. *Ultrasound Med Biol* (1978) **4**: 111–123.

Hawkes JJ, Coakley WT. A continuous flow ultrasonic cell-filtering system. *Enzyme Microbiol Tech* (1996) **19**: 57–62.

Henriques FC, Jr. Studies of thermal injury. *Arch Pathol* (1947) **43**: 489–502.

Herrick JF. Pearl chain formation, in *Proc of the Second Tri-Service Conference on Biological Effects of Microwave Energy* (1958).

Hill CR, Rivens I, Vaughan MG, ter Haar GR. Lesion development in focused ultrasound surgery: A general model. *Ultrasound Med Biol* (1994) **20**: 259–269.

Hill CR, Bamber JC, ter Haar G, (eds.), *Physical Principles of Medical Ultrasonics*, 2nd edition. (2004) John Wiley & Sons: Chichester.

Holt RG, Roy RA. Measurements of bubble-enhanced heating from focused, MHz-frequency ultrasound in a tissue-mimicking material. *Ultrasound Med Biol* (2001) **27**: 1399–1412.

Holtzmark J, Johnsen I, Sikkeland T, Skavlem SJ. Boundary layer flow near a cylindrical obstacle in an oscillating incompressible fluid. *J Acoust Soc Am* (1954) **26**: 26–39.

Hu J. A π-shaped ultrasonics tweezers concept for manipulation of small particles. *IEEE Trans Ultrason Ferroelec Freq Control* (2004) **51**: 1499–1707.

Hughes DE, Nyborg WL. Cell disruption by ultrasound. *Science* (1962) **138**: 108–114.

Hwang JH, Brayman AA, Reidy MA, Matula TJ, Kimmey MB, Crum LA. Vascular effects induced by combined 1-MHz ultrasound and microbubble contrast agent treatments *in vivo*. *Ultrasound Med Biol* (2005) **31**: 553–564.

de Jong N, Hoff L, Skotland T, Bom N. Absorption and scatter of encapsulated gas filled microspheres: Theoretical considerations and some measurements. *Ultrasonics* (1962) **30**: 95–103.

Kudo N, Miyaoka T, Okada K, Yamamoto K. Study on mechanism of cell damage caused by microbubbles exposed to ultrasound. 2002 IEEE Ultrasonics Symposium-1351.

Lehmann JF (ed.) *Therapeutic Heat and Cold*, 4th edition. Baltimore. Williams & Wilkins, 1990.

Leighton TG. The Acoustic Bubble. Academic Press: London, 1994.

Lindner JR, Coggins MP, Kaul S, Klibanov AL, Brandenburger GH, Ley K. Microbubble persistence in the microcirculation during ischemia/reperfusion and inflammation is caused by integrin- and complement-mediated adherence to activated leukocytes. *Circulation* (2000) **101**: 668–675.

Lizzi FL, Coleman DJ, Driller J, Franzen LA, Leopold M. Effects of pulsed ultrasound on ocular tissue. *Ultrasound Med Biol* (1981) **7**: 245–252.

Lizzi FL, Ostromogilsky M. Analytical modelling of ultrasonically induced tissue heating. *Ultrasound Med Biol* (1987) **13**: 607–618.

Marmottant P, Hilgenfeldt S. Controlled vesicle deformation and lysis by single oscillating bubbles. *Nature* (2003) **423**: 153–156.

Marsh JN, Hall CS, Hughes MS, Mobley J, Miller JG, Brandenburger GH. Broadband through-transmission signal loss measurements of Albunex® suspensions at concentrations approaching *in vivo* doses. *J Acoust Soc Am* (1997) **101**: 1175–1161.

Michlovitz SL, (ed.) *Thermal Agents in Rehabilitation*, 3rd edition. (1996) F.A. Davis Co.: Philadelphia.

Mihran RT, Barnes FS, Wachtel H. Temporally-specific modification of myelinated axon excitability *in vitro* following a single ultrasonic pulse. *Ultrasound Med Biol* (1990) **16**: 297–309.

Miller DL. An instrument for microscopical observation of the biophysical effects of ultrasound. University of Vermont (1976) Ph.D. thesis.

Miller DL. A review of the ultrasonic bioeffects of microsonation, gas-body activation, and related cavitation-like phenomena. *Ultrasound Med Biol* (1987) **13**: 443–470.

Miller DL. Particle gathering and microstreaming near ultrasonically activated gas-filled micropores. *J Acoust Soc Am* (1988) **84**: 1378–1387.

Miller DL, Dou C. Membrane damage thresholds for pulsed or continuous ultrasound in phagocytic cells loaded with contrast agent gas bodies. *Ultrasound Med Biol* (2004a) **30**: 405–411.

Miller DL, Dou C. Membrane damage thresholds for 1- to 10-MHz pulsed ultrasound exposure of phagocytic cells loaded with contrast agent gas bodies *in vitro*. *Ultrasound Med Biol* (2004b) **30**: 973–977.

Miller DL, Williams AR. Bubble cycling as the explanation of the promotion of ultrasonic cavitation in a rotating tube exposure system. *Ultrasound Med Biol* (1989) **17**: 641–648.

Miller DL, Thomas RM. The role of cavitation in the induction of cellular DNA damage by ultrasound and lithotripter shock waves *in vitro*. *Ultrasound Med Biol* (1996) **22**: 681–687.

Miller DL, Thomas RM, Williams AR. Mechanisms for hemolysis by ultrasonic cavitation in the rotating exposure system. *Ultrasound Med Biol* (1991) **17**: 171–178.

Miller MW, Ziskin MC. Biological consequences of hyperthermia. *Ultrasound Med Biol* (1989) **15**: 707–722.

Miller MW, Miller DL, Brayman AA. A review of *in vitro* bioeffects of inertial ultrasonic cavitation from a mechanistic perspective. *Ultrasound Med Biol* (1996) **22**: 1131–1154.

Miller MW, Sherman TA, Brayman AA. Comparative sensitivity of human and bovine erythrocytes to sonolysis by 1 MHz ultrasound. *Ultrasound Med Biol* (2000) **26**: 1317–1326.

Minnaert M. On musical air-bubbles and sounds of running water. *Phil Mag* (1933) **16**: 235–248.

Mitragotri S, Edwards DA, Blankschtein D, Langer R. A mechanistic study of ultrasonically-enhanced transdermal drug delivery. *J. Pharm Sci* (1995) **84**: 697–706.

Morse PM. *Vibration and Sound* (1981) Acoustical Society of America: Melville, New York.

NCRP. Exposure criteria for medical diagnostic ultrasound. I. Criteria based on thermal mechanisms. National Council on Radiation Protection and Measurements Report No.113. Bethesda MD: NCRP Publications, 1992.

NCRP. Exposure criteria for medical diagnostic ultrasound. II. Criteria based on all known mechanisms. National Council on Radiation Protection and Measurements Report No.140. Bethesda MD: NCRP Publications, 2002.

Nightingale KR, Kornguth PJ, Trahey GE. The use of acoustic streaming in breast lesion diagnosis: A clinical study. *Ultrasound Med Biol* (1999) **25**: 75–87.

Noltingk BE, Neppiras EA. Cavitation produced by ultrasonics. *Proc Phys Soc B (London)* (1950) **63B**: 674–685.

Nyborg WL. Acoustic streaming, in Mason WP, (ed.), Physical Acoustics, Vol II — Part B. Properties of polymers and nonlinear acoustics (1965) Academic Press: New York, pp. 265–331.

Nyborg WL. Heat generation by ultrasound in a relaxing medium. *J Acoust Soc Am* (1981) **70**: 310–312.

Nyborg WL. Sonically produced heat in a fluid in a fluid with bulk viscosity and shear viscosity. *J Acoust Soc Am* (1986) **80**: 1133–1139.

Nyborg WL. Solutions of the bio-heat transfer equation. *Phys Med Biol* (1988) **33**: 785–792.

Nyborg WL. Theoretical criterion for acoustic aggregation. *Ultrasound Med Biol* (1989) **15**: 93–99.

Nyborg WL. Acoustic streaming, in Hamilton MF, Blackstock DT (eds.) *Nonlinear Acoustics* (1998) Academic Press: San Diego, pp. 207–231.

Nyborg WL. Biological effects of ultrasound: Development of safety guidelines. Part II: General review. *Ultrasound Med Biol* (2001) **27**: 301–333.

Nyborg WL, Gershoy A. Microsonation of cells under near-threshold conditions in International Congress Series No. 309. *Ultrasonics in Medicine, Proc Second World Congress on Ultrasonics in Medicine*, Rotterdam, 4–8 June 1973, Excerpta Medica — Ansterdam 1974, pp. 360–365.

Nyborg WL, Miller DL. Biophysical implications of bubble dynamics. *Appl Sci Res* (1982) **38**: 17–24.

Nyborg WL, Steele B. Nearfield of a piston source of ultrasound in an absorbing medium. *J Acoust Soc Am* (1985) **78**: 1882–1891.

Pennes HH. Analysis of tissue and arterial blood temperatures in the resting forearm. *J Appl Physiol* (1948) **1**: 93–122.

Pierce AD. *Acoustics. An Introduction to Its Physical Principles and Applications* (1994) 3rd edition. Acoustical Society of America: Melville, New York.

Plesset MS, Chapman RB. Collapse of an initially spherical vapor cavity in the neighborhood of a solid boundary. *J Fluid Mech* (1971) **47**: 283–290.

Pohlmann R. Die Ultraschalltherapie. (1951) Bern, Switzerland: Hans Huber Verlag.

Raney WP, Corelli JC, Westervelt PJ. Acoustical streaming in the vicinity of a cylinder. *J Acoust Soc Am* (1954) **26**: 1006–1014.

Rayleigh, Lord. *The Theory of Sound*. New York, Dover Publications, 1945.

Rooney JA. Hemolysis near an ultrasonically pulsating gas bubble. *Science* (1970) **169**: 869–871.

Sapareto SA, Dewey WC. Thermal dose determination in cancer therapy. *Int J Oncol Biol Phys* (1984) **10**: 787–800.

Schwan HP. Nonthermal cellular effects of electromagnetic fields: AC-field induced ponderomotoric forces. *Br J Cancer* (1982) **45(Suppl V)**: 220–224.

Sheikov N, McDannold N, Vykhodtseva N, Jolesz F, Hynynen K. Cellular mechanisms of the blood-brain barrier opening induced by ultrasound in the presence of microbubbles. *Ultrasound Med Biol* (2004) **30**: 979–989.

Siegel RJ, (ed.), *Ultrasound Angioplasty* (1996) Kluwer Academic Publishers: Boston.

Siegel RJ, Steffen W, Luo H, Marzelle J, Fishbein MC. High-intensity, low-frequency, catheter-delivered ultrasound for thrombus dissolution, in Siegel RJ (ed.) *Ultrasound Angiography* (1996) Kluwer Academic Publishers: Boston, pp. 135–150.

Spengler JK, Coakley WT. Microstreaming effects on particle concentration in an ultrasonic standing wave. *AICE J* (2003) **49**: 2773–2782.

Starritt HC, Duck FA, Humphrey VF. An experimental investigation of streaming in pulsed diagnostic ultrasound beams. *Ultrasound Med Biol* (1989) **15**: 363–373.

Starritt HC, Duck FA, Humphrey VF. Forces acting in the direction of propagation in pulsed ultrasound fields. *Phys Med Biol* (1991) **36**: 1465–1474.

Stavros AT, Dennis MA. The ultrasound of breast pathology in Parker SH, Jobe WE (eds.) *Percutaneous Breast Biopsy* (1993) Raven Press Ltd.: New York.

Suslick KS. *Ultrasound: Its Chemical, Physical and Biological Effects* (1988) VCH Publishers: New York.

Suslick KS, Kemper KA. The effect of fluorocarbon gases on sonoluminescence: A failure of the electrical hypothesis. *Ultrasonics* (1993) **31**: 463–465.

Swindell W, Roemer RB, Clegg ST, Temperature distributions caused by dynamic scanning of focused ultrasonic transducers, in *Proc 1982 IEEE Ultrasound Symposium*, IEEE Inc. (1982) pp. 750–753.

Tachibana K, Tachibana S, Prototype therapeutic ultrasound emitting catheter for accelerating thrombolysis. *J Ultrasound Med* (1997) **16**: 529–535.

Tsirulnikov EM, Vartanyan IA, Gersuni GV, Rosenblyum AS, Pudov VI, Gavrilov LR. Use of amplitude-modulated focused ultrasound for diagnosis of hearing disorders. Rise in a tissue-mimicking material generated by unfocused and focused ultrasonic transducers. *Ultrasound Med Biol* (1988) **14**: 277–285.

Wang CY. Acoustic streaming of a sphere near an unsteady source. *J Acoust Soc Am* (1982) **71**: 580–584.

Wang TG, Lee CP. Radiation pressure and acoustic levitation, in Hamilton MF, Blackstock DT, (eds.), *Nonlinear Acoustics*. San Diego, Academic Press, (1998) pp. 177–205.

Ward M, Wu J, Chiu JF. Ultrasound-induced cell lysis and sonoporation enhanced by contrast agents. *J Acoust Soc Am* (1999) **105**: 2951–2957.

Ward M, Wu J, Chiu JF. Experimental study on effects of Optison concentration on sonoporation *in vitro*. *Ultrasound Med Biol* (2000) **26**: 1169–1175.

Weiser MA, Apfel RE. Extension of acoustic levitation to include the study of micron-sized particles in a more compressible host liquid. *J Acoust Soc Am* (1982) **71**: 1261–1268.

Westervelt PJ. Acoustic streaming near a small obstacle. *J Acoust Soc Am* (1953) **25**: 1123.

Westervelt PJ. Acoustic streaming near a small obstacle. *J Acoust Soc Am* (1955) **27**: 379.

Whitworth G, Coakley WT. Particle column formation in a stationary ultrasonic field. *J Acoust Soc Am* (1992) **91**: 79–85.

Williams AR, Hughes DE, Nyborg WL. Hemolysis near a transversely oscillating wire. *Science* (1970) **169**: 871–873.

Williams AR. *Ultrasound: Biological Effects and Potential Hazards* (1983) Academic Press: London.

Williams AR, McHale J, Bowditch M, Miller DL, Reed B. Effects of MHz ultrasound on electrical pain threshold perception in humans. *Ultrasound Med Biol* (1987) **13**: 249–258.

Wu J. Acoustical tweezers. *J Acoust Soc Am* (1991) **89**: 2140–2143.

Wu J. Calculation of acoustic radiation force generated by focused beams using the ray acoustics approach. *J Acoust Soc Am* (1995) **97**: 2747–2750.

Wu J. Temperature rise generated by ultrasound in the presence of contrast agent. *Ultrasound Med Biol* (1998) **24**: 267–274.

Wu J. Theoretical study on shear stress generated by microstreaming surrounding contrast agents attached to living cells. *Ultrasound Med Biol* (2002) **28**: 125–129.

Wu J, Chase JD, Zhu Z, Holzapfel TP. Temperature rise in a tissue-mimicking material generated by unfocused and focused ultrasonic transducers. *Ultrasound Med Biol* (1992) **18**: 495–512.

Wu J, Cubberley F, Gormley G, Szabo TL. Temperature rise generated by diagnostic ultrasound in a transcranial phantom. *Ultrasound Med Biol* (1995) **21**: 561–568.

Wu J, Winkler AJ, O'Neill TP. Effect of acoustic streaming on ultrasonic heating. *Ultrasound Med Biol* (1994) **20**: 195–201.

Wu J, Ross JP, Chiu J-F. Reparable sonoporation generated by microstreaming. *J Acoust Soc Am* (2002) **111**: 1460–1464.

Young FR. *Cavitation* (1989) McGraw-Hill: New York.

Young FR. *Sonoluminescence* (2005) CRC Press: London.

Zderic V, Clark JI, Vaezy S. Drug delivery into the eye with the use of ultrasound. *J Ultrasound Med* (2004) **23**: 1349–1359.

III

ULTRASOUND-MEDIATED GENE THERAPY

Douglas L. Miller

Ultrasound owes its capability for gene therapy to the nonthermal bio-effects of sonoporation. Sonoporation has been demonstrated by a wide range of ultrasound sources including sonication probes, lithotripters, low intensity therapeutic ultrasound and diagnostic imaging ultrasound. This effect involves transient permeabilization of individual cells by ultrasonic cavitation activity. Large molecules may be loaded into cells, which may then reseal and survive. If the molecule is an active DNA vector, then this phenomenon can subsequently modify the gene expression of the cells. Thus, the combination of ultrasound with cavitation enhancement and DNA vectors has created a new therapeutic regimen of potentially wide applicability. *In vitro* results for ultrasound-mediated gene transfer have seemed quite promising, but have proven difficult to translate for tissues *in vivo*. *In vivo* situations typically show minimal cavitation activity due to a dearth of cavitation nucleation sites; however, by augmenting nucleation with air or ultrasound contrast agents, sonoporation and DNA delivery have been demonstrated in several different tissues. Several studies of ultrasound-mediated gene therapy have been published including potential therapies for cancer, myocardial infarction, restenosis, transplant rejection, renal fibrosis and stem cell stimulation for dental wound repair. Research into the complexities of the method, including the most appropriate ultrasound modes, nucleation agents, gene vectors, and disease targets is steadily improving results. Prospects appear bright for clinical application of this emerging therapeutic ultrasound technology.

                              D. L. Miller

1. Introduction

The concept of gene therapy is a product of modern medical research, unimaginable a few decades ago. The realization that genetic material could be dissected, recombined and packaged into artificial vectors presents a seemingly miraculous means of therapy and healing. Many diseases have a genetic basis which could be treated by corrective genes, and many medicinal foreign proteins could be introduced by reprogramming the cells of patients to produce curative drugs *in situ*. The prospect is compeling and has generated an ongoing wave of research into therapeutic genes and gene delivery methods. This review is concerned primarily with the gene delivery method of how a therapeutic gene can be placed at the right place at the right time to effect treatment?

Therapeutic genes can be packaged in several different ways in order to allow for the transfer of the large charged molecules into the interior of the cells. The simplest form may be the bacteria-derived plasmid. These large molecules of DNA contain a specific gene or genes, plus promoter sequences to yield expression of the gene by production of the coded protein. Plasmids are typically adjusted in size for insertion into a cell by having a circular form, plus coiling or packaging. Packaging can be accomplished by the condensation of the plasmid DNA by various molecules such as lipids or polylysine. Some types of cationic liposomes can be used to deliver DNA into the cells by facilitating passage through the cell membrane. The most highly developed gene packages are viruses, which insert themselves inside the cells and program their replication. For gene therapy, viruses are modified to inactivate replication, to include the therapeutic genetic material, and to moderate the toxicity of the virus. Virus forms, which have received considerable attention, include adenoviruses used in gene therapy of cardiovascular disease, and retroviruses used especially for cancer therapy. When the functioning DNA reaches the inside of the cell, the protein can be expressed for some time. For stable transfection, the gene is actually incorporated into the genome, and thus becomes a permanent feature of the genetic make up of the cells. Stable transfection may be the ideal for treating genetic disease, such as for inserting missing genes, but it can be difficult to achieve safely. Transient transfection represents a simpler and safer means of gene therapy, for which the therapeutic gene is not integrated into the chromosomes and expression declines over days or weeks.

Viral-mediated transfection allows high transfection rates when compared with DNA alone, and numerous gene therapy strategies have reached the stage of clinical trials. These clinical trials have not been greatly successful and no gene therapy products are presently approved for sale. Unfortunately, there have been failures, including death of patients due to problems with the gene delivery methods. The major concerns related to potential toxicity involve several adverse effects. One problem is the non-specific action of some vectors, which can deliver the genetic material to tissues such as liver, rather than to the desired regions. In addition, there is a potential for development of severe immunological reactions, particularly for adenoviruses. This can cause inflammatory responses, and largely prevents re-use of the vector. There is also some concern that a viral vector, once active in the patient, could regain its ability to cause disease. The stable transfection strategies using retroviruses to treat genetic diseases, also carry the potential for induction of new mutations when the genetic material is randomly inserted into the genome, leading to new disease.

The problems with viral gene therapy have motivated a vigorous search for non-viral methods. There are several potential candidates, including lipofection, electroporation, particle bombardment, and sonoporation. Lipofection is one of the most widely used non-viral methods of transferring genetic material to cells. In this method, cationic lipids encapsulate the negatively charged DNA and allow transfer of the DNA through the cell membrane. This method allows high transfection rates with minimal cellular toxicity, particularly *in vitro*. However, this method shares some problems with the viral vectors, such as the poor control of spatial delivery to the desired tissue. Electroporation utilizes high voltage electric fields to open pores in cell membranes, allowing the transfer of DNA to the interior. This method affords some degree of spatial targeting, but the placement of electrodes *in vivo* is challenging and invasive. A straightforward method involves bombardment of tissue by particles to inject foreign DNA into cells. This "gene gun" method provides for highly accurate delivery to targeted tissue, but presently appears to be limited to surface applications such as the treatment of skin cancer.

The possibility of ultrasound-mediated gene transfer has been discovered relatively recently. Acoustic cavitation, the predominant nonthermal mechanism of ultrasound bioeffects (See Chap. II), provides localized mechanical perturbation of cell membranes. This mechanical process appears to stress the membranes, opening pores and allowing the transfer of material into and out of the cell. Owing to the similarity to electroporation, the method is known as sonoporation. Sonoporation refers to transient permeabilization, in which large molecules can be trapped inside surviving cells, in contrast to the commonly-noted permanent permeabilization of nonviable cells indicated by vital stains such as trypan blue or propidium iodide.

Sonoporation was initially demonstrated using 20 kHz ultrasound exposure of ameboid cells using a "sonicator" cavitation device (Fechheimer *et al.*, 1986). Sonication treatment was also used to load mammalian cells with large fluorescent Dextran molecules (Fechheimer *et al.*, 1987). Following the development of lithotripsy for the treatment of kidney stones, research on lithotripsy shock waves quickly broadened to encompass a variety of biological effects (Delius, 1994). In treating cell suspensions, some cells were found to be transiently permeabilized, allowing them to take up large molecules normally excluded by the cell membrane Gambihler *et al.* (1994). This discovery was quickly recognized as a new treatment tool, and lithotripter shock wave (LSW) treatment was proposed as a means of gene therapy (Delius *et al.*, 1995). Although LSWs reliably initiate cavitation activity *in vitro* and sometimes *in vivo*, other ultrasound modes can also generate cavitational effects. At least five research groups demonstrated simultaneously and independently the ultrasound-mediated cellular uptake of both DNA and other macromolecules (Kim *et al.*, 1996; Bao *et al.*, 1997; Tata *et al.*, 1997; Wyber *et al.*, 1997; Lauer *et al.*, 1997). The findings of this research demonstrated a new means for non-viral gene transfer and gene therapy. Ultrasound contrast agents, which consist of stabilized microbubbles, are capable of nucleating acoustic cavitation at specific sites. Ultrasound focused on the region of interest can even provide feedback in the form of diagnostic images and reception of cavitation-produced acoustic emissions. Conceptually, simple plasmids could be mixed with ultrasound contrast agents, injected into the circulation or directly into tissues and precisely transferred into cells by focused ultrasound treatment. Furthermore, ultrasound-mediated gene therapy appears to reduce or eliminate the risk of systemic gene transfer to the wrong tissue, immune responses to viral vectors and potential problems with repeated treatments or invasive procedures.

These promising indications led to a substantial burst of research activity, which is the subject of this review. There have been a number of previous reviews (Porter and Xie, 2001; Newman *et al.*, 2001; Unger *et al.*, 2001a; Unger *et al.*, 2001b; Miller *et al.*, 2002; Hosseinkhani *et al.*, 2003; McCreery *et al.*, 2004; Dijkmans *et al.*, 2004; Feril and Kondo, 2004; Wells, 2004). However, most of the research has been basic *in vitro* and *in vivo* research, and only a few publications report actual attempts at ultrasound-mediated gene therapy with laboratory animals. This present review draws heavily on Miller *et al.* (2002), but is updated with the research findings of the last few years. First of all, the basic biophysical foundations of the method, primarily derived from *in vitro* research, are briefly presented. Research on the translation of the encouraging *in vitro* results into a viable *in vivo* treatment modality is then examined as applied to various tissues. The publications presently available which report ultrasound treatment using actual therapeutic genes to effect gene therapy are then reviewed. Finally, the entire body of research findings is critically discussed, with the emphasis on both the identification of problems which have been encountered, and on prospects for successful and medically useful ultrasound-mediated gene therapy.

2. Biophysical Foundations

2.1. *Bioeffects of ultrasound*

As an ultrasound wave propagates, the simple oscillation of the medium generally does not directly cause bioeffects. The primary mechanisms for bioeffects of ultrasound are heating and cavitation (NCRP, 2002). Heating occurs as the ultrasonic energy is absorbed in a medium, and can be important for high time-average intensities. Absorption in tissue can be quite important in biomedical applications, particularly above 1 MHz, and is related to ultrasound intensity (typical units of W/cm^2). The absorption coefficient of many tissues increases with frequency, and is about 0.44 dB/(cm MHz) for many soft tissues (see Chap. II). The absorbed energy appears as the heating of the tissue, and resulting physiological responses depend on the temperature and duration of temperature elevations. Acoustic cavitation is the interaction between a propagating ultrasound wave and gaseous inclusions in aqueous media. The pressure amplitude, especially the rarefactional pressure amplitude (RPA with a typical unit of MPa), is the primary exposure parameter for cavitation (See Chap. II). Intensity is proportional to the square of the acoustic pressure amplitude with 1 MPa equivalent to about 33 W/cm^2 in water. Another quantity used as an exposure parameter is the Mechanical Index, which is a measure or estimate of the peak RPA in the region of interest divided by the square root of the ultrasonic frequency (in MHz). In general, tissue heating necessarily occurs, but tissue temperature elevations can be insignificant for pulsed ultrasound exposure with substantial cavitational activity. For low pressure amplitudes, gas bubble pulsation depends strongly on bubble size relative to the ultrasound frequency, and is maximized at the resonance frequency of the bubble. At 1 MHz, a resonance size bubble in water is about 7 microns in diameter. Large bubbles or air-water interfaces act as reflective surfaces for ultrasound waves under most conditions. At higher pressure amplitudes, transformation of cavitation nuclei (See Chap. II), which are normally inactive and difficult to detect, into active cavities and bubbles gives the appearance of a threshold for vigorous cavitation. However, if suitable bodies of gas are present initially, then these will respond at any amplitude. At lower amplitudes, it represents a non-threshold form of cavitation activity, termed gas-body activation. In addition, proliferation of bubble populations by breaking up larger bubbles can multiply cavitation effectiveness. Inertial cavitation occurs above specific physical thresholds when bubbles collapse into minute sites of intense heat, for which free radical production and shockwave generation can introduce additional mechanisms for bioeffects.

The concentration of ultrasonic energy by cavitation bubbles yields a potential for biological effects in their vicinity whenever bubbles or cavitation nuclei are present in a biological medium exposed to ultrasound. Cavitation bioeffects can be confusing and elusive to study owing to the requirement of pre-existing gaseous inclusions. Thresholds for cavitation are difficult to predict without knowledge of the nuclei present. In some *in vitro* situations, cavitation readily occurs at modest pressure amplitudes, due to the presence of cavitation nuclei on surfaces or as suitably sized bubbles. In contrast, *in vivo* conditions in mammals typically minimize populations of cavitation nuclei because of active filtering by the circulation and sterilization by the mononuclear phagocyte system. Cavitation causes mechanical perturbation in the vicinity of active bubbles, which include the production of direct stresses due to pulsation, and indirect stresses due to time averaged forces or fluid flow (See Chap. II). The effects on cell membranes range from deformation and sonoporation, which is the transient opening of holes in the membrane, to cell lysis or even fragmentation. Sonoporation is the phenomenon of interest in this chapter, because the effected cells exchange molecules with the surrounding medium but reseal and survive. If viable genetic material diffuses into the cell during sonoporation, then the material can be trapped and subsequently lead to expression of the gene-encoded protein.

2.2. *Methods for ultrasound-mediated gene transfer*

There are three elements needed for successful ultrasound-mediated gene transfer: the ultrasound exposure, the means of cavitation initiation, and the genetic material configuration.

2.2.1. *Ultrasound exposure systems*

Therapeutic applications often exploit the heating effects of ultrasound. In low intensity therapeutic ultrasound (LITU), continuous (or burst) mode ultrasound with slow heating of large regions of tissue using a hand-held applicator is used for the physical therapy of muscle and joint disease. High intensity focused ultrasound (HIFU) can be used to rapidly heat and destroy tissue. For example, HIFU systems are used for treating cancer tumors, benign prostate hyperplasia, and other localized volumes, usually under the guidance of diagnostic ultrasound imaging or other modalities (See Chap. VIII).

Nonthermal mechanisms are also of value for therapeutic applications. Low frequency (*e.g.*, 20 kHz) ultrasound probes are used for cavitation-induced lysis and the disruption of cells. Although laboratory sonicators are for disruption of cell suspensions, similar medical systems can be applied to tissue removal, such as in liposuction and angioplasty (See Chap. II). Focused high amplitude shockwaves are used for lithotripsy of kidney and gall bladder stones. These lithotripter shockwaves (LSW) typically involve single cycle pulses of about 100 kHz ultrasound with RPA values in excess of 5 MPa in magnitude. The extreme tensile stresses produced in solid stones by these high amplitude pulses fracture the stones and gradually reduce them to fine particles.

In diagnostic ultrasound, frequencies from about 1.2 to 12 MHz are used under conditions of minimal bioeffects. Blood flow or other tissue motion is detected by the Doppler effect using either continuous or pulsed ultrasound. Pulse-echo systems with scanned beams of ultrasound are used for medical imaging in obstetrics, cardiology and radiology. Typically, pulsed ultrasound has relatively low time averaged intensity, leading to relatively low heating. Although the pulses can have relative high RPA (greater than 2 MPa in magnitude), the relative lack of cavitation nuclei *in vivo* leads to relatively low risk of cavitational bioeffects. The exception to this rule can occur if use is made of ultrasound contrast agents, consisting of suspensions of stabilized gas bodies.

Each of these ultrasound exposure systems has been used for ultrasound-mediated gene transfer, and examples of each are listed in Table 1. All these ultrasound methods require water, or other suitable medium for the transmission of the ultrasonic waves from the source to the tissue or cells that are to be exposed. When a suspension of cells is to be exposed to ultrasound with an *in vitro* system, the vessel containing the suspension would normally be immersed in a water bath. *In vitro* methods are sometimes difficult to arrange for well-defined exposure parameters. For example, the culture dish system with a physical therapy applicator aimed upward from below will involve reflection of the ultrasound. These reflections make the exact RPA at the cell monolayer virtually impossible to know, since it depends on the precise distance between the applicator and the dish, the thickness of the dish bottom and the thickness of the liquid layer in the dish. The sonicator, culture dish, chamber and rotating tube methods are used mainly for *in vitro* research on cell suspensions. The diagnostic scanner, LITU, HIFU and LSW devices can be used *in vivo*, and would be considered for medical application. These systems can sometimes be applied directly to an animal; however, well defined acoustical conditions in small animals also require placement in a water bath. There are few direct comparisons of the different methods. The use of LSW was compared with focused ultrasound at 1.18 MHz for the transfection of cultured cells (Huber *et al.*, 1999). The focused ultrasound was significantly better in terms of reduced cell killing and higher transfection percentages.

Table 1. Ultrasound exposure systems for gene transfer with examples of their reported use (LITU = low intensity therapeutic ultrasound, HIFU = high intensity focused ultrasound).

Ultrasound Source	Field Configuration	Frequency Range MHz	Intensity or RPA	*in vitro*		*in vivo*	
				System	Citation	Tissue	Citation
Sonicator	point source	0.02–0.04	cavitating	suspension	Wyber *et al.*, 1997	none	
Lithotripter	focused shock waves	0.1–0.3	up to ~10 MPa	fixed chamber suspension	Lauer *et al.*, 1997	malignant tumor	Song *et al.*, 2002
LITU	unfocused beam	0.5–3.0	0.5–5.0 W/cm^2	culture dish monolayer	Kim *et al.*, 1996	skeletal muscle	Taniyama *et al.*, 2002
Laboratory	unfocused beam	0.5-3.0 typical	0.8 MPa	rotating tube suspension	Bao *et al.*, 1997	rotation not applicable	
Pulsed HIFU	focused beam	0.75–3	up to ~15 MPa	fixed chamber suspension	Huber *et al.*, 1999	carotid artery	Huber *et al.*, 2003
Diagnostic imager	scanned focused	1.3–13	1.9 $\sqrt{f}$ MPa	chamber monolayer	Miller *et al.*, 2003	myocardium	Shohet *et al.*, 2000

2.2.2. *Means of cavitation enhancement*

Cavitation activity is necessary for sonoporation and ultrasound-mediated transfection. This has been demonstrated many times using *in vitro* systems (Bao *et al.*, 1997; Greenleaf *et al.*, 1998; Ward *et al.*, 1999; Koch *et al.*, 2000; Deng *et al.*, 2004). Cavitation can be a complex phenomenon involving both mechanical and chemical mechanisms for bioeffects (See Chap. II). For sonoporation, free radical production does not appear to be necessary (Lawrie *et al.*, 2003). Sonication and LSW exposure systems *in vitro* can typically initiate vigorous cavitation activity without nucleation enhancement. However, in many situations with less powerful ultrasound treatment, cavitation initiation can be problematic resulting in widely varying effects. For example, cell culture media is clean and sterile, minimizing the presence of cavitation nuclei, unless special arrangements are used.

A common exposure system used for *in vitro* research on cavitation bioeffects is the rotating tube system. Cells in suspension are affected by bubbles which cycle back and forth across the tube as it rotates (Miller and Williams, 1989). This is an efficient process which includes the proliferation of the microbubbles. The culture dish system also has a mechanism for cavitation initiation and enhancement (Chen *et al.*, 2004). When the ultrasound aimed at the dish from below encounters the interface between the culture medium and air, there is a strong reflection of the beam. This causes disturbance of the surface. For only moderate levels of exposure, this disturbance evolves into surface wave agitation, local field enhancement and even air bubble entrapment. This foaming agitation provides a rich supply of cavitation bubbles and reliably causes bioeffects on the cells growing in the dish.

Ultrasound contrast agents contain stabilized microbubbles for the enhancement of blood echogenicity. Soon after the commercial development of ultrasound contrast agents, their ability to nucleate cavitation activity was demonstrated (Miller and Thomas, 1995). This property of the stabilized microbubbles has been a boon to sonoporation and transfection research. Even for the rotating tube system, the addition of these cavitation nuclei improves results (Bao *et al.*, 1997). During cavitation activity, the stabilized microbubbles become destabilized. For *in vivo* diagnostic applications of pulsed ultrasound modes, the gas bodies must typically be replenished, for example, by intermittent triggering of image frame sequences to allow blood perfusion to refill a tissue volume with gas body-containing blood.

Tissues *in vivo* are also generally clean and sterile so that cavitation nucleation is problematic even for LSW, with a threshold estimated to be 4 MPa in tissue (Coleman *et al.*, 1995). In arterial blood, cavitation could not be detected even after prolonged LSW treatment (Williams *et al.*, 1989). For sonoporation and transfection studies *in vivo*, enhancement of cavitation nucleation is crucial for robust results. Transfection has been enhanced for tumor treatment *in vivo* by simply injecting air (Miller *et al.*, 1999). However, contrast agents are the nucleation agents of choice, since these are developed and produced for use *in vivo*. The object of adding contrast agents to the test specimen is to nucleate cavitation and most agents will fill this role. The newer agents using perfluorocarbon gases to improve microbubble persistence appear to be more effective. The air-filled microbubbles in Albunex® (Mallinckrodt Medical Inc., St. Louis MO) were shown to be less effective for the sonoporation of cultured cells than the octafluoropropane microbubbles in Optison® (Amersham Health Inc., Princeton NJ) (Ward *et al.*, 1999). This observation also applies to *in vivo* applications. Levovist® (Schering AG, Berlin) and Albunex® were much less effective for the transfection of muscle cells with LITU than Optison® (Li *et al.*, 2003).

2.2.3. *Genetic material configuration*

The gene carrier is the final component in ultrasound-mediated transfection. Most commonly, marker plasmids have been used for exploratory research. These plasmids can simply be purchased and grown up to the desired quantity in bacteria. Plasmids coding for luciferase are useful for gauging the overall transfection and gene expression level in a cell culture or treated tissue. In a typical experiment, the cells are lysed, luciferin is added and the resulting light emission is measured in a luminometer. Plasmids coding for green (or other color) fluorescent protein are useful for determining the fraction of cells which are transfected, or for locating transfected cells in tissue. Typically, the cells are observed using a fluorescence microscope or flow cytometer. Another useful marker is the lac Z gene coding for the β-galactosidase enzyme. Cell extracts can be assayed for overall activity or individual cells can be stained for enzyme expression. Many other research gene systems are also possible and therapeutic gene vectors are monitored by measuring the gene expression products, as well as by observing the therapeutic response.

Plain or "naked" plasmids are simple to use *in vitro*. Adding some contrast agent and some plasmids to a cell suspension, followed by brief ultrasound exposure, is all that is needed for demonstrating ultrasound-mediated gene transfection (see, *e.g.*, Bao *et al.*, 1997). Naked plasmids are also useful *in vivo* even though DNAases can rapidly break down the plasmids. This method is most useful for tissue injection such as in tumors (Miller *et al.*, 1999) or muscle (Taniyama *et al.*, 2002a). However, there are many possible variations. Modifications of the DNA by commercially available lipid preparations can be used to transfect cells without ultrasound. However, the transfection ability of lipid formulas can be enhanced by ultrasound (Unger *et al.*, 1997; Lawrie *et al.*, 1999; Koch *et al.*, 2000). Other possibilities include the packaging of the desired genetic material by polymers (Kuo *et al.*, 2003), in viruses (Shohet *et al.*, 2000), as stabilized DNA polyplexes with prolonged circulation times (Zhou *et al.*, 2005), or even in artificial chromosomes (Oberle *et al.*, 2004).

One strategy for improving the delivery of genes to cells using contrast agent microbubbles is to attach the DNA to the stabilizing shell. This scheme was tested as a means of delivering antisense oligonucleotides to tissue by using diagnostic ultrasound to destabilize the microbubbles at the desired location (Porter *et al.*, 1996). For gene transfer, several schemes have been tried. Plasmids can be attached to albumin-stabilized microbubbles by sonication of the plasmid with the albumin solution and used to trans-fect cultured cells (Frenkel *et al.*, 2002). The expression of the luciferase reporter gene was significantly higher than for microbubbles mixed with plasmid. Plasmid loaded microbubbles have also been applied to coro-nary arteries *ex vivo* and activated by diagnostic ultrasound to transfect the endothelium (Tuepe *et al.*, 2002). Lipid-plasmid complexes were linked to lipid stabilized microbubbles and were used to transfect canine heart cells with 1.3 MHz diagnostic ultrasound (Vannan *et al.*, 2002). Although trans-fection was targeted to the heart by the ultrasound scanning, transfection was also found to occur in other organs, including lung, liver and kidney. Polymer-DNA complexes have been used to construct stabilized microbub-bles, in which the shell consists of the complexes (Seemann *et al.*, 2002).

Viruses can also be exploited in this strategy. Modified adenovirus coding for β-galactosidase was attached to albumin stabilized microbubbles by mixing for 2 hours (Shohet *et al.*, 2000). The destruction of the microbubbles in the heart by diagnostic ultrasound produced a 10-fold increase in enzyme expression, compared with controls.

2.3. *Basic in vitro research*

In vitro studies of sonoporation and ultrasound-mediated transfection provide useful insights into the basic biophysical process. In this section, some of these studies will be reviewed briefly in regard to the phenomenon of sonoporation, transfection, and of the relevance of the *in vitro* research to *in vivo* transfection and gene therapy.

2.3.1. *Sonoporation*

Sonoporation was initially demonstrated using 20 kHz sonication (Fechheimer *et al.*, 1986), although this finding was not immediately noted as a new ultrasound bioeffect (it was intended as a method for intracellular pH measurement). Ameboid mold cells were sonicated in the presence of large fluorescent Dextran molecules. Cell recovery was ~40% of the original number, and 10% of these were loaded with the large molecules. Sonication treatment (20 kHz) also permeabilizes mammalian cells (Fechheimer *et al.*, 1987). 10 to 20% of sonicated hepatoma, mouse myeloma, HeLa and fibroblast cell lines were found to take up 40 kD fluorescent Dextran. Johannes and Obe (1997) showed that 20 kHz sonication of cultured CHO cells in the presence of endonuclease enzymes caused chromosome aberrations in ~20% of subsequently cultured cells. Observations of calcein uptake using 20–100 kHz sonication correlated with cavitation noise, but not subharmonic signals, suggested that inertial cavitation was primarily responsible for the sonoporation (Sundaram *et al.*, 2003). The effects on viability and permeability could be modeled using exponential functions of the energy density, similar to the functions noted below for LSW.

Following the development of lithotripsy using high amplitude shock waves, research on lithotripsy-mode ultrasound broadened to include a variety of potential applications. For *in vitro* exposure, some cells were found to be transiently permeabilized, and to take up large molecules normally excluded by the cell membrane. Gambihler *et al.* (1994) evaluated the accumulation of fluorescein-labeled Dextran (3,900 to 2 million molecular weight) in L1210 cells exposed in the presence of the Dextran. The large molecules were found in the surviving cells with a diffuse distribution within the cytoplasm. These observations led to the suggestion that LSW could be used for gene therapy (Delius *et al.*, 1995).

Sonoporation of red blood cells by LSW was examined in whole blood (Miller *et al.*, 1998). Fluorescent Dextran (580 kDa) was added to the suspensions of canine erythrocytes and the mixture was exposed to LSW in small chambers. An air bubble was needed in the chamber to obtain substantial effects. Hemolysis increased with increasing numbers of shockwaves, but the numbers of cells with fluorescent dextran uptake remained fairly constant for 250 to 1,000 shockwaves. Thus, the sonoporated cells represented an increasing percentage of the surviving cells. These trends could be modeled by the simple theory for random interaction of the cells with bubbles. The number of cells S, of the original number S_0, surviving n shockwaves declines exponentially at a rate of a per shockwave, is given by

$$S = S_0 e^{-an} \tag{1}$$

The number of fluorescent cells F arising at a rate b from the surviving cells, and lysed at rate a, is then given by

$$F = S_0 e^{-an}(1 - e^{-bn}) \tag{2}$$

This model predicts that more of the survivors will eventually become loaded with fluorescent molecules, as n increases toward infinity, but this number will be a decreasing fraction of the original number. This theory fitted actual measurements reasonably well (Miller *et al.*, 1998), as shown in Fig. 1. Approximately one cell became fluorescent for every three cells lysed. The percentage of survivors which were fluorescent, plotted in the lower panel of Fig. 1, was calculated as F/S times 100%. Due to these trends, it appears that sonoporation efficiency cannot be greatly improved simply by increasing ultrasound exposure.

Sonoporation by LSW has also been demonstrated by Zhong *et al.* (1999). Mouse lymphoid cells were treated in the presence of fluorescent

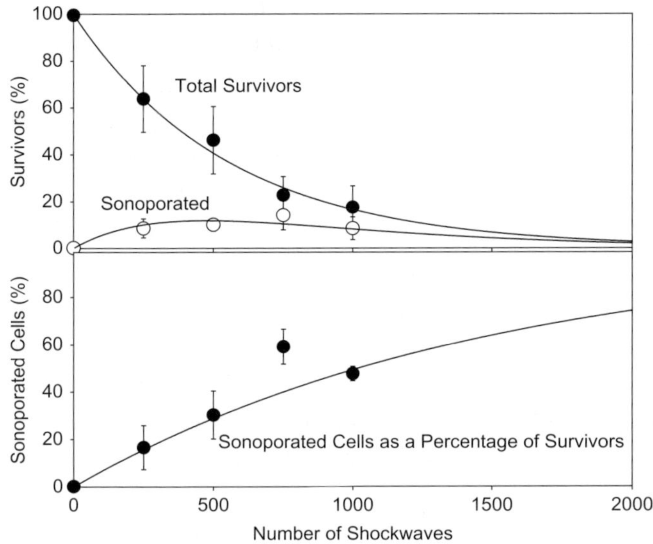

Fig. 1. The percentage of erythrocytes lysed and sonoporated (upper panel) for lithotripter shock wave treatment of whole blood with an air bubble and added fluorescent Dextran. The lower panel shows the percentage of sonoporated survivors. The plotted curves represent a theoretical model of the dose-response, which was fitted to the data (see text). Reproduced with permission from Miller *et al.*, 1998.

Dextran, and the percentage of transiently permeabilized cells reached 11.2% after 100 shockwaves. The effects were associated with acoustic emissions indicative of cavitation. High speed photography was used to show creation and collapse of bubbles with maximum sizes in the range of 100 to 200 μm, which emitted shockwaves upon creation and collapsed up to 1 ms later.

LSW are not needed for sonoporation, and higher frequency ultrasound with cavitation enhanced by contrast agents readily induces a range of effects on cells. Sonoporation of cultured cells was demonstrated with the rotating tube system using fluorescent Dextran (Bao *et al.*, 1997). Chinese hamster ovary cells were exposed to 2.25 MHz ultrasound in sterile 4.5 ml polyethylene chambers and tested for cell lysis, sonoporation and DNA transfection. 10% of Albunex[®], a gas-body-based ultrasound contrast agent, was added to ensure cavitation nucleation, and the chambers were rotated at 60 rpm during the 1 min exposures. Sonoporation

     D. L. Miller

was observed for spatial peak pressure amplitudes as low as 0.1 MPa, and significant lysis occurred above 0.2 MPa. Up to half of the surviving cells were fluorescent after exposure at 0.8 MPa. The ultrasonic frequency has an important role in sonoporation (Miller *et al.*, 1999). After continuous wave exposure at frequencies of 1.0, 1.68, 2.25, 3.3, 5.3 and 7.15 MHz, sonoporation was noted above 0.1 MPa up to 3.3 MHz, but only above 0.39 MPa at 7.15 MHz. The fluorescent cell count increased approximately in proportion to increasing Albunex® concentration. The sonoporation effect represents a form of membrane damage, and although the cells survive, they appear to have a poor proliferation ability in culture. The plating efficiency of cells exposed to 0.28 MPa at 2.25 MHz, and sorted by a flow cytometer were only 19% (3.6% standard deviation) for fluorescent cells, compared with 67% (1% s. d.) for non-fluorescent exposed cells.

Ward *et al.* (1999) observed ultrasound induced cell lysis and sonoporation for 2 MHz, 0.2 MPa exposure of cell suspensions in a 200 rpm rotating tube system. Addition of ultrasound contrast agent was essential for effects and Optison® provided greater enhancement of effects than Albunex®. In further work with Optison® (Ward *et al.*, 2000), the expected mean spacing between bubbles and cells had an important role in the magnitude of effects. The spacing was inferred from a static model (*i.e.*, neglecting ultrasonic forces on the bubbles or between cells and bubbles) for different cell and bubble concentrations. The percentage of effected cells declined approximately as the inverse third power of the static spacing, which is related to the concentration.

The interaction between cells and contrast agent microbubbles can occur even for short pulses of ultrasound, if the cells and microbubbles are in contact. Sonoporation was demonstrated for monolayer cells in contact with Optison® gas bodies for 3.5 MHz diagnostic ultrasound (Miller and Quddus, 2000). Up to 10% of the cells in a 1 mm field of view had an uptake of fluorescent dextran after 1 minute exposure. Pressure amplitudes of 0.23 MPa in Doppler mode (5 μs pulses) and 0.39 MPa (0.46 μs pulses) in scan mode were almost equally effective. This result suggests that diagnostic ultrasound scanners might be useful for gene therapeutic applications, particularly with the guidance of treatment afforded by the imaging mode.

There are many factors which influence the phenomenon of sonoporation. Using 500 kHz ultrasound with an exposure chamber system, Guzman *et al.* (2001a, 2001b) examined the importance of pulsing parameters on cell viability and the uptake of calcein, a relatively small fluorescent molecule. The effects increased strongly with RPA and time, but were not strongly influenced by variation in pulse duration or duty cycle for a given on-time. Similar results were seen for 24 kHz sonication (Keyhani *et al.*, 2001). Although exposure was uniform over the chamber, the cells showed a wide range of effects, which reflected the highly variable individual interaction of cells and bubbles. However, the overall effect tended to increase in proportion to the acoustic energy delivered. The size of molecules used to observe sonoporation was not a strong factor in results for a range of sizes from calcein (623 Da) to albumin and large fluorescent dextran molecules (464 kDa) (Guzman *et al.*, 2002).

Deng *et al.* (2004) examined the permeabilization of relatively large "cells", which were Xenopus oocytes, using voltage clamp techniques. Optison® and 0.96 MHz exposure were both required for sonoporation, indicated by transient membrane currents which increased with pressure amplitude from 0.29 to 0.6 MPa. The transient currents recovered in 3–10 s for surviving cells, as shown in Fig. 2. Resealing required the presence of calcium in the medium, and did not occur for relatively high exposure levels such as 0.7 MPa for 0.5 s.

2.3.2. *Transfection*

Sonication treatment (20 kHz) has been used to transfect cells with plasmid DNA (Fechheimer *et al.*, 1987). Murine fibroblasts lacking the gene for the production of the enzyme thymidine kinase were used as the target cells for "therapy" with a plasmid (pPVTK4) coding for the enzyme. After sonication treatment in the presence of the plasmid, survival was ∼70%. Stable transfection was demonstrated by culture with medium containing hypozanthine, aminopterin and thymidine (HAT) to select against colonies lacking the thymidine kinase gene. An average of 23 transformed colonies were counted per million viable cells, and repeated passage of selected cells indicated that stable transfection had occurred.

Wyber *et al.* (1997) reported a 20-fold enhancement of transfection for 20 kHz sonication of yeast cells together with LEU2 reporter gene plasmids,

     D. L. Miller

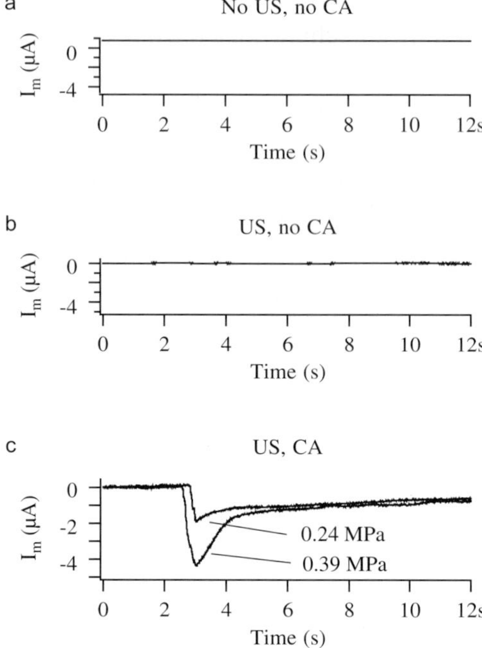

Fig. 2.   Ultrasound was applied for 1 s to a voltage-clamped oocyte. No change was normally observed in the ionic transmembrane current (a). Ultrasound alone did not induce a change in the ionic current (b). Application of ultrasound in the presence of Optison® contrast agent gas bodies produced a transient change in ionic current, which was dependent on exposure amplitude (c). The current gradually returned to normal as the membrane resealed. Reproduced with permission from Deng *et al.*, 2004.

plus salmon sperm DNA (as a carrier DNA) relative to controls. Cavitation activity was measured by the iodine release assay, and was correlated with the loss of cell colony forming units (viability). Sonication induced transfection was examined using the GFP plasmid *in vitro* by Wei *et al.* (2004). Up to 35% transfection was achieved with 90% viability, with relatively low amplitudes at 31.5 kHz.

Sonoporation by LSW is also effective for *in vitro* transfection of cell suspensions. Expression of β-galactosidase gene in a reporter plasmid was observed in 0.1 to 0.5% of viable plated cells after 48 hours (Lauer *et al.*, 1997). The expression increased with increasing concentration of DNA during exposure and with increasing numbers of shockwaves. Transfection was suppressed by application of 10 MPa over-pressure, which implicates cavitation activity as the mechanism for the bioeffect. The method was applicable to many different cultured cell lines including HeLa cells, mouse L-M fibroblasts, monkey kidney cells, and L1210 mouse leukemia cells. The GFP reporter plasmid was utilized by Miller *et al.* (1999) to investigate LSW transfection. Plasmid solution was added to the B16 melanoma cell suspension at 20 μl/ml and 0.2 ml of air was retained in the 1.2 ml exposure chambers. After 800 SW, cell counts after two days of culture were only 5.3% of shams, with 1.4% of the cells expressing GFP.

The transfection efficacy of LSWs was compared to 1.18 MHz focused ultrasound exposure by Huber *et al.* (1999). While lithotripter shock waves induced up to an eight-fold increase in marker gene expression, relative to controls with 5% viability, focused ultrasound induced up to an 80-fold increase with 45% viability. Viability decreased and DNA transfer increased for increasing pressure amplitude up to 5 MPa at 40% duty cycle, and increasing sonication time up to 10 minutes. Huber and Pfisterer (2000) compared transfection by 1.18 MHz focused ultrasound on prostate tumor cells *in vitro* and *in vivo* (see below for *in vivo* results). *In vitro*, 1 MPa exposures with 4 ms burst duration and 100 Hz PRF produced 55 to 220 fold increases in β-galactosidase expression in different cell lines, including human melanoma and Dunning rat prostate tumor cells.

Several research groups almost simultaneously reported that LITU could be used to transfect cells with marker plasmids. Kim *et al.* (1996) developed an exposure system with a 1 MHz ultrasound beam aimed into culture dishes. Primary fibroblasts were exposed with a β-galactosidase control vector or with a plasmid (pMC1neo poly(A)) containing an antibiotic resistance gene. Variations in transfection efficiency were found with temperature, pressure amplitude above 0.2 MPa, exposure duration and on-off timing. Highest transfection rates were found for $\sim$0.4 MPa and 20 sec exposures, with $\sim$50% survival. Stable transfection rates averaged 0.34% of surviving cells. The involvement of cavitation was demonstrated by augmenting nucleation with Albunex® ultrasound contrast agent (Greenleaf *et al.*, 1998). A human condrocyte cell line was exposed with a GFP marker plasmid and transfection increased above an apparent threshold of 0.12 MPa (spatially averaged over the culture dish) and reached $\sim$50% of viable cells at 0.41 MPa for 20 s exposure duration.

Seeding of the medium with 10% Albunex® was required to promote transfection of CHO cells at low amplitudes in the rotating tube exposure system (Bao *et al.*, 1997). Luciferase reporter plasmid at 20 μg/ml was added to the suspension during exposure. Cells were assayed for proliferation ability and for luciferase gene expression two days after exposure. Cell proliferation was greatly reduced above the cavitation threshold and luciferase production was significant for 0.20 MPa exposure, reaching 0.33 ng per 10^6 cells for 0.8 MPa exposure. The luciferase production was greater for cells exposed in medium supplemented with serum than for cells exposed in serum-free medium.

Tata *et al.* (1997) examined GFP marker plasmid transfer in two human cancer cell lines, LnCap and PC-3. Ultrasound treatment was at 932 MHz frequency with a 20% duty cycle directed upward into culture dishes, with an average intensity of 0.33 W/cm^2. Loss of cell viability and uptake of fluorescent-labeled plasmids into viable cells were greatest for continuous or low pulse repetition frequency (PRF) exposure. Gene expression followed a similar pattern, with maximal expression for 50 to 150 Hz PRF, and no increase in GFP expression for a PRF of 1 kHz. This response pattern possibly reflects the variation in occurrence and the amount of cavitation activity in this exposure system.

The sonoporation method might be useful for cardiovascular applications of gene therapy. Lawrie *et al.* (1999) cultured porcine vascular smooth muscle cells and endothelial cells, and compared luciferase marker plasmid transfer with naked or lipid-DNA complexes with 1 MHz ultrasound. The transfection period was 3 hours in duration, with ultrasound applied at 0.4 W/cm^2 for 60 s, 30 minutes into the transfection period. Ultrasound exposure enhanced subsequent luciferase expression by 7.5 times for naked DNA, 2.4 times for lipid-DNA in the muscle cells, and 3.3 times for lipofection of endothelial cells. Involvement of the cavitational mechanism was confirmed in experiments with 10% added Albunex® or Optison® ultrasound contrast agents (Lawrie *et al.*, 2000). Up to 300 fold enhancement over naked DNA transfection was obtained for ultrasound treatment. The addition of Optison® also enhanced transfection with lipofection (Tfx-50 lipoplexes) and with polyplexes (LT-1) of the smooth muscle cells.

Cultured endothelial and smooth muscle cells were treated in culture dishes with an unspecified ultrasound system using luciferase marker plasmids and Optison® (Taniyama *et al.*, 2002b). Ultrasound increased the transfection relative to plasmid alone, and addition of Optison® produced a further increase for both cell types. Scanning electron microscopy revealed holes in cell membranes for ultrasound and ultrasound plus Optison® specimens. Interpretation of the exact relationship of the holes to the gene transfer is problematical, since the freeze dried preparations used for electron microscopy are prone to artifact.

Manome *et al.* (2000) have examined transfer of naked DNA into tumor cells *in vitro* and *in vivo* using 1 MHz continuous ultrasound (see below for *in vivo* results). *In vitro*, 30 s ultrasound treatment enhanced β-galactosidase and antibiotic-resistance reporter gene expression in mouse adenocarcinoma cells, both in transient and stable transfection assays. Stable transfection for ten days of culture with geneticin selection averaged 34 per 10^6 cells for 30 s ultrasound exposure.

A clinical spectral Doppler ultrasound system, as well as a laboratory ultrasound exposure system, was used by Koch *et al.* (2000) to enhance transfection by cationic liposomes. The GFP reporter plasmid was used with rodent and canine glioma cells. For the clinical system, exposure was performed at 2 MHz with 0.5 W/cm^2 average intensity in 12 well culture plates. Up to 32.7% transfection was obtained at 24 hours for 90 s exposure, compared with 7.4% in controls. For the laboratory system, no transfection was seen at 0.6 MPa, unless Levovist® ultrasound contrast agent was added. Ultrasound-mediated transfection in cultured cells by 1 MHz ultrasound with Levovist® was enhanced by addition of lidocaine or by heating to 42–44°C (Nozaki *et al.*, 2003). These effects were thought to result from alterations in membrane fluidity.

Pislaru *et al.* (2003) also examined the potential for transfection using luciferase plasmid and the contrast agents Optison® and PESDA, made in the laboratory by sonication of albumin solutions. Ultrasound from a 1.7 MHz diagnostic scanner or 1 MHz continuous wave (CW) system were used with the culture dish arrangement. PESDA gave higher luciferase expression in vascular smooth muscle cells and in human vascular endothelial cells than Optison®, but both generated a similar dose response in cell loss. The different ultrasound modes gave similar results.

Observations of the transfer of GFP and luciferase plasmids into cultured cells with 500 kHz focused ultrasound, showed that less than one fourth of the cells with plasmid uptake went on to exhibit marker gene expression (Zarnitsyn and Prausnitz, 2004). Although overall luciferase expression was many fold that of sham exposed cells, the number of cells expressing the GFP marker was only a few percent of the original number treated. The reduced incidence of gene expression may reflect cellular injury or the lack of sufficient numbers of transferred gene vectors.

Packaging of the DNA in stabilized polyplexes can help to protect it from degradation *in vivo*. This could allow prolonged circulation times for treatment, but may reduce transfection performance. Zhou *et al.* (2005) have demonstrated gene transfer *in vitro* with stabilized polyplexes, comparable to that with naked plasmids. This indicates a potential for improved *in vivo* results using this packaging strategy.

The culture dish exposure system has been a popular research tool for ultrasound-mediated transfection. A puzzling aspect of some reports of transfection using this system was that cavitation activity often did not need to be enhanced, for example, by addition of contrast agents. Chen *et al.* (2004) observed that transfection of GFP plasmids by 1 MHz ultrasound was accompanied by agitation of the surface of the medium covering the cell monolayer. Covering of the surface with a thin membrane inhibited the agitation and the transfection. Apparently, the agitation resulted in bubble generation and cavitation activity either by foaming of the surface or by the creation of high pressure amplitude (above the cavitation threshold) regions, by reflections from the distorted surface.

Cultured myoblast cells were exposed to 1 MHz ultrasound in the culture dish system with GFP plasmid (Liang *et al.*, 2004). The results were similar to or lower than those for the other cells in this system and surface agitation was noted. Optimum conditions at 0.5 to 1 W/cm^2 gave a 4.5% transfection efficiency with 83% viability. The overall transfection, measured as average fluorescence, was proportional to the logarithm of plasmid concentration, which is consistent with a passive diffusion process.

Ultrasound contrast agents were developed for use with diagnostic ultrasound. The stabilized microbubbles were specifically created for strong activation using imaging pulses, and, as noted above, can produce enhanced sonoporation and gene transfer. The question arises as to whether contrast-aided diagnostic ultrasound exposures could be used for therapy.

Teupe *et al.* (2002) used microbubbles generated with plasmid DNA, so that the plasmids were attached to the stabilizing shells. Using 5 s of 2.2 MHz diagnostic ultrasound in harmonic imaging mode produced observable transfection in porcine coronary arteries *in vitro*. The endothelial cells were transfected with the lac-Z gene without impairment of vasoreactivity. Frenkel *et al.* (2002) also utilized plasmid loaded albumin microbubbles to transfect cells suspended in a test tube with 1.3 MHz diagnostic ultrasound. Microbubbles loaded with plasmids produced 5 times more expression of luciferase than unattached plasmids. As noted above, Pislaru *et al.* (2003) showed that diagnostic ultrasound produced results similar to LITU treatment in a culture dish. Diagnostic ultrasound was also used to transfect monolayer cells with the GFP plasmid using Optison® microbubbles in contact with the cells, but not loaded with the plasmid (Miller *et al.*, 2003). The 1.5 MHz scan head was aimed upward at a culture chamber and moved to scan the entire chambers. GFP was expressed by 3.7% of the treated cells, compared with 0.4% for controls for 2.3 MPa RPA, as shown in Fig. 3. This effect was accompanied by cell killing, with 28.6% dead cells after scanning, compared with 3.4% in shams. Thus, even for low-power diagnostic ultrasound, the potential therapeutic effect of gene transfer imaging mode produced with a loss of cell viability.

2.3.3. *Relevance of in vitro tests to in vivo conditions*

The study of ultrasound-mediated transfection *in vitro* has produced a basic body of knowledge, which is useful for devising and interpreting *in vivo* experiments. The most important factor is that the ultrasound effect results from the cavitation mechanism. Due to the involvement of this mechanism, effects are highly non-uniform in a population of cells, even for well controlled and uniform ultrasound exposure. The effect is also enhanced by cavitation nucleation. The sonoporation effect represents cell injury, and ultrasound induced transfection has been repeatedly associated with the loss of cell viability, which is often greater in terms of cell numbers than the transfection effect. Finally, the involvement of cavitation reduces the direct relevance of many *in vitro* studies to *in vivo* conditions, i.e., the cell-microbubble interaction can be very efficient *in vitro*, owing to the small number of cells and the vigorous promotion of cavitation activity in liquids.

                                   D. L. Miller

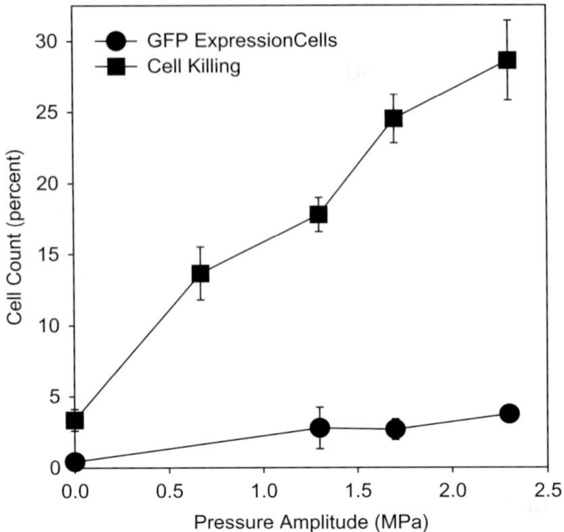

Fig. 3. Epidermoid cell monolayers were exposed to diagnostic ultrasound in the presence of GFP marker plasmid and 2% Optison®. Cell killing increased with increasing RPA of the pulses delivered by the ultrasound scanner up to the maximum available. The transfection was a small but significant percentage of the cells for the higher RPAs. Reproduced with permission from Miller *et al.* (2003).

In vivo conditions are quite different, *e.g.*, conditions in the rotating tube system or the dish system with agitating surface, cannot be duplicated in living animals. The *in vitro* research, while valuable for basic insights, cannot be used to predict *in vivo* outcomes.

3. Ultrasound-mediated Gene Transfer *In Vivo*

The observation of permeabilization by shockwaves led to a suggestion by Delius *et al.* (1995) that extracorporeal shockwave lithotripsy might be useful for gene therapy. Based on *in vitro* results at higher frequencies, and even diagnostic ultrasound with contrast agents, many forms of ultrasound appear to be capable of DNA transfer to varying degrees, depending on the cavitation activity obtained. *In vivo* testing has been performed in reference to several tissue applications including cancer, myocardium, endovascular tissue, skeletal muscle, and so forth.

3.1. *Cancer*

Malignant tumors may be good candidates for ultrasound-mediated gene therapy. There has been extensive research on effective therapeutic genes for cancer treatment. In addition, the expected cell killing side effect by ultrasonic cavitation activity might be acceptable or even desirable for cancer treatment. Simple intratumor injection of plasmids has been shown to produce some gene transfer in tumors (Yang and Huang, 1996), which may also be a propitious indication for ultrasound-mediated cancer gene therapy.

In vivo testing of LSW for enhanced cancer gene transfer was performed using the luciferase marker plasmid in the B16 mouse melanoma tumor by Bao *et al.* (1998). Luciferase reporter vector was injected with a concentration of 2 mg/ml at 10% of the tumor volume, after mixing with air at 10% of tumor volume to enhance acoustic cavitation activity. LSW were applied at 5.2 MPa peak negative pressure amplitude to tumors on the hindlimbs of mice placed in a waterbath. For cells harvested from tumors immediately after exposure, luciferase production was significantly increased, relative to shams, occurring for 200, 400, 800 and 1200 shockwaves with plasmid and air injection. Expression was enhanced roughly 15-fold relative to direct injection alone, and air injection gave a further 7-fold increase. Cells isolated one day after exposure gave increased luciferase production for 100 and 400 shockwave exposure, without and with air injection. For this delayed isolation, a 350-fold enhancement was found for 400 SW plus air, compared with simple direct injection. The GFP reporter plasmid was utilized to elucidate the numbers of B16 melanoma tumor cells undergoing transfection (Miller *et al.*, 1999). The plasmid solution was injected intratumorally at 0.2 mg DNA per ml of tumor, after mixing with air at 10% of tumor volume. For 400 SW exposure, viable cell recovery from excised tumors was reduced to 4.2% of shams, indicating substantial cell killing. Cell transfection was enhanced by a factor of about eight, reaching 2.5% of viable cell counts. These results indicated that tumor ablation by cell killing, plus enhancement of transfection in the remaining viable tumor cells, can be accomplished simultaneously for LSW treatment of tumors.

An important consideration *in vivo* is the enhancement of cavitation nucleation. Several cavitation nucleation strategies were compared for the transfection of tumor tissue using LSW (Miller and Song, 2002). Four strategies were compared, namely, saline injection, direct injection of air, Optison® contrast agent, and perfluorocarbon microdroplets, which can be locally vaporized by ultrasound inside the tumor itself, before or during exposure. The RENCA tumor model was used with cells implanted and grown to $\sim 300\,\mu l$ tumor volumes on the hind legs of mice. Prior to treatment, a cavitation agent, together with a DNA plasmid coding for marker proteins, was injected into the tumor. For sham exposure, tumor volume increased by a factor of 3.6 in four days. With 500 LSW treatment, all the nucleation agents reduced four-day tumor growth of approximately the same amount (to factors of 1.2 to 1.9). β-galactosidase marker gene expression, visualized by staining of fresh tumor cross-sections, was generally localized to the region around the needle injection path. All the agents, except saline, produced statistically significant increases of 11.8 to 14.6 fold in luciferase expression after two days, relative to sham exposure. Intravenous injection of Optison® or droplet nucleation agents prior to LSW treatment reduced tumor growth to factors of 1.0 and 0.7, but did not increase transfection for injection of the plasmid suspension into the tumor.

The LSW method was tested in the Dunning rat prostate cancer model (Michel *et al.*, 2003). Subcutaneous tumors were injected with a plasmid solution at 10% of tumor volume plus an equal volume of air. After treatment, cells were harvested from excised tumors and cultured for 24 hours. The cell transfection rate was significantly increased from 0.3% to 4.6% for treatments with 2000 LSWs.

Huber and Pfisterer (2000) evaluated 1 MHz focused ultrasound enhancement of transfection of the β-galactosidase reporter plasmid into Dunning prostate tumors implanted in rats. Rats were exposed in a water tank to 1 MPa burst mode ultrasound (4 ms duration, 100 Hz PRF), after injection of $10\,\mu g$ of the plasmid DNA. Staining of sections of exposed tumor revealed areas of β-galactosidase positive (blue stained) cells. DNA injection plus ultrasound produced a 10-fold increase in positive cells, compared with intratumoral DNA injection alone, and a 15-fold enhancement in β-galactosidase protein assayed by ELISA. No transfection of tumor cells was obtained for intravenous injection of $100\,\mu g$ of plasmid DNA, with or without ultrasound exposure.

Manome *et al.* (2000) followed up on *in vitro* results with *in vivo* testing in colon carcinoma tumors implanted in mice. The tumors were injected with $200\,\mu g$ β-galactosidase reporter plasmid and exposed to 1 MHz ultrasound at 10 to $20\,\text{W/cm}^2$ ten minutes later. Relative β-galactosidase activity 48 hours after treatment increased approximately 3-fold for ultrasound, and was higher at the higher intensity. Expression peaked for 30 s exposure and declined for longer exposures up to 2 minutes. The mechanism of the enhanced transfection was not examined, but the intensities employed were sufficient for possible induction of some cavitation activity at the injection site.

LITU treatment was used to enhance transfection of tumor cells by cationic lipids *in vivo* (Anwer *et al.*, 2000). Without ultrasound, most transfection obtained with CAT reporter or interleukin-12 coding plasmids complexed to cationic liposomes occurred in the lungs. Ultrasound treatment of the tumor before or after intravenous injection of the plasmid complex resulted in up to 270 fold enhancement of gene transfer to the tumor, depending on the conditions. The tumor DNA delivery increased with increasing DNA dose, and increasing exposure duration. The effect was maximized for ultrasound treatment up to $1.5\,\text{W/cm}^2$ about 1 minute after injection of the DNA complexes. By immunostaining of histological sections taken 15 minutes after treatment, the DNA delivery was localized to the endothelium within the tumor. The ultrasound treatment was termed sonoporation; however, the mechanism for this *in vivo* effect is not completely clear, because no cavitation enhancement was employed.

The use of HIFU with a cavitation nucleation agent for ultrasound enhanced cancer gene therapy was tested using the RENCA tumor (Miller and Song, 2003). A diagnostic ultrasound system was used to obtain 10 MHz images of the tumors to aim the 1.55 MHz HIFU focus. Optison® ultrasound contrast agent was mixed with the plasmid solution and injected into the tumor. Treatment consisted of multiple 100 ms bursts aimed to cover the entire tumor using a square grid at 2 mm spacing (equal to the $-6\,\text{dB}$ beam width). Bursts at 8 MPa RPA interrupted tumor growth during the four-day observation period, compared with a 2.8 fold growth in shams. β-galactosidase staining showed transfected cells scattered in the tissue. Using the luciferase plasmid, gene expression was about 60 times greater for 2 MPa HIFU than in shams with plasmid injection only. Longer bursts or higher pressure amplitudes led to decreased tumor growth without increases in transfection, as shown in Fig. 4. The effect of pulsing conditions was

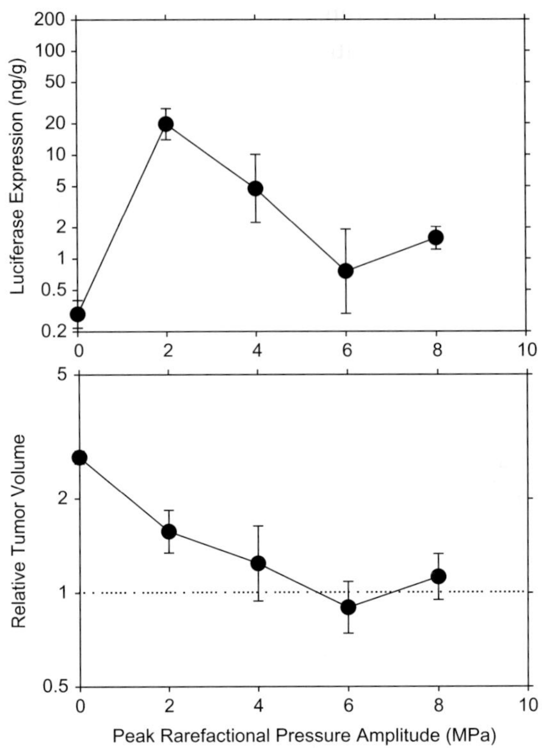

Fig. 4. Pulsed HIFU was used to transfect cells in subcutaneously implanted renal carcinoma tumors injected with Optison® and a luciferase marker plasmid. The anti tumor effect of the treatment increased with increasing RPA with two-day tumor growth stopped for the higher RPAs. In contrast, the luciferase expression measured in excised tumor tissue was maximal at the lowest RPA and decreased for higher values. This suggested that the tumoricidal effect also killed many transfected cells, which resulted in reduced gene expression. Reproduced with permission from Miller and Song (2003).

tested using similar methods (Miller and Song, 2004). Pulsed HIFU treatment at 1.55 MHz consisted of 1 s duration exposures with 100 μs pulses and 1 kHz PRF. Tumor growth tended to decline with increasing peak RPA and was essentially stopped at 8 MPa. Luciferase expression was variable, but was significantly elevated for 2, 4, 6, and 8 MPa.

Dittmar *et al.* (2005) exposed squamous cell carcinoma tumors to pulsed HIFU without enhancement of cavitation nucleation. Bursts of 1 MHz ultrasound were delivered at a 4.5% duty cycle for 2 minutes to tumors on one flank, while tumors implanted on the other flank served as controls. Following the ultrasound exposure, GFP marker plasmids were injected *via* a tail vein. GFP expression after 1 day was observed in frozen sections of the treated tumor, but not the controls. Quantitative measurements by Western blot analysis indicated significantly greater GFP expression by about a factor of 9 in treated tumors relative to controls. Other tissues were not analyzed. The treated tumors did not show evidence of focal lesions or other damages. Since both cavitation and heating were apparently absent or minimal, the mechanism for this effect was uncertain.

The possible use of LITU for gene transfer into bladder cancer cells was investigated by Ogawa *et al.* (2004). For *in vivo* tests, human prostate or bladder cancer cell suspensions were injected into the bladders of rats and treated transabdominally by 1 MHz ultrasound at 0.78 W/cm^2. Levovist$^®$ was used for cavitation nucleation and the luciferase gene was used to indicate transfection. After treatment, the cell suspension was removed and cultured. Increasing Levovist$^®$ doses produced increased gene expression after one day. Heating the animals in a 42°C water bath or adding lidocane to the cell suspension enhanced results. Since the cells were in suspension within the bladder, essentially used as an exposure chamber, it is unclear whether the results would be similar for bladder tumors.

3.2. *Endovascular tissue*

Gene transfer to endovascular tissue might be of value for the treatment of vascular injury or disease. Amabile *et al.* (2001) used a special catheter based ultrasound exposure system to effect gene transfer to rabbit femoral arteries injured by overdilation. Both adenoviral and plasmid-lipoplex vectors containing the blue fluorescence protein (BFP) gene were perfused into the arteries. One artery received endovasular ultrasound at 2 MHz and 50 W/cm^2 (approximately equivalent to 1.2 MPa) in burst mode (1 ms bursts at 30 Hz) for 16 minutes, whilst the collateral artery did not. The ultrasound treatment greatly increased the BFP expression after 7 days by 12 to 19 fold over the simple perfusion procedure for both gene vectors. Some loss of cell viability was observed for the ultrasound with adenovirus. The mechanism of this gene transfer effect is uncertain, since cavitation activity was not enhanced by contrast agents; however, the long bursts at moderate intensity may have been sufficient to produce some cavitation activity in the injected fluid.

Rat carotid artery was injured by inflation of a balloon catheter and then treated with contrast aided ultrasound and plasmid DNA in suspension (Taniyama *et al.*, 2002b). The injured region was isolated by ligation and treated with an unspecified ultrasound system for 2 minutes. Two days after treatment, luciferase activity was greater than 1000 times more for the ultrasound with plasmid and Optison® than with plasmid alone. This strategy was also tried with a therapeutic gene as described below.

High intensity focused ultrasound (HIFU) was tested as a means to transfect cells in the carotid arteries of rabbits (Huber *et al.*, 2003). Segments of the carotid arteries were isolated by ligations, and injected with β-galactosidase plasmid or plasmid plus Optison® mixtures. The 0.85 MHz focused ultrasound with 50 ms bursts and 5% duty cycle was delivered for 1 minute. HIFU at 6.3 MPa enhanced gene expression after 2 days by 8 times, increasing to 17.5 fold with Optison®. The effects increased with increasing pressure amplitude up to 15 MPa, although hemorrhages were observed on the vessel surface for treatment with Optison® above 6.3 MPa.

3.3. *Skeletal muscle*

Skeletal muscle cells can be transfected by simple injection of plasmid solutions (Wolff *et al.*, 1990), which might make this tissue a good prospect for nonviral ultrasound methods. Schratzberger *et al.* (2002) explored the use of 0.3 or 1 MHz ultrasound to enhance the lac-Z marker gene transfection in rabbit hind limb muscles. Simple injection of the plasmid produced some β-galactosidase expression after 5 days. At an equivalent MI of 1.8 and 30 cycle pulses with 6% duty cycle, the 1 MHz ultrasound gave approximately a 20-fold increase in expression. The 0.3 MHz ultrasound yielded the same result. When ultrasound was applied before injecting the plasmid, the effect was reduced but not eliminated. For histochemical staining, many more nuclei were seen to be expressing the marker enzyme for ultrasound exposure. This method was also tested for the possible use of therapeutic genes for neo-vascularization (described below).

Muscular dystrophy could be amenable to treatment by gene therapy. Danialou *et al.* (2002) studied the transfection of the lacZ reporter gene into the muscles of normal and dystrophic mice. LITU at 1 MHz and 1.5 W/cm^2 was used with a 3 ms on, 7 ms off duty cycle. In normal mice, ultrasound without or with added Definity$^®$ (Bristol-Myers Squibb Medical Imaging, Inc. N. Billerica MA) contrast agent had little effect on the number of fibers expressing β-galactosidase 5 days after treatment. However, in the dystrophic MDX mice, ultrasound plus Definity$^®$ increased the numbers of positive fibers and gave a 22-fold increase in the amount of protein expression over injection without ultrasound. No histologically definable muscle damage was found to be induced by any of the treatments.

Cationic lipid-DNA complexes incorporated into microbubbles have also been tested for transfection of the skeletal muscle (Christiansen *et al.*, 2003). Diagnostic ultrasound at 1.75 MHz was used for treatment in B-mode with *in situ* RPA values of 1.04–1.14 MPa. The pulsing interval was each 7 s for 15 minutes. Infusion of the agent was by femoral artery or by femoral vein, with 10 times the microbubbles to compensate for the loss in the lungs relative to intra-arterial (IA) infusion. The luciferase marker gene was used and transfection assessed after 4 days. Intramuscular injection of plasmid alone produced strong gene expression, matched by the IA treatment with plasmid loaded microbubbles and ultrasound. Intra-venous (IV) infusion greatly reduced the effect in skeletal muscle, but was more efficacious in the treatment of the heart. No transfection was seen outside the ultrasound treated region, neither in the liver or lung tissue, nor in muscle treated with ultrasound and plasmid IA, without enhancement of cavitation by added microbubbles.

Optison$^®$ was used with tone burst 1 MHz ultrasound of 20% duty cycle and peak intensity of 3 W/cm^2 (equivalent to $\sim$0.3 MPa pressure amplitude) for transfection of mouse skeletal muscle with GFP reporter plasmids (Lu *et al.*, 2003). The plasmids were used with or without polymer condensation with polyethylenimine (PEI). GFP expression was evaluated after 1 week. Injection of the plasmid DNA produced minimal transfection of the muscle fibers. This was significantly enhanced by injection of the plasmids with Optison$^®$ even without ultrasound, and the extent of muscle injury was reduced. The addition of ultrasound treatment did not further improve the result. Addition of PEI to the tests produced a similar trend, and once again ultrasound failed to improve the transfection outcome. The lack of ultrasound enhancement of the effect with added microbubbles might have been due to difficulty in maintaining microbubble stability during intramuscular injection and continuous ultrasound exposure.

The commercially available contrast agents Levovist®, Albunex® and Optison® were compared with respect to their enhancement of the GFP gene transfer into the mouse skeletal muscle (Li *et al.*, 2003). LITU at 1 MHz was applied at 2 W/cm^2 for 2 minutes after IM injection of the plasmid and agent mixture. GFP expression was evaluated after 7 days. The use of the air based agents Albunex® and Levovist® had no enhancement effect with ultrasound over that of simple IM injection. However, the perfluorocarbon based Optison® plus ultrasound produced a significant 10-fold enhancement in transfection. The reason for the apparently different outcome from the Lu *et al.* (2003) study is uncertain, since Li *et al.* (2003) did not report results of a control test with Optison® without ultrasound.

Pislaru *et al.* (2003) also examined the potential for transfection of the skeletal muscle. The contrast agent PESDA was used with ultrasound either from a 1.7 MHz diagnostic scanner or a 1 MHz continuous wave (CW) system. The agent and luciferase plasmid or plasmid coding for the secreted product tissue factor pathway inhibitor (TFPI) were injected into rat muscles IM or delivered intra arterially. *In vivo*, the diagnostic scanner produced somewhat greater luciferase expression than the CW system. The expression with ultrasound was also better than simple IM injection. An adenovirus gave higher luciferase expression in the IM tests, but also caused transfection in the liver. Different muscles produced different results, and the triceps brachii gave higher luciferase expression than did treatment of the hindlimb (gastrocnemius) muscle. Intra-arterial injection into the femoral artery gave variable results. The TFPI plasmid yielded a dose dependent increase in plasma TFPI, which was significantly different from no-ultrasound controls after 5 days as shown in Fig. 5. This result suggests that transfection of the skeletal muscle could yield systemic treatment by secreted therapeutic proteins.

3.4. *Myocardium*

Gene delivery to the myocardium of rats was obtained with harmonic mode diagnostic ultrasound, a microbubble contrast agent and a viral β-galactosidase vector (Shohet *et al.*, 2000). The contrast agent was prepared

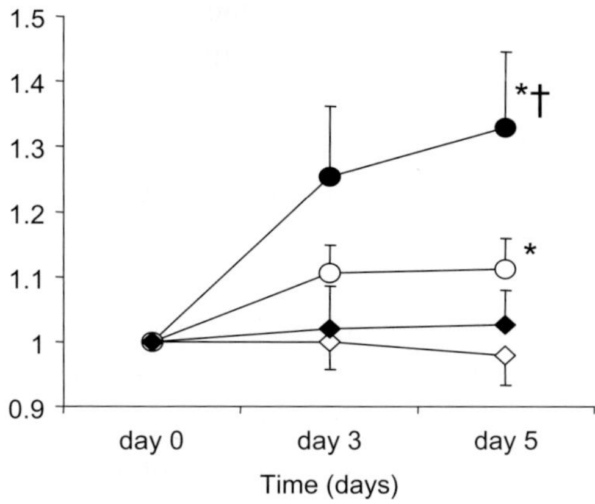

Fig. 5. Normalized plasma TFPI activity up to 5 days after sonoporation into the triceps brachii. Controls (open diamonds) or 400 μg (filled diamonds) plasmid without ultrasound showed no effect. The ultrasound plus contrast agent with 200 μg (open circles) or 400 μg (filled circles) plasmid produced significant (*) elevations in circulating TFPI. Reproduced with permission from Pislaru *et al.* (2003).

in the laboratory and was processed with the vector to attach the virus particles to the microbubbles. For exposure, 2 ml of this preparation was infused over a 30-minute period via the jugular vein. Three frames from a 1.3 MHz transducer destroyed the microbubbles evident in the second-harmonic image, and three frame bursts were triggered intermittently to allow refill of the tissue between scans. After four days, expression of the reporter gene was assayed in histological sections and measurement of enzyme activity. Staining and enzyme activity was detected in the myocardium for echocardiographic destruction of the microbubbles plus viral vector at $\sim$10 times the levels found for bubble destruction without the vector, microbubbles plus vector without ultrasound, and vector alone without ultrasound (although β-galactosidase was found in the livers of all animals receiving the viral vector). Since the procedure involved destruction of contrast agent microbubbles, cavitation activity was clearly responsible for the effect; however, it was uncertain whether the viral vector was delivered by mechanical sonoporation or by some other process. Echocardiographic microbubble destruction followed by vector infusion produced approximately twice the gene expression of controls, suggesting that disruption of the endothelial barrier during microbubble destruction might have been a factor in the enhanced viral transduction.

Vannan *et al.* (2002) used cationic microbubble linked plasmids with diagnostic ultrasound to induce transfection in dog hearts with the chloramphenicol acetyltransferase (CAT) marker gene. The diagnostic ultrasound was delivered in anesthetized, closed chest dogs at 1.3 MHz and the highest power settings. Multiple frames were triggered at each 4–6 cardiac cycles in an apical four chamber view. The triggered imaging allows for refill of the myocardium with the microbubble agent after destruction of the microbubbles by the ultrasound pulses of the previous frames. The specially prepared microbubbles were injected into a cephalic vein. Tissue samples were taken 48 hours after treatment and tested for CAT content by ELISA assay and by histochemical staining. There was no discernable CAT expression in the heart for microbubbles with no ultrasound or ultrasound without microbubbles. For ultrasound with the plasmid-loaded microbubbles, CAT expression was found in several regions of the heart with 303 ng/g in myocardium for four dogs. In addition, for the ultrasound treatment of the heart only, CAT expression was found in distant tissues of the lungs, liver, kidney and skeletal muscle. This may have resulted from the release of active cationic lipid-DNA complexes upon microbubble activation, and presents a problem in terms of targeting specificity.

The transfection of cardiac tissue was also demonstrated using albumin and lipid microbubbles containing luciferase plasmid (Bekeredjian *et al.*, 2003). The agents were infused for 20 minutes through the jugular vein of anesthetized rats, and the hearts were scanned with a 1.3 MHz cardiac ultrasound machine. Luciferase expression after 4 days was primarily detected in the heart, with some transfection occurring in the liver for the albumin microbubbles and in the pancreas for the lipid microbubbles. The cardiac luciferase expression declined after 4 days, but could be repeatedly delivered to the heart to obtain a longer duration of gene expression. The opportunity for multiple treatment repetitions represents an advantage for ultrasound-mediated transfection of plasmids, relative to, for example, virus-based vectors which can elicit a strong immune response upon retreatment.

The echocardiographic treatment parameters were varied to find the optimum treatment conditions for the adenoviral or plasmid modified contrast agent microbubbles (Chen *et al.*, 2003). Cardiac scanning was performed in anesthetized rats to transfer the luciferase plasmid. Triggered imaging was more effective than continuous imaging for gene transfer to the heart, since it allows refill of the myocardium. The lowest frequency of 1.3 MHz was most effective, compared with 5 MHz and 12 MHz. The harmonic B-scan mode and Doppler modes were equally effective. Diagnostic ultrasound is designed and regulated for diagnostic applications, and some modification of treatment parameters might be useful for therapeutic applications. An increase of the Mechanical Index from the normal maximum of 1.6 for the diagnostic machine used in the study to 2.0, produced significantly more transfection (the FDA guideline upper limit for diagnostic ultrasound is MI = 1.9). The adenovirus method apparently produced higher luciferase expression in the heart. However, the adenovirus preparation resulted in substantial gene transfer and expression in the liver, while the plasmid microbubble preparation was specific to the heart.

Transfection of marker plasmids into mouse myocardium was reported by Guo *et al.* (2004). An albumin microbubble preparation was mixed with the plasmid solution at a concentration of 15% and injected via tail vein at a volume of 1.0–1.2 ml into the 18–22 gm mice. Cardiac diagnostic ultrasound was applied to the thorax at an MI of 1.5. Significant expression of the exogenous gene for luciferase was found in the heart. Several plasma enzyme levels were significantly increased by the treatment including alkaline phosphatase and creatine kinase. The elevated enzymes were indicative of cardiac injury, possibly related to the relatively high doses of contrast agent used for the treatment.

3.5. *Other potential applications*

Kim *et al.* (1996) tested the possible extension of their *in vitro* experiments to *in vivo* conditions. The β-galactosidase reporter plasmid was injected into both knee joints of rats, and one joint was treated with 1 MHz plus 30 kHz ultrasound at 0.4 MPa and 40 kPa respectively for 1 minute. Three of the four treated knees showed reporter gene expression after four days, while none was detected in the unexposed joints.

Gene therapy of the fetus could be a means to treat genetic diseases. To test this possibility, marker plasmids together with Optison® were injected into the amniotic cavity, into the pleural or peritoneal cavities, or into the ventricles of the fetuses of pregnant mice (Endoh *et al.*, 2002). The uterus was exteriorized and treated with 1 MHz ultrasound for 10 s at about 0.6 MPa. Luciferase expression in the fetal skin occurred for intra-amniotic injection and was enhanced 1,000-fold for ultrasound with plasmid and contrast agent relative to plasmid injection alone. Scanning electron microscopy revealed skin injury due to the treatment. Luciferase expression was also detected in the brain, lung, heart, liver and gut, as well as the skin, for each of the injection sites. Use of GFP or β-galactosidase reporter plasmids and fluorescent labeled oligonucleotides revealed a scattered distribution of transfected cells. The expression appeared to be transient, and there was no indication of transmission to the offspring.

Ultrasound-mediated transfection in the central nervous system of rats was tested by Shimamura *et al.* (2004). Luferase plasmids with Optison® were injected into the brain or into the subarachnoid space fluid and treated with 1 MHz LITU at up to 0.55 MPa. For the subarachnoid injection, the measured luciferase expression in the brain after 1 day increased with Optison® concentration, ultrasound intensity and exposure duration. Gene expression was limited to the brainstem and cerebellum, and decreased to essentially zero after 1 week. Similar trends were seen with injection of the material into the striatum, except that gene expression remained detectable after 2 weeks. Several methods were applied to detect tissue damage, including histological staining and a search for the leakage of fluorescent albumin. Body weight was decreased for a few days after treatment, and there was no persistent difference between the groups. There was no detectable histological damage or albumin leakage after treatment, except at the injection needle track for intrastriatal injection.

Gene transfer into injured spinal cord could enhance the possibility of healing, but safety of direct injection is uncertain. Shimamura *et al.* (2005) injected naked plasmid DNA into the cerebrospinal fluid and then exposed the spinal cord to 1 MHz LITU *via* a window created by removing the dorsal portion of the T_{9-10} vertebra. The plasmid was mixed with Optison® before injection. The ultrasound treatment enhanced luciferase marker gene expression by 15–60 fold at the treatment site. The transfected cells were found to be mostly meningeal cells on the surface of the spinal cord using a fluorescent marker plasmid. Gene transfer was also obtained in injured spinal cord, and no functional neurological deficit was associated with the treatment.

The transfection of the brain tissue was explored by Manome *et al.* (2005) in neonatal mice, after testing with cultured brain slices indicated positive results. A luciferase marker plasmid with or without added Levovist® was injected into the right hemisphere. LITU treatment utilized a relatively low frequency of 0.21 MHz at 5 W/cm². Plasmid and plasmid plus Levovist had insignificant transfection. Ultrasound for 5 s induced some transfection, which was increased 4.6 fold by combining with the contrast agent.

Transfection of kidney cells was explored using the luciferase and GFP plasmids and Optison® with 1 MHz CW ultrasound (Koike *et al.*, 2005). A volume of 0.5 ml of the plasmids and Optison® were injected into the left renal artery of rats. Ultrasound treatment using a commercial LITU device was delivered to the kidney for 1 minute, but the exposure level in terms of intensity or RPA was unspecified (a 5% power setting was employed). Luciferase expression increased with increasing Optison® concentration, varied up to 100% with a constant 50 μg of plasmid. Histological damage of the glomeruli was seen for 50% and 100% Optison®, for both kidneys. However, no perturbations of plasma levels of aspartate aminotransferase, alanine aminotranserase, blood urea nitrogen or creatinine were detected after 4 days. For 25% Optison®, transfection declined each week for 3 weeks. GFP was detected both in the glomeruli and in other parts of the kidney tissue. The ultrasound-mediated gene transfection was significantly better than transfection by a virus based liposome vector.

4. Ultrasound-Mediated Gene Therapy

In Sec. 2, basic research conducted *in vitro* to assess sonoporation and gene transfer by ultrasound was reviewed. Research on *in vivo* transfection aided by ultrasound was reviewed in Sec. 3, which included a wide range of results for various tissues. Although many of these reports are quite encouraging for eventual clinical application, the ability to generate a therapeutic response remains the ultimate goal. Several studies of ultrasound treatment using actual therapeutic gene strategies have been published, including potential therapies for cancer, myocardial infarction, restenosis, transplant rejection,

renal fibrosis and stem cell stimulation for dental wound repair as listed in
Table 2. In this section, these studies are reviewed to assess the current state
of ultrasound-mediated gene therapy.

4.1. *Cancer*

As noted above, cancer may be a particularly suitable target for ultrasound-
mediated gene therapy. The concept of LSW application for tumor treatment had been explored in the early 1990s, and the possibility of LSW gene
therapy was suggested by Delius *et al.* (1995). The efficacy of ultrasound
enhanced cancer gene therapy during lithotripsy shockwave (LSW) treatment was tested with interleukin-12 (IL-12) immunotherapy (Song *et al.*,
2002a). An established cancer treatment method of IL-12 immunotherapy
was utilized for this study, because this method tends to illicit an antitumor response against surviving tumor cells, even for metastases at distant
sites. The strategy was therefore to destroy much of the tumor tissue with
LSW enhanced by cavitation, and simultaneously stimulate the immune
system by the gene-transfer and expression of IL-12 at the exposure site.
The effects of LSW, recombinant interleukin-12 (rIL-12) protein and DNA
plasmids coding for interleukin-12 (pIL-12) were investigated on two established mouse tumor models, B16 melanoma and RENCA renal carcinoma.
Cultured tumor cells were implanted on the hind legs of syngeneic mice
to grow tumors. Prior to treatment, mice were anesthetized, and the tumor
region was shaved and depilated, which is an important step to avoid entrapment of air in the fur. A volume of phosphate buffered saline, equivalent
to 10% of tumor volume, either with nothing extra or with rIL-12 (0.5 μg)
for immunotherapy or pIL-12 (2 mg/ml) for immuno-gene therapy was
injected into the tumor. An equal volume of air mixed with the saline was
injected into the tumor at the same time to augment *in vivo* nucleation of
acoustic cavitation. A spark gap lithotripter was used to treat the tumors
with 500 LSWs at 7.4 MPa RPA. Tumor size was measured every other day
and tumor growth was statistically modeled as an exponentially increasing volume with a possible growth interruption due to treatment. Sham
exposure with only injection of saline and air bubbles produced no effect
on tumor growth. LSW with air injection interrupted tumor growth for a
few days immediately after exposure. Immunotherapy with rIL-12 injection alone tended to produce a growth rate reduction. Intratumor rIL-12

injection combined with LSW enhanced the effect on tumor progression, to the extent that a statistically significant increase in survival was realized in both tumor models. One mouse with B16 melanoma survived more than 30 days (before euthanasia), with apparently complete tumor regression. For immuno-gene therapy, pIL-12 injection alone provided no detectable tumor-growth inhibition. The combination of LSW and pIL-12 injection provided a statistically significant inhibition of tumor growth, relative to LSW alone for both tumor models. Results for RENCA tumors are shown in Fig. 6. The LSW with air produced an interruption in tumor growth, which is indicative of tumor ablation. Extrapolation of the exponential growth curves, after tumor growth had resumed, back to the initial treatment day suggests that ~50% of the tumor may have been destroyed. The IL-12 treatment tended to produce a reduction in the rate of growth, indicative of an immune response causing inhibition of tumor progression. The combination of the two anti-tumor effects, growth delay and rate reduction, was

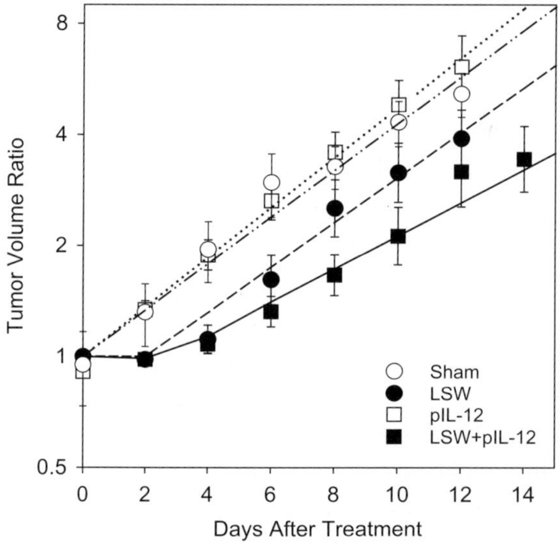

Fig. 6. Mouse renal carcinoma tumor progression after sham exposure, LSW only, intra-tumor interleukin-12 plasmid injection or LSW plus plasmid. The LSW treatment produced a delay in tumor growth for about 2 days, and the IL-12 immunogene therapy gave an additional significant reduction in tumor growth after 10 days. Reproduced with permission from Song *et al.* (2002a).

therefore not a simple addition, but rather a cooperative interaction between the mechanical damage and the physiological immune response.

IL-12 expression due to LSW induced gene transfer was confirmed by ELISA assays of excised tumor tissue in 4 groups of 4 mice for each tumor model (Song *et al.*, 2002a). After two days, the pIL-12 injection gave slight increases of 1.3 times for RENCA and 5.2 times for B16 melanoma, relative to the amount of IL-12 present in controls. The LSW treatment by itself yielded larger increases of 3.3 and 3.1 times for RENCA and B16 melanoma respectively. LSW combined with pIL-12 resulted in increases of 11 and 36 times for RENCA and B16 melanoma respectively, relative to controls. Nevertheless, the therapeutic effect for LSW with pIL-12 gene therapy was less than for LSW with the three doses of rIL-12, and seems to indicate an insufficient expression of the therapeutic gene.

As discussed in Sec. 3, LSW are not necessary for transfection *in vivo*. Sakakima *et al.* (2005) utilized a 1 MHz LITU system at $2\,\text{W/cm}^2$ to treat subcutaneous human hepatic cancer tumors implanted in nude mice. Plasmids coding for GFP or for a therapeutic Interferon β gene were injected directly into the tumors, after mixing with the contrast agent BR14 (Bracco Research SA, Switzerland). Expression of the GFP gene was detected one day after treatment with both the plasmid and contrast agent. In the therapy group, 12 of 20 tumors regressed by 4 weeks (2 recurred), compared with no regressions in 20 tumors injected but not treated with ultrasound. The relative growth of the treated group was reduced to approximately a quarter of the untreated group after 4 weeks, and remained reduced to approximately one third after 6 weeks. The action of the Interferon β was somewhat uncertain, but staining for apoptotic cells showed induction of apoptosis in treated but not untreated tumors.

A diagnostic ultrasound machine was used for cancer gene therapy by Hauff *et al.* (2005). Nude mice were implanted subcutaneously with human pancreatic adenocarcinoma (Capan-1) tumor, which lack a tumor suppressor gene (p16). A plasmid encoding the p16 gene, which was stabilized with polylysine and encapsulated to form gas filled microparticles as described by Seeman *et al.* (2002), was used for antitumor therapy. For ultrasound treatment, the diagnostic ultrasound probe (unspecified frequency) was applied via a 2 cm standoff at the maximum MI of 1.5 in color Doppler mode. Three 45 s IV infusions of the plasmid construct were performed using the Doppler image as a guide to the destruction of the gas filled microparticles over a total treatment time of about 12 minutes. Mice were treated once a week for 5 weeks, and tumor growth was monitored at intervals of 14 days. The therapeutic treatment produced a growth reduction relative to controls for plasmid without ultrasound, control plasmid with ultrasound or ultrasound alone. The modest effect was statistically significant for the second and third evaluation intervals. The third interval indicated an increase in the tumor doubling time of about a factor of two.

4.2. *Muscular ischemia*

Disease associated with ischemia presents a difficult medical problem which may be amenable to treatment by gene therapy. Microbubble destruction with 1 MHz ultrasound in skeletal muscle has been shown to stimulate arteriogenesis, apparently by stimulating natural repair processes (Song *et al.*, 2002b). Hepatocyte growth factor (HGF) stimulates angiogenesis and can be produced *in situ* by transferring the gene coding for this factor. Taniyama *et al.* (2002a) tested the feasibility of ultrasound-mediated transfer of the HGF coding plasmids in a model of ischemia in the rabbit hindlimb. Ten days after surgical preparation of the rabbit ischemic hindlimb model, the naked HGF or control plasmids with or without Optison® were injected directly into the muscle. LITU at 1 MHz was applied for 1 minute at 2.5 W/cm^2. Angiography was used to quantify circulation, and numbers of blood vessels and blood flow were characterized. Compared with controls, injection of HGF plasmid alone produced a significant improvement in the measured parameters and HGF plasmid plus Optison® and ultrasound gave a significant further increase.

Schratzberger *et al.* (2002) followed research with marker plasmids (noted above) with tests of VEGF gene therapy in the rabbit hindlimb ischemia model. Thirty-cycle bursts of 950 kHz ultrasound at 100 W/cm^2 were applied to the muscle immediately after plasmid injection. The treatment yielded a significant increase in the capillary/myocyte ratio after 30 days, as shown in Fig. 7. Improvement was also seen in the blood flow and angiographic score. The role of cavitation in these results is uncertain; however, the ultrasound intensity was sufficient to allow for possible cavitation activity in the injected liquid.

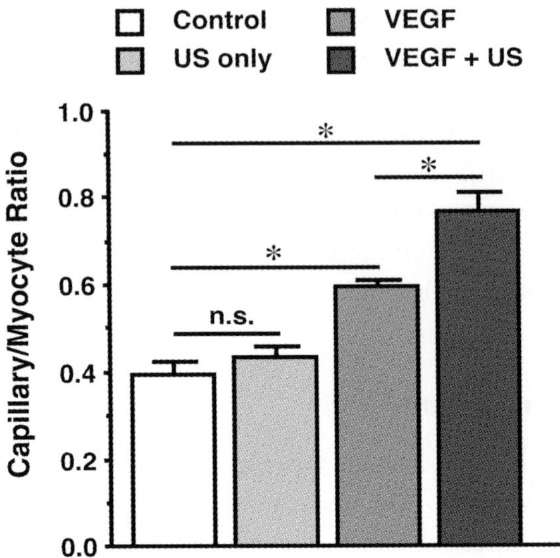

Fig. 7. Angiogenesis induced in ischemic hind limb muscles of rabbits 30 days after therapy by injection of a VEGF plasmid and ultrasound treatment. Statistically significant comparisons are denoted by (*). Reproduced with permission from Schratzberger *et al.* (2002).

4.3. *Myocardial infarction*

Myocardial infarction might be treated by gene therapy designed to induce formation of new blood vessels. Zhigang *et al.* (2004) used the ultrasound method to transfect myocardial tissue with a gene vector coding for vascular endothelial growth factor (VEGF). An albumin based contrast agent was mixed with plasmid and incubated to attach the plasmid to the microbubbles. Rats were prepared by ligation of the left anterior descending coronary artery to create an infarct. Three days after infarction, the plasmid vehicle was injected *via* tail vein and targeted to the heart by 1.8 MHz echocardiography with ECG triggering each 6–8 beats. After 2 weeks, the hearts were removed for immunohistochemical measurement of protein expression, which was quantified by image analysis, and for the determination of microvascular density. Few VEGF positive particles were found in controls or hearts treated without ultrasound, compared with the plasmid plus ultrasound treatment. In addition, a statistically significant increase in the microvascular density in the ischemic myocardium was found in the ultrasound plus plasmid group. The apparent promotion of the proliferation of endothelial cells induced by the expression of VEGF may aid in the remodeling of the injured myocardium.

The rat model of myocardial infarction was also used by Kondo *et al.* (2004) to test the efficacy of gene therapy by hepatocyte growth factor (HGF). Cardiomyocytes appear to have HGF receptors, and treatment by HGF improves the response to ischemia reperfusion injury. The naked plasmid coding for HGF was injected through a catheter inserted into the left ventricle, while the femoral vein was used to infuse Optison® microbubbles. After creation of a myocardial infarction by ligation of the left coronary artery, myocardial contrast echocardiography (MCE) was performed to determine the size of the area at risk, using a 5–12 MHz cardiac probe at MI = 1.1 with 1:4 end systole triggering and infusion of 10% Optison® at 0.2 ml/minute for 3 minutes. Four treatment groups were set up: (i) HGF plasmid plus microbubbles plus ultrasound, (ii) control plasmid plus microbubble plus ultrasound, (iii) HGF plasmid plus ultrasound, and (iv) HGF plasmid alone. The treatment consisted of slow injection of 1.5 mg of plasmid with 20% Optison® infusion at 0.2 ml/minute for 5 minutes and 1.3 MHz ultrasound triggered in 3 frame bursts 1:8 at end systole. The peak RPA was 2.16 MPa applied *via* an agar standoff, which eliminated all microbubble contrast visible in the left ventricle. Half the rats in each group (n = 6–8) were used to measure HGF expression after 7 days, and the other half had assessment of LV function for three weeks prior to sacrifice for histologic examination. Some HGF expression was found in groups 3 and 4, but the score for group 1 with ultrasound plus microbubble plus HGF plasmid was significantly higher. LV remodeling was reduced, and geometric and functional parameters significantly improved for group 1. The capillary density in the area around the infarct was 50% greater in group 1 than in the other groups, but similar in the more remote regions. Staining for scar formation showed a significantly smaller scar area in sections from group 1, as shown in Fig. 8. In addition, the numbers of small arteries was increased, indicating that the ultrasound-mediated HGF gene therapy had enhanced angiogenesis and arteriogenesis in the infarct border zone. The mortality rate was similar for all the groups, suggesting that adverse effects of the cavitational activity were not prohibitive. The possible transfection and HGF expression in other organs was not assessed.

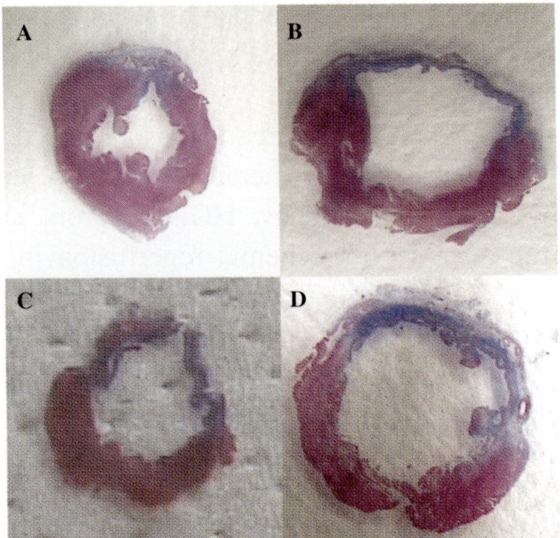

Fig. 8.   Slices of infarcted rat hearts stained with Azan-Mallory stain to show scar formation (blue). The rat treated using a plasmid coding for hepatocyte growth factor together
with diagnostic ultrasound plus Optison® (A) had a reduced scar formation relative to plasmid alone (D), plasmid plus diagnostic ultrasound (C) or control plasmid with diagnostic
ultrasound plus Optison® (B). Reproduced with permission from Kondo *et al.* (2004).

4.4. *Vascular restenosis*

Gene therapy for restenosis after angioplasty is an active area of gene
delivery research. Taniyama *et al.* (2002b) examined the possible use of
ultrasound-mediated gene therapy with the P53 anti-oncogene in carotid
artery of rats. Injury of the carotid artery was accomplished with a balloon
catheter. The artery was temporarily isolated by ligation and infused with
Optison® plus P53 plasmid or a control plasmid. Ultrasound treatment was
for 2 minutes at 2.5 W/cm^2, with an unspecified LITU device. After 5 days,
the P53 expression was significantly greater in the treatment group than in
controls. Two weeks after injury, the neointimal formation, which reduces
the lumen of the artery, was significantly reduced for the treated group.

   A similar study was conducted using decoy oligodeoxynucleotides
(ODN) to reduce activity of transcription factor E2F, which alters gene transcription and activation of genes mediating cell cycle progression (Hashiya
et al., 2004). After balloon injury, the region was isolated and treated with

Optison® plus decoy or control ODN and LITU (1 MHz, 2.5 W/cm²). Fluorescent labeled ODN was found in the vessel walls after transfection. After one week, the treated groups had reduced DNA synthesis in the vessel walls. After two weeks, the ratio of intimal to medial area measured in cross sections was significantly reduced in the group treated with the combination of E2F decoy ODN, ultrasound and Optison® compared with groups with no treatment, ultrasound plus Optison®, E2F decoy ODN alone, or combined control ODN (mismatched decoy), ultrasound and Optison®. This method of inhibiting re-stenosis is attractive since it may be applicable at the time of angioplasty with minimal added difficulty.

Although angioplasty has become a common procedure, saphenous vein grafts are often required for coronary artery bypass. *Ex vivo* gene transfer of the inhibitor of metalloproteinase 3 (TIMP-3) can reduce narrowing and occlusion of the graft during remodeling. Akowuah *et al.* (2005) utilized this strategy with ultrasound-mediated gene transfer. TIMP-3 plasmids, 1 MHz ultrasound (MI = 1.8, 6% duty cycle) and BR14 contrast agent microbubbles were used to treat saphenous vein grafts to the carotid artery of Yorkshire White pigs. After 28 days, the vessel size was significantly greater in the TIMP-3 group than in controls without transfection or transfection with a lacZ marker gene.

4.5. *Transplant rejection*

The *ex vivo* transfection strategy noted above for simple heterotropic grafting (Sec. 4.4) may also prove valuable for improving allogeneic organ transplantation outcome, since only a few extra steps would be needed at the time of transplant. Organ transplantation often requires immune suppression for successful outcome, a potential application of gene therapy. One factor in the complex phenomenon of organ rejection is nuclear factor 6κB (NFκB). Azuma *et al.* (2003) assessed the possible inhibition of NFκB as a means to prolong graft survival by using ultrasound-mediated transfer of a decoy oligo DNA. A rat model involved transplantation of a Wistar rat kidney into Lewis rats, which had bilateral nephrectomy. The treatment was optimized using transfection of luciferase plasmid, and the decoy DNA was labeled with a fluorescent marker for determining its location in tissue. Treatment consisted of injecting a plasmid and Optison® mixture into the renal artery of the excised kidneys and applying 2 MHz LITU at 2.5 W/cm^2 (approximately 0.26 MPa), before completing the transplantation into the Lewis rat recipient. Graft function was evaluated in collected urine samples and morphology was observed by histology. Immune response was assessed by immunohistochemistry for inflammatory cells and cytokines. Optimization tests showed that ultrasound significantly enhanced transfection up to 1 minute, but for longer treatment times or high Optison® concentrations (25%) tissue injury was evident. The results were similar for the fluorescent labeled decoy DNA. Therapeutic treatment then involved injection of 100 μg of the decoy DNA with 10% Optison® and 1 minute of ultrasound. Five groups of rats included the various control tests, such as the use of a control oligo. The ultrasound-mediated gene therapy produced a significant increase in animal survival relative to all the other groups (14.2 $\pm$ 5.2, compared with 7.1 $\pm$ 1.2 days, $P < 0.01$). Some rats survived more than 20 days, compared with less than 10 days for no treatment, or treatment with the control decoy DNA, as shown in Fig. 9. The treatment also improved graft function and histological structure, while decreasing expression of NFκB regulated cytokines and inflammatory cell infiltration for 2–6 days

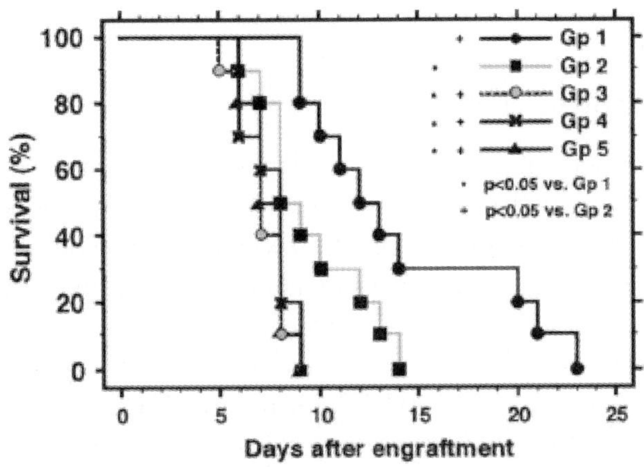

Fig. 9. Survival of rats with transplanted kidneys. For groups 1 and 2, the excised kidneys were treated with ultrasound and a decoy oligonucleotide for nuclear factor κB with (Group 1) or without (Group 2) Optison®. Groups 3 and 4 were treated similarly but with a control oligonucleotide and Group 5 received no treatment. Reproduced with permission from Azuma *et al.* (2003).

after transplantation. This approach only involves a relatively simple additional step in the transplantation procedure, and therefore may be valuable for transplantation of other organs.

4.6. *Renal fibrosis*

Progressive tubulointerstitial fibrosis is a factor in end stage renal disease, which might be ameliorated by inhibiting mediators of fibrosis. One strategy involves the inhibition of transforming growth factor β (TGF-β), which has been shown to be involved in fibrosis, by overexpression of the protein Smad7. Lan *et al.* (2003) have applied the ultrasound gene transfer method to inhibit renal fibrosis using this strategy. The gene construct involved the combination of a Smad7 expressing plasmid with an inducible vector controlled by doxycycline. The use of inducible vectors allows an additional means for control of the expression of the gene products, beyond the general control by plasmid dose, cavitation nucleation agent and ultrasound exposure. A unilateral ureteral obstruction model was created in rats by ligation of the left ureter. For treatment immediately after obstruction, plasmids mixed with Optison® were injected into the renal artery, whilst temporally isolating the kidney, and 1 MHz LITU (at an unspecified power output) was applied to both sides of the kidney. Doxycyline was then administered by an injection into the peritoneum followed by addition to the drinking water for 7 days in order to induce and regulate the expression of the Smad7 gene. The ultrasound treatment did not appear to cause any abnormal histologic or functional changes. The gene therapy significantly reduced the expression of renal alpha smooth muscle actin (α-SMA) and collagen type I and III, which are indicative of fibrosis, relative to ureteral obstructed kidneys treated with a control vector (non-therapeutic). A similar strategy was used to reduce fibrosis in a rat remnant kidney model (Hou *et al.*, 2005). In this model of kidney failure, 5/6 subtotal nephrectomy was performed, leading to progressive renal failure. These were treated with the doxycyline inducible Smad7 plasmid mixed with Optison® using 1 MHz LITU. Results were assessed by measuring functional variables including blood pressure, proteinuria, serum creatinine and creatinine clearance for 4 weeks after treatment. Independent of the increased blood pressure which occurs in this model, the Smad7 gene therapy significantly reduced proteinuria and serum creatinine, and increased creatinine clearance, relative to control rats at 4 weeks. This favorable result was related to a reduction in fibrosis, indicated by reduced α-SMA and collagen expression, and a reduction in the vascular damage evident in kidneys treated with a control vector.

4.7. *Dental injury*

Many types of tissue injury might benefit from stimulation of stem cells to reform specific tissues. Nakashima *et al.* (2003) utilized a bone morphogenic protein, growth/differentiation factor 11 (Gdf11) for the stimulation of dentin repair in teeth by ultrasound-mediated gene transfer. Testing was conducted with reporter plasmids and a therapeutic plasmid containing the sequence for Gdf11 was constructed. The plasmid solution with Optison® was applied to teeth cut down to expose the pulp and treated with 1 MHz ultrasound. In preliminary tests, the pulp tissue was isolated and cultured and the optimal treatment conditions were at $0.5 \, \text{W/cm}^2$ for 30 s using 5% Optison®, for which transfection efficiency was nearly 50%. Higher Optison® concentrations, ultrasound intensities or exposure durations reduced the effect. *In vivo* tests were conducted in dog teeth with exposed pulp tissue. For treatment, $40 \, \mu\text{g}$ of plasmid in saline with 5% Optison® was applied and treated with ultrasound through ultrasound transmission gel. After treatment, the cavity was filled and the teeth extracted for analysis after 4 weeks. Extensive reparative dentin formation was found covering the pulp with odontoblasts extending into the dentin for the treated teeth, but not in controls. Thus, the ultrasound treatment appeared to induce the desired differentiation of the pulp cells and the reparative dentin formation. This ultrasound-mediated gene therapy for dental repair was superior to previous tests of electroporation mediated gene therapy, with reduced pulp injury and more uniform gene expression.

5. Problems and Prospects

5.1. *Problems*

The ultrasound method of gene therapy has several potential limitations. As for all forms of gene therapy, the compelling rationale for use of gene transfer, as opposed to a more direct medication, must be carefully considered. Non-viral ultrasound-mediated gene therapy primarily produces a transient response of therapeutic gene expression, which limits its applicability. Ultrasound treatment can be restricted to selected tissues, which are accessible to illumination by ultrasound beams. For example, heart, liver and kidney are generally accessible to ultrasound, while lung, brain, intestine, spine or bone marrow are difficult targets. In addition, the method involves a complex combination of gene vector, cavitation nucleation, ultrasound exposure and tissue properties. Control of the many parameters involved in this combination, in order to produce a desired medicinal effect, presents a formidable research problem.

The process of ultrasound-mediated gene transfer has most often been reported to require cavitation activity. The primary interaction is between a cell and a microbubble, with the gene vector entering the cell by sonoporation. This process results in a wide range of effects on individual cells, even for uniformly treated homogenous cell suspensions. The desired localized gene transfer is therefore removed further away from direct control by the practitioner manipulating the ultrasound exposure parameters. This problem emerges most clearly when results *in vitro*, where cavitation activity can be relatively easy to initiate and control, are compared with *in vivo* results, where cavitation is difficult to initiate and is confined by tissue structures. A fundamental problem, shared by many therapeutic regimens, is that an injurious process is used for the gene transfer. Sonoporation is injurious to cells, and cavitation can lead to additional tissue injury. Therefore, planning of gene therapy protocols using ultrasound mediation tends to require counter-intuitive strategies. For example, simply increasing the power level can produce severely damaging side effects and result in lesser gene expression.

Examples of the problems, which can be encountered when applying ultrasound mediated gene therapy, arose for the apparently promising application of lithotripter shock waves (LSW) to cancer gene therapy. LSW had been shown capable of directly treating tumors. DNA can be injected into tumors and cavitation, particularly with augmentation by gas bubbles, is very vigorous with LSW even *in vivo*. Any concomitant malignant tumor debulking by cell destruction might be considered to be a welcome simultaneous tumor treatment. This strategy of ultrasound-mediated gene therapy was tried using the IL-12 immunogene method (Song *et al.*, 2002a), and a small but statistically significant reduction in tumor progression was demonstrated. However, animal survival was not increased. The LSW-induced cavitation produced substantial hemorrhage and significant mortality of mice, in which cavitation initiation was enhanced with ultrasound contrast agents (Miller and Song, 2002). The direct injection of material into the tumors restricted much of the effect to the needle track. In fact, direct injection of the active IL-12 protein combined with LSW produced better results than the indirect method of LSW gene transfer and subsequent IL-12 expression. Finally, the cavitation damage to the tumor vasculature appeared to release tumor cells from the tumor, increasing the metastatic spread of the cancer (Miller *et al.*, 2004). It should be noted that most of these problems are unique to LSW treatment, and may not be applicable to the other ultrasound treatment modes.

5.2. *Prospects*

A clear need in gene therapy is for novel vector delivery methods and several non-viral gene delivery methods are now under active research development. These include direct plasmid injection (Wolff *et al.*, 1990; Yang and Huang, 1996), "gene gun" delivery of DNA on particulate projectiles (Rakhmilevich *et al.*, 1996), *in vivo* electroporation with implanted electrodes (Nishi *et al.*, 1996), and ultrasound-mediated gene transfer. The ultrasound method has inherent advantages which may be transcendent in many applications. These include the ability to target deep tissues, a minimally invasive treatment protocol, with a possibility for repeated treatment, and a variable degree of simultaneous cell lysis. The work reviewed here indicates that better results are obtained with relatively low power therapeutic ultrasound (LITU), reduced power pulsed HIFU or even diagnostic ultrasound, than for LSW or typical HIFU treatment. Use of relatively large doses of plasmid and contrast agent seem to work better than disabled virus or lipid-DNA complexes, which tend to induce transfection at distant sites, thus abrogating the specific targeting ability of ultrasound. Research has produced promising results for several applications, including treatment of cancer (Sakakima *et al.*, 2005), myocardial infarct (Kondo *et al.*, 2004) and restenosis (Hashiya *et al.*, 2004).

Table 2. Research reports of potential applications of ultrasound mediated gene therapy.

Application	Subject	Ultrasound	Nucleation	DNA Vector	Strategy	Gene	Reference
Cancer	mouse tumor	lithotripter shock waves	air bubbles intratumor	plasmid intra-tumor	immuno-therapy	interleukin-12	Song *et al.*, 2002
Cancer	human tumor nude mouse	low intensity therapeutic	BR14	plasmid intra-tumor	apoptosis	interferon β	Sakakima *et al.*, 2005
Cancer	human tumor nude mouse	diagnostic scanner	gasesous microparticle	plasmid-microparticle IV	supressor gene	p16	Hauff *et al.*, 2005
Muscular ischemia	rabbit hindlimb	low intensity therapeutic	Optison® intra-muscular	plasmid intra-muscle	angiogenesis	hepatocyte growth factor	Taniyama *et al.*, 2002
Myocardial infarction	rat myocardium	diagnostic scanner	albumin agent tail vein	plasmid intra-venous	revascula-rization	VEGF	Zhigang *et al.*, 2004
Myocardial infarction	rat myocardium	diagnostic scanner	Optison® femoral vein	plasmid left ventricle	improved healing	hepatocyte growth factor	Kondo *et al.*, 2004
Vascular injury	rat carotid artery	low intensity therapeutic	Optison® artery segment	plasmid isolated seg-ment	reduced restenosis	P53	Taniyama *et al.*, 2002
Vascular injury	rat carotid artery	low intensity therapeutic	Optison® artery segment	decoy oligo isolated seg-ment	reduced restenosis	targeted E2F	Hashiya *et al.*, 2004

Table 2. (*Continued*)

Application	Subject	Ultrasound	Nucleation	DNA Vector	Strategy	Gene	Reference
Vascular graft	pig carotid artery	low intensity therapeutic	BR14 vein segment	plasmid, *ex vivo* vein segment	reduced occlusion	TIMP-3	Akowuah *et al.*, 2005
Organ transplant	excised rat kidney	low intensity therapeutic	Optison® renal artery	decoy oligo intra-artery	reduced rejection	targeted nuclear factor κB	Azuma *et al.*, 2003
Renal fibrosis	rat ureteral obstruction	low intensity therapeutic	Optison®, renal artery	plasmid IA	reduced fibrosis	inducible Smad7	Lan *et al.*, 2003
Renal fibrosis	5/6 rat nephrectomy	low intensity therapeutic	Optison®, renal artery	plasmid IA	reduced fibrosis	inducible Smad7	Hou *et al.*, 2005
Dental injury	dog teeth	low intensity therapeutic	Optison® tooth cavity	plasmid intra- cavity	dentin formation	growth factor Gdf11	Nakashima *et al.*, 2003

5.3. *Conclusion*

Ultrasound can cause biological effects under some conditions by the non-thermal mechanism of acoustic cavitation. Sonoporation is one such effect, which involves cell membrane perturbation to an extent which is survivable. This process is injurious to the cells, but affords an opportunity to deliver large molecules from the extracellular medium to the cytoplasm. Gene transfer is accomplished by adding DNA coding for proteins to be expressed by the affected cells to the surrounding medium, thus creating the possibility of ultrasound-mediated gene therapy.

Sonoporation has been demonstrated by a wide range of ultrasound sources including 20 kHz sonication probes, lithotripter shockwaves (LSW), low intensity therapeutic ultrasound (LITU), diagnostic ultrasound scanners and high intensity focused ultrasound (HIFU). *In vitro* results for ultrasound-mediated gene transfer have seemed quite promising, but have proven difficult to translate into robust results for *in vivo* tissues. Concomitant cell killing or tissue injury distort the overall picture in many instances. Although improvements in transfection of marker plasmids, such as luciferase-coding plasmids, have produced large increases in marker gene expression relative to controls, these findings have uncertain predictive value relative to transfection of therapeutic genes, with critical levels of subsequent protein expression required for treatment efficacy. Several tests of actual ultrasound-mediated gene therapy have been attempted for cancer, ischemia, myocardial infarction, restenosis, transplant rejection, renal fibrosis and stem cell stimulation for dental wound repair. Problems have been encountered, but encouraging results have been reported as well. Research into the complexities of the ultrasound method, into the most appropriate genes, and into the most propitious disease targets will steadily improve results. Prospects for eventual clinical application of this nascent technology will brighten, as improved results fulfil expectations from the inherent advantages of ultrasound-mediated gene therapy.

Acknowledgments

I am indebted to Prof James Greenleaf and Dr Sorin Pislaru, Department of Physiology and Biophysics, Mayo Foundation, Rochester MN, for contributions to our previous review of sonoporation (Miller *et al.*, 2002), which aided the present review. This work was supported in part by the National Institutes of Health via grant number EB00338.

References

Akowuah EF, Gray C, Lawrie A, Sheridan PJ, Su CH, Bettinger T, Brisken AF, Gunn J, Crossman DC, Francis SE, Baker AH, Newman CM, Ultrasound-mediated delivery of TIMP-3 plasmid DNA into saphenous vein leads to increased lumen size in a porcine interposition graft model. *Gene Ther* (2005) **12**: 1154–1157.

Amabile PG, Waugh JM, Lewis TN, Elkins CJ, Janas W, Dake MD, High-efficiency endovascular gene delivery via therapeutic ultrasound. *J Am Coll Cardiol* (2001) **37**: 1975–1980.

Anwer K, Kao G, Proctor B, Anscombe I, Florack V, Earls R, Wilson E, McCreery T, Unger E, Rolland A, Sullivan SM, Ultrasound enhancement of cationic lipid-mediated gene transfer to primary tumors following systemic administration. *Gene Ther* (2000) **7**: 1833–1839.

Azuma H, Tomita N, Kaneda Y, Koike H, Ogihara T, Katsuoka Y, Morishita R, Transfection of NFκB-decoy oligodeoxynucleotides using efficient ultrasound-mediated gene transfer into donor kidneys prolonged survival of rat renal allografts. *Gene Ther* (2003) **10**: 415–425.

Bao S, Thrall BD, Gies RA, Miller DL, *In vivo* transfection of melanoma cells by lithotripter shockwaves. *Cancer Res* (1998) **58**: 219–221.

Bao S, Thrall BD, Miller DL, Transfection of a reporter plasmid into cultured cells by sonoporation *in vitro*. *Ultrasound Med Biol* (1997) **23**: 953–959.

Bekeredjian R, Chen S, Frenkel PA, Grayburn PA, Shohet RV, Ultrasound-targeted microbubble destruction can repeatedly direct highly specific plasmid expression to the heart. *Circulation* (2003) **108**: 1022–1026.

Chen S, Shohet RV, Bekeredjian R, Frenkel P, Grayburn PA, Optimization of ultrasound parameters for cardiac gene delivery of adenoviral or plasmid deoxyribonucleic acid by ultrasound-targeted microbubble destruction. *J Am Coll Cardiol* (2003) **42**: 301–308.

Chen WS, Lu X, Liu Y, Zhong P, The effect of surface agitation on ultrasound-mediated gene transfer *in vitro*. *J Acoust Soc Am* (2004) **116**: 2440–2450.

Christiansen JP, French BA, Klibanov AL, Kaul S, Lindner JR, Targeted tissue transfection with ultrasound destruction of plasmid-bearing cationic microbubbles. *Ultrasound Med Biol* (2003) **29**: 1759–1767.

Coleman AJ, Kodama T, Choi MJ, Adams T, Saunders JE, The cavitation threshold of human tissue exposed to 0.2-MHz pulsed ultrasound: Preliminary measurements based on a study of clinical lithotripsy. *Ultrasound Med Biol* (1995) **21**: 405–417.

Danialou G, Comtois AS, Dudley RW, Nalbantoglu J, Gilbert R, Karpati G, Jones DH, Petrof BJ, Ultrasound increases plasmid-mediated gene transfer to dystrophic muscles without collateral damage. *Mol Ther* (2002) **6**: 687–693.

Delius M, Medical applications and bioeffects of extracorporeal shockwaves. *Shockwaves* (1994) **4**: 55–72.

Delius M, Hofschneider P, Lauer U, Messmer K, Extracorporeal shock waves for gene therapy? *Lancet* (1995) **345**: 1377.

Deng CX, Sieling F, Pan H, Cui J, Ultrasound-induced cell membrane porosity. *Ultrasound Med Biol* (2004) **30**: 519–526.

Dijkmans PA, Juffermans LJ, Musters RJ, van Wamel A, ten Cate FJ, van Gilst W, Visser CA, de Jong N, Kamp O, Microbubbles and ultrasound: From diagnosis to therapy. *Eur J Echocardiogr* (2004) **5**: 245–256.

Dittmar KM, Xie J, Hunter F, Trimble C, Bur M, Frenkel V, Li KC, Pulsed high-intensity focused ultrasound enhances systemic administration of naked DNA in squamous cell carcinoma model: Initial experience. *Radiology* (2005) **235**: 541–546.

Endoh M, Koibuchi N, Sato M, Morishita R, Kanzaki T, Murata Y, Kaneda Y, Fetal gene transfer by intrauterine injection with microbubble-enhanced ultrasound. *Mol Ther* (2002) **5**(Pt 1): 501–508.

Fechheimer M, Denny D, Murphy RF, Taylor DL, Measurement of cytoplasmic pH in Dictyostelium discoideum by using a new method for introducing macromolecules into living cells. *Eur J Cell Biol* (1986) **40**: 242–247.

Fechheimer M, Boylan JF, Parker S, Sisken JE, Patel GL, Zimmer SG, Transfection of mammalian cells with plasmid DNA by scrape loading and sonication loading. *Proc Natl Acad Sci USA* (1987) **84**: 8463–8467.

Feril LB, Kondo T, Biological effects of low intensity ultrasound: The mechanism involved, and its implications on therapy and on biosafety of ultrasound. *J Radiat Res (Tokyo)* (2004) **45**: 479–489.

Frenkel PA, Chen S, Thai T, Shohet RV, Grayburn PA, DNA loaded albumin microbubbles enhance ultrasound-mediated transfection *in vitro*. *Ultrasound Med Biol* (2002) **28**: 817–822.

Gambihler S, Delius M, Ellwart JW, Permeabilization of the plasma membrane of L1210 mouse leukemia cells using lithotripter shock waves. *J Membrane Biol* (1994) **141**: 267–275.

Greenleaf WJ, Bolander ME, Sarkar G, Goldring MB, Greenleaf JF, Artificial cavitation nuclei significantly enhance acoustically induced cell transfection. *Ultrasound Med Biol* (1998) **24**: 587–595.

Guo DP, Li XY, Sun P, Wang ZG, Chen XY, Chen Q, Fan LM, Zhang B, Shao LZ, Li XR, Ultrasound/microbubble enhances foreign gene expression in ECV304 cells and murine myocardium. *Acta Biochim Biophys Sin (Shanghai)* (2004) **36**: 824–831.

Guzman HR, Nguyen DX, Khan S, Prausnitz MR, Ultrasound-mediated disruption of cell membranes. I. Quantification of molecular uptake and cell viability. *J Acoust Soc Am* (2001a) **110**: 588–596.

Guzman HR, Nguyen DX, Khan S, Prausnitz MR, Ultrasound-mediated disruption of cell membranes. II. Heterogeneous effects on cells. *J Acoust Soc Am* (2001b) **110**: 597–606.

Guzman HR, Nguyen DX, McNamara AJ, Prausnitz MR, Equilibrium loading of cells with macromolecules by ultrasound: Effects of molecular size and acoustic energy. *J Pharm Sci* (2002) **91**: 1693–1701.

Hashiya N, Aoki M, Tachibana K, Taniyama Y, Yamasaki K, Hiraoka K, Makino H, Yasufumi K, Ogihara T, Morishita R, Local delivery of E2F decoy oligodeoxynucleotides using ultrasound with microbubble agent (Optison®) inhibits intimal hyperplasia after balloon injury in rat carotid artery model. *Biochem Biophys Res Commun* (2004) **317**: 508–514.

Hauff P, Seemann S, Reszka R, Schultze-Mosgau M, Reinhardt M, Buzasi T, Plath T, Rosewicz S, Schirner M Evaluation of gas-filled microparticles and sonoporation as gene delivery system: Feasibility study in rodent tumor models. *Radiology* (2005) **236**: 572–578.

Hosseinkhani H, Aoyama T, Ogawa O, Tabata Y, Ultrasound enhances the transfection of plasmid DNA by non-viral vectors. *Curr Pharm Biotechnol* (2003) **4**: 109–122.

Hou CC, Wang W, Huang XR, Fu P, Chen TH, Sheikh-Hamad D, Lan HY, Ultrasound-microbubble-mediated gene transfer of inducible Smad7 blocks transforming growth factor-beta signaling and fibrosis in rat remnant kidney. *Am J Pathol* (2005) **166**: 761–771.

Huber PE, Pfisterer P, *In vitro* and *in vivo* transfection of plasmid DNA in the Dunning prostate tumor Rss27-AT1 is enhanced by focused ultrasound. *Gene Ther* (2000) **7**: 1516–1525.

Huber PE, Jenne J, Debus J, Wannenmacher MF, Pfisterer P, A comparison of shock wave and sinusoidal focused ultrasound induced localized transfection of HeLa cells. *Ultrasound Med Biol* (1999) **25**: 1451–1457.

Huber PE, Mann MJ, Melo LG, Ehsan A, Kong D, Zhang L, Rezvani M, Peschke P, Jolesz F, Dzau VJ, Hynynen K, Focused ultrasound (HIFU) induces localized enhancement of reporter gene expression in rabbit carotid artery. *Gene Ther* (2003) **10**: 1600–1607.

Johannes C, Obe G, Ultrasound permeabilizes CHO cells for endonucleases AluI and benson nuclease. *Mutat Res* (1997) **374**: 245–251.

Keyhani K, Guzman HR, Parsons A, Lewis TN, Prausnitz MR, Intracellular drug delivery using low-frequency ultrasound: Quantification of molecular uptake and cell viability. *Pharm Res* (2001) **18**: 1514–1520.

Kim HJ, Greenleaf JF, Kinnick RR, Bronk JT, Bolander ME, Ultrasound-mediated transfection of mammalian cells. *Hum Gene Ther* (1996) **7**: 1339–1346.

Koch S, Pohl P, Cobet U, Rainov NG, Ultrasound enhancement of liposome-mediated cell transfection is caused by cavitation effects. *Ultrasound Med Biol* (2000) **26**: 897–903.

Koike H, Tomita N, Azuma H, Taniyama Y, Yamasaki K, Kunugiza Y, Tachibana K, Ogihara T, Morishita R, An efficient gene transfer method mediated by ultrasound and microbubbles into the kidney. *J Gene Med* (2005) **7**: 108–116.

Kondo I, Ohmori K, Oshita A, Takeuchi H, Fuke S, Shinomiya K, Noma T, Namba T, Kohno M, Treatment of acute myocardial infarction by hepatocyte growth factor gene transfer: The first demonstration of myocardial transfer of a "functional" gene using ultrasonic microbubble destruction. *J Am Coll Cardiol* (2004) **44**: 644–653.

Kuo JH, Jan MS, Sung KC. Evaluation of the stability of polymer-based plasmid DNA delivery systems after ultrasound exposure. *Int J Pharm* (2003) **257**: 75–84.

Lan HY, Mu W, Tomita N, Huang XR, Li JH, Zhu HJ, Morishita R, Johnson RJ, Inhibition of renal fibrosis by gene transfer of inducible Smad7 using ultrasound-microbubble system in rat UUO model. *J Am Soc Nephrol* (2003) **14**: 1535–1548.

Lauer U, Burgelt E, Squire Z, Messmer K, Hofschneider PH, Gregor M, Delius M, Shock wave permeabilization as a new gene transfer method. *Gene Ther* (1997) **4**: 710–715.

Lawrie A, Briskin AF, Francis SE, Tayler DI, Chamberlain DC, Crossman DC, Cumberland DC, Newman CM, Ultrasound enhances reporter gene expression after transfection of vascular cells *in vitro*. *Circulation* (1999) **99**: 2617–2620.

Lawrie A, Briskin AF, Francis SE, Cumberland DC, Crossman DC, Newman CM, Microbubble-enhanced ultrasound for vascular gene delivery. *Gene Ther* (2000) **7**: 2023–2027.

Lawrie A, Brisken AF, Francis SE, Wyllie D, Kiss-Toth E, Qwarnstrom EE, Dower SK, Crossman DC, Newman CM, Ultrasound-enhanced transgene expression in vascular cells is not dependent upon cavitation-induced free radicals. *Ultrasound Med Biol* (2003) **29**: 1453–1461.

Li T, Tachibana K, Kuroki M, Kuroki M, Gene transfer with echo-enhanced contrast agents: comparison between Albunex®, Optison®, and Levovist® in mice-initial results. *Radiology* (2003) **229**: 423–428.

Lu QL, Liang HD, Partridge T, Blomley MJ, Microbubble ultrasound improves the efficiency of gene transduction in skeletal muscle *in vivo* with reduced tissue damage. *Gene Ther* (2003) **10**: 396–405.

Manome Y, Nakamura M, Ohno T, Furuhata H, Ultrasound facilitates transduction of naked plasmid DNA into colon carcinoma cells *in vitro* and *in vivo*. *Hum Gene Ther* (2000) **11**: 1521–1528.

Manome Y, Nakayama N, Nakayama K, Furuhata H, Insonation facilitates plasmid DNA transfection into the central nervous system and microbubbles enhance the effect. *Ultrasound Med Biol* (2005) **31**: 693–702.

McCreery TP, Sweitzer RH, Unger EC, Sullivan S, DNA delivery to cells *in vivo* by ultrasound. *Meth Mol Biol* (2004) **245**: 293–298.

Michel MS, Erben P, Trojan L, Schaaf A, Kiknavelidze K, Knoll T, Alken P, Acoustic energy: A new transfection method for cancer of the prostate, cancer of the bladder and benign kidney cells. *Anticancer Res* (2004) **24**: 2303–2308.

Michel MS, Erben P, Trojan L, Knoll T, Alken P, Prostate cancer transfection by acoustic energy using pEGFP-N1 as reporter gene in the solid Dunning R-3327-MatLu tumor. *Prostate Cancer Prostat Dis* (2003) **6**: 290–293.

Miller DL, Quddus J, Sonoporation of monolayer cells by diagnostic ultrasound activation of contrast-agent gas bodies. *Ultrasound Med Biol* (2000) **26**: 661–667.

Miller DL, Song J, Lithotripter shock waves with cavitation nucleation agents produce tumor growth reduction and gene transfer *in vivo*. *Ultrasound Med Biol* (2002) **28**: 1343–1348.

Miller DL, Song J, Tumor growth reduction and DNA transfer by cavitation enhanced high intensity focused ultrasound *in vivo*. *Ultrasound Med Biol* (2003) **29**: 887–893.

Miller DL, Song J, Tumor growth reduction and DNA transfer by cavitation enhanced pulsed high intensity focused ultrasound, in JY Chapelon and C Lafon (eds.) *Proc 3rd Intl Symp Therapeutic Ultrasound* (INSERM, France) (2004) pp. 119–123.

Miller DL, Thomas RM, Ultrasound contrast agents nucleate inertial cavitation *in vitro*, *Ultrasound Med Biol* (1995) **21**: 1059–1065.

Miller DL, Williams AR, Bubble cycling as the explanation of the promotion of ultrasonic cavitation in a rotating tube exposure system. *Ultrasound Med Biol* (1989) **15**: 641–648.

Miller DL, Williams AR, Morris JE, Chrisler WB, Sonoporation of Erythrocytes by Lithotripter Shockwaves *in vitro. Ultrasonics* (1998) **36**: 947–952.

Miller DL, Bao S, Morris JE, Sonoporation of cultured cells in the rotating tube exposure system. *Ultrasound Med Biol* (1999a) **25**: 143–149.

Miller DL, Bao S, Gies RA, Thrall BD, Ultrasonic enhancement of gene transfection in murine melanoma tumors. *Ultrasound Med Biol* (1999b) **25**: 1425–1430.

Miller DL, Pislaru SV, Greenleaf JF, Sonoporation: Mechanical DNA delivery by ultrasonic cavitation. *Somat Cell Mol Genet* (2002) **27**: 115–134.

Miller DL, Dou C, Song J, DNA transfer and cell killing in epidermoid cells by diagnostic ultrasound activation of contrast agent gas bodies *in vitro. Ultrasound Med Biol* (2003) **29**: 601–601.

Miller DL, Dou C, Song J, Lithotripter shockwave-induced enhancement of mouse melanoma lung metastasis: Dependence on cavitation nucleation. *J Endourol* (2004) **18**: 925–929.

Nakashima M, Tachibana K, Iohara K, Ito M, Ishikawa M, Akamine A, Induction of reparative dentin formation by ultrasound-mediated gene delivery of growth/differentiation factor 11. *Hum Gene Ther* (2003) **14**: 591–597.

NCRP. *Biological Effects of Ultrasound: Mechanisms and Clinical Implications* (1983) (Report No. 74, National Council on Radiation Protection and Measurements, Bethesda, MD.).

Newman CM, Lawrie A, Brisken AF, Cumberland DC, Ultrasound gene therapy: On the road from concept to reality. *Echocardiography* (2001) **18**: 339–347.

Nishi T, Yoshizato K, Yamashrio S, Takeshima H, Sato K, Hamada K, Kitamura I, Yoshimura T, Saya H, Kuratsu J, Ushio Y, High-efficiency *in vivo* gene transfer using intraarterial plasmid DNA injection following *in vivo* electroporation. *Cancer Res* (1996) **56**: 1050–1055.

Nomura T, Nkajima S, Kawabata K, Yamashita F, Takakura Y, Hashida M, Intratumoral pharmacokinetics and *in vivo* gene expression of naked plasmid DNA and its cationic liposome complexes after direct gene transfer. *Cancer Res* (1997) **57**: 2681–2686.

Oberle V, de Jong G, Drayer JI, Hoekstra D, Efficient transfer of chromosome-based DNA constructs into mammalian cells. *Biochim Biophys Acta* (2004) **1676**: 223–230.

Ogawa R, Kagiya G, Feril LB Jr, Nakaya N, Nozaki T, Fuse H, Kondo T, Ultrasound mediated intravesical transfection enhanced by treatment with lidocaine or heat. *J Urol* (2004) **172**: 1469–1473.

Pislaru SV, Pislaru C, Kinnick RR, Singh R, Gulati R, Greenleaf JF, Simari RD, Optimization of ultrasound-mediated gene transfer: Comparison of contrast agents and ultrasound modalities. *Eur Heart J* (2003) **24**: 1690–1698.

Porter TR, Xie F, Therapeutic ultrasound for gene delivery. *Echocardiography* (2001) **18**: 349–353.

Porter TR, Iversen PL, Li S, Xie F, Interaction of diagnostic ultrasound with synthetic oligonucleotide-labeled perfluorocarbon-exposed sonicated dextrose albumin microbubbles. *J Ultrasound Med* (1996) **15**: 577–584.

Rakhmilevich AL, Turner J, Ford MJ, McCabe D, Sun WH, Sondel PM, Grota K, Yang N, Gene gun-mediated skin transfection with interleukin 12 gene results in regression of established primary and metastatic murine tumors. *Proc Natl Acad Sci USA* (1996) **93**: 6291–6296.

Sakakima Y, Hayashi S, Yagi Y, Hayakawa A, Tachibana K, Nakao A, Gene therapy for hepatocellular carcinoma using sonoporation enhanced by contrast agents. *Cancer Gene Ther* (2005), in press.

Schratzberger P, Krainin JG, Schratzberger G, Silver M, Ma H, Kearney M, Zuk RF, Brisken AF, Losordo DW, Isner JM, Transcutaneous ultrasound augments naked DNA transfection of skeletal muscle. *Mol Ther* (2002) **6**: 576–583.

Seemann S, Hauff P, Schultze-Mosgau M, Lehmann C, Reszka R, Pharmaceutical evaluation of gas-filled microparticles as gene delivery system. *Pharm Res* (2002) **19**: 250–257.

Shimamura M, Sato N, Taniyama Y, Yamamoto S, Endoh M, Kurinami H, Aoki M, Ogihara T, Kaneda Y, Morishita R, Development of efficient plasmid DNA transfer into adult rat central nervous system using microbubble-enhanced ultrasound. *Gene Ther* (2004) **11**: 1532–1539.

Shimamura M, Sato N, Taniyama Y, Kurinami H, Tanaka H, Takami T, Ogihara T, Tohyama M, Kaneda Y, Morishita R, Gene transfer into adult rat spinal cord using naked plasmid DNA and ultrasound microbubbles. *J Gene Med* (2005).

Shohet RV, Chen S, Zhou Y, Wang Z, Meidell RS, Unger RH, Grayburn A, Echocardiographic destruction of albumin microbubbles directs gene delivery to the myocardium. *Circulation* (2000) **101**: 2554–2556.

Song J, Tata D, Li L, Taylor J, Bao S, Miller DL, Combined shockwave and immunogene therapy of mouse melanoma and renal carcinoma tumors. *Ultrasound Med Biol* (2002a) **28**: 957–964.

Song J, Qi M, Kaul S, Price RJ, Stimulation of arteriogenesis in skeletal muscle by microbubble destruction with ultrasound. *Circulation* (2002b) **106**: 1550–1555.

Sundaram J, Mellein BR, Mitragotri S, An experimental and theoretical analysis of ultrasound-induced permeabilization of cell membranes. *Biophys J* (2003) **84**: 3087–3101.

Taniyama Y, Tachibana K, Hiraoka K, Aoki M, Yamamoto S, Matsumoto K, Nakamura T, Ogihara T, Kaneda Y, Morishita R, Development of safe and efficient novel nonviral gene transfer using ultrasound: Enhancement of transfection efficiency of naked plasmid DNA in skeletal muscle. *Gene Ther* (2002a) **9**: 372–380.

Taniyama Y, Tachibana K, Hiraoka K, Namba T, Yamasaki K, Hashiya N, Aoki M, Ogihara T, Yasufumi K, Morishita R, Local delivery of plasmid DNA into rat carotid artery using ultrasound. *Circulation* (2002b) **105**: 1233–1239.

Tata DB, Dunn F, Tindall DJ, Selective Clinical Ultrasound Signals Mediate Differential Gene Transfer and Expression in Two Human Prostate Cancer Cell Lines: LnCap and PC-3. *Biochem Biophys Res Comm* (1997) **234**: 64–67.

Teupe C, Richter S, Fisslthaler B, Randriamboavonjy V, Ihling C, Fleming I, Busse R, Zeiher AM, Dimmeler S, Vascular gene transfer of phosphomimetic endothelial nitric oxide synthase (S1177D) using ultrasound-enhanced destruction of plasmid-loaded microbubbles improve vasoreactivity. *Circulation* (2002) **105**: 1104–1109.

Unger EC, McCreery TP, Sweitzer RH, Ultrasound enhances gene expression of liposomal transfection. *Invest Radiol* (1997) **32**: 723–727.

Unger EC, Hersh E, Vannan M, McCreery T, Gene delivery using ultrasound contrast agents. *Echocardiography* (2001a) **18**: 355–361.

Unger EC, Hersh E, Vannan M, Matsunaga TO, McCreery T, Local drug and gene delivery through microbubbles. *Prog Cardiovasc Dis* (2001b) **44**: 45–54.

Vannan M, McCreery T, Li P, Han Z, Unger E, Kuersten B, Nabel E, Rajagopalan S, Ultrasound-mediated transfection of canine myocardium by intravenous administration of cationic microbubble-linked plasmid DNA. *J Am Soc Echocardiogr* (2002) **15**: 214–218.

Ward M, Wu J, Chiu J, Ultrasound-induced cell lysis and sonoporation enhanced by contrast agents. *J Acoust Soc Am* (1999) **105**: 2951–2957.

Ward M, Wu J, Chiu J, Experimental study of the effects of Optison® concentration on sonoporation *in vitro*. *Ultrasound Med Biol* (2000) **26**: 1169–1175.

Wei W, Zhengzhong B, Yongjie W, Lafeng Y, Yalin M, A novel approach to quantitative ultrasonic naked gene delivery and its non-invasive assessment. *Ultrasonics* (2004) **43**: 69–77.

Wells DJ, Gene therapy progress and prospects: Electroporation and other physical methods. *Gene Ther* (2004) **11**: 1363–1369.

Williams AR, Delius M, Miller DL, Schwarze W, Investigation of cavitation in flowing media by lithotripter shock waves both *in vitro* and *in vivo. Ultrasound Med Biol* (1989) **15**: 53–60.

Wolff JA, Malone RW, Williams P, Chong W, Acsadi G, Jani A, Felgner PL, Direct gene transfer into mouse muscle *in vivo. Science* (1990) **247**: 1465–1468.

Wyber JA, Andrews J, D'Emanuele A, The use of sonication for the efficient delivery of plasmid DNA into cells. *Pharmaceutical Res* (1997) **14**: 750–756.

Yang JP, Huang L, Direct gene transfer to mouse melanoma by intratumor injection of free DNA. *Gene Ther* (1996) **3**: 542–548.

Zarnitsyn VG, Prausnitz MR, Physical parameters influencing optimization of ultrasound-mediated DNA transfection. *Ultrasound Med Biol* (2004) **30**: 527–538.

Zhigang W, Zhiyu L, Haitao R, Hong R, Qunxia Z, Ailong H, Qi L, Chunjing Z, Hailin T, Lin G, Mingli P, Shiyu P, Ultrasound-mediated microbubble destruction enhances VEGF gene delivery to the infarcted myocardium in rats. *Clin Imag* (2004) **28**: 395–398.

Zhong P, Haifan L, Xi X, Zhu S, Bhogte ES, Shock wave-inertial microbubble interaction: Methodology, physical characterization, and bioeffect study. *J Acoust Soc Am* (1999) **105**: 1997–2009.

Zhou QH, Miller DL, Carlisle RC, Seymour LW, Oupicky D, Ultrasound-enhanced transfection activity of HPMA-stabilized DNA polyplexes with prolonged plasma circulation. *J Control Rel* (2005) **106**: 416–427.

IV

EMERGING TECHNOLOGIES USING ULTRASOUND FOR DRUG DELIVERY

Katsuro Tachibana and Shunro Tachibana

Therapeutic ultrasound has mainly been applied for its thermal or mechanical effects. Medical applications of high-energy ultrasound to ablate cancers are now under investigation. Recently, there have been numerous reports on the application of non-thermal ultrasound energy for treating various diseases in combination with drugs. Furthermore, the introduction of microbubbles and nanobubbles as carriers/enhancers of drugs has added a whole new dimension to therapeutic ultrasound. Progress in the past decade from the pharmaceutical side has further added much excitement in applying this technology especially in the field of molecular biology, gene therapy and regenerative medicine. Alternatively, from the device side, therapeutic ultrasound catheters and extracorporeal ultrasound probes are under development specifically for this purpose, with some already in clinical trials. Examples such as enhancement of thrombolytic agents by ultrasound have proven to be beneficial for patients with acute strokes and peripheral arterial occlusions. Non-invasive focused ultrasound in conjunction with anti cancer drugs may help to reduce tumor size and lessen recurrence, as well as reduce severe drug side effects. Chemical activation of drugs by ultrasound energy for the treatment of atherosclerosis and tumors is another new field recently termed as "Sonodynamic Therapy". Lastly, advances in molecular imaging have also initiated great expectations in applying ultrasound for both diagnosis and therapy at the same time. Microbubbles or nanobubbles targeted at the molecular level will permit medical doctors to make a final diagnosis of a disease by ultrasound and immediately proceed to therapeutic ultrasound. This chapter will put emphasis on emerging technologies in therapeutic ultrasound related to the above topics.

1. Introduction

A completely new concept of using non-thermal ultrasound in conjunction with drug has broadened the scope of therapeutic ultrasound. Characterized ultrasound thermal bioeffects and their application have been studied previously, but relatively few researchers have investigated the possibility of using nonthermal ultrasound as a means to enhance the effectivity of drugs until recently. Non-thermal mechanisms include various forms of energy such as cavitation, acoustic streaming, micro jets and radiation force which increases possibilities for targeting tissue with drugs and enhancing drug effectiveness or even chemically activating certain materials. In these applications, the ultrasound itself produces only minimal damage to tissues; the bioeffects that occur lead to a beneficial outcome for drug therapy.

In order to discuss the significance of ultrasound application in conjunction with drugs, one must understand the pharmacological background involved. Although there are thousands of types of drugs available for use today, the number of drugs that never reached the market may be ten-fold or even a hundred-fold greater. These types of drugs either had severe side effects or proven to be ineffective during the preclinical or early clinical trials. The various agents for cancer chemotherapy are of these types. Some of these agents administered systemically can kill solid tumors, but severely damage healthy tissues and organs at the same time too. Renal or heart failure and liver dysfunction are not rare among cancer patients treated with these highly toxic chemotherapeutic agents. A tumor site-specific drug is definitely needed in this case. On the other hand, drugs for hypertension require a 24-hour elevated drug concentration level in order to maintain stable blood pressure. As still another requirement, intermittent insulin injection is needed after each meal for diabetic patients. A new drug release system which could eliminate frequent oral administration of the drug is desired. These issues have been a major limitation and a challenge to pharmacologists for many years. Pharmaceutical companies have attempted to address these problems by suggesting the concept or strategy termed "drug delivery system (DDS)" since the 70s. The two keywords for DDS are "targeting" and "controlled release". The major goal was to avoid severe side effects by reducing the total dosage, but at the same time concentrating the drug at the target site. Additionally, controlled drug release permits more control over the amount of drug administered in a certain time frame. Recent progress in the application of ultrasound energy for DDS has demonstrated it to be a promising modality for both "targeting" and "controlled release" of drugs.

The application of nonthermal ultrasound for DDS can be classified into three major categories. Firstly, ultrasound energy can actually help agents penetrate through various tissues. It has been demonstrated that acoustic pressure can "push" materials into the skin (please see Chap. VII), blood clots or other tissues. Secondly, ultrasound can have a direct effect on the membrane and change the permeability or absorption of the drug into cells (please see Chap. VI) and tissues. Lastly, ultrasound can "release" drugs from a certain drug carrier or change the chemical properties of the drug itself at localized site (Fig. 1). For a general discussion of mechanisms for

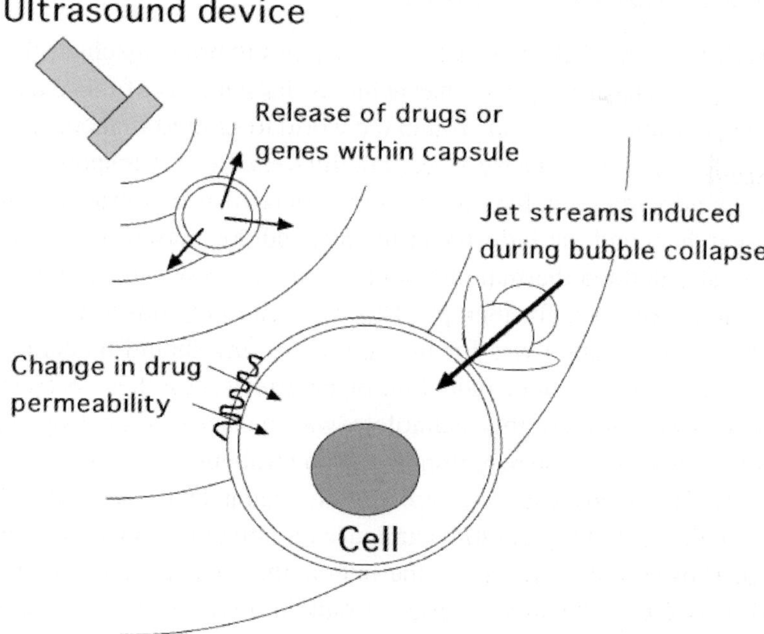

Fig. 1.   Major mechanism believed to be involved in drug delivery by ultrasound.

biological effects of ultrasound, please refer to Chap. II. Microbubbles and nanobubbles can carry and release a certain drug at a specific target site and a particular time by ultrasound. Ultrasound-sensitive materials such as hematoporphyrin, a nontoxic agent, can also be activated by ultrasound at a localized lesion and can thus result in killing cancer cells. A wide variety of applications for drug delivery with ultrasound are currently under investigation in many fields. The most futuristic investigation under progress is the use of ultrasound for gene therapy (please see Chap. III). The DNA can be injected through the cell membrane as if a "micro syringe" were used and induce transfection with ultrasound energy. Induction of gene transfer by ultrasound to the cell could result in regeneration of blood vessels, nerves or any other tissue. With the help of microbubbles or nanobubbles, it is possible to change the permeability of drugs in the microscopic cell membrane level. Recent experimental data using ultrasound for gene therapy suggests that this technology could prove to be critical for some of the emerging "next generation" drugs in the clinical context.

2. Historical Background

Although the potential of ultrasound, with nonthermal mechanism, as a means to deliver various drugs has achieved its status as of this date, with many papers appearing from around the world to support it, the ultrasound medical society and industry were initially very slow in responding, and at times coldly rejecting the concept itself. In retrospect, ultrasound imaging researchers and the industry in the 80s and 90s may or may not have intentionally defined thermal ultrasound as the main or only cause of bioeffects and applicable for therapy. This resulted in the misperception that non-thermal ultrasound was for imaging alone and should be completely harmless and safe without induction of bioeffects. Another obstacle that hampered recognition of this technology was the lack of knowledge on the pharmaceutical side, where nothing was known about devices such as those that are used in medical ultrasound. *Vice versa*, the device side knew nothing about drugs. Finally, multidisciplinary research programs were needed to understand the mechanism of the interaction between drugs and ultrasound, as well as the final biological outcome. These types of research was not frequent in those days. Investigational research on ultrasound-drug relationships was not an easy task for both acoustic physicists or biologists.

The complexity of the technology also prevented venture companies and investment from developing products, fearing lengthy approval rounds with the FDA. Within the FDA, the approval process was completely separate between the medical device and the pharmaceutical division which prevented rapid penetration of this technology into the medical market. The rare exception of FDA approval of a device-drug combination therapy product occurred in the early 90s. This product was the combination of a photosensitive drug and lasers that chemically activate it for early lung and gastric cancer (photodynamic therapy, PDT). Meanwhile, a handful of diligent scientists continued to produce ultrasound/drug related papers over the years and finally brought the technology to its broader scope today.

In 1976, Kremkau *et al.* were the first to study the cytotoxic effects of various anti cancer drugs, such as nitrogen mustard, to mouse leukemia L1210 in combination with ultrasound irradiation. Although ultrasound energy clearly enhanced the cytotoxicity of drugs, it was not determined if this enhancement was due to ultrasound or hyperthermic effect on the cells. It was later discovered from the experiments that the increase in drug efficiency cannot be completely explained by mere temperature elevation induced by ultrasound treatment. A nonthermal effect of ultrasound that interacts with drugs was suggested to be the mechanism involved. Saad *et al.* (1989) demonstrated, in a temperature-controlled experimental system, that synergistic cytotoxicity can be obtained by anti cancer drugs and ultrasound that was unrelated to hyperthermia. Experiments performed by Harrison *et al.* (1991) using low-intensity ultrasound without any temperature increase showed similar results. It was pointed out that low-level ultrasound may have altered the cell membrane, thus changing its permeability to the drug. Marked enhancement by ultrasound of the cytotoxicity of adriamycin and amphotericin B against Chinese hamster ovary cells HA1 at lower energies has been demonstrated by Harrison.

Tachibana *et al.* (1981) and Furuhata *et al.* (1989) discovered in the early 80s that the time needed to dissolve blood clots by lytic agents was significantly reduced when clots were irradiated with low intensity, nonthermal ultrasound. This finding led to much excitement in the treatment for acute myocardial and brain infarction, because shortening the duration of blood vessel occlusion by clots is a critical factor for better prognosis. Figure 2 shows the classical test tube experiment with the artificial fibrin

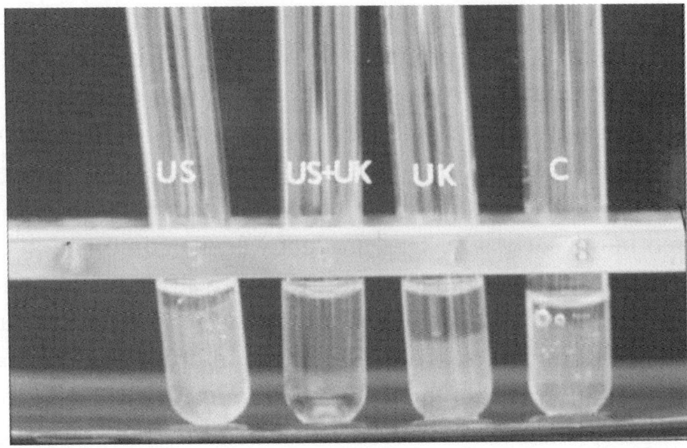

Fig. 2. Early experiments show evidence of ultrasound accelerated thrombolysis. Arificial thrombus (white area) was produced in test tubes. Each test tube was irradiated by ultrasound (50 kHz, 2 W/cm^2, 5 min) with or without thromobolytic drug (urokinase; UK). All test tubes were incubated (37°C) for 4 hours. Far right: control, no US, no UK; second from right: UK, no US; far left: US, no UK.

clots and lytic agents. The clots added with drug and treated with ultrasound showed acceleration of lysis, compared with the control. Tachibana *et al.* (1981) first introduced the concept of the therapeutic ultrasound device, of which this phenomenon could be used clinically for stroke patients (Fig. 3). Ultrasound could either be applied from outside the skull or with a miniature ultrasound emitting catheter from within. Catheters for mere drug delivery were just beginning to be used in coronary arteries for thrombolysis at that time.

One of the successful forms of DDS first introduced commercially in the 80s was the delivery of systemic drugs through the skin. The merit of transdermal delivery is that drugs can be administered systemically without interference of hepatic first pass metabolism and also at stabilized dose levels. Various types of drugs are currently available such as nicotine or estrogen patches that could be placed on the skin. However, these are among the few because of the low skin permeability to relatively large molecules such as proteins. This low permeability is mainly attributable to the stratum corneum, the outermost skin layer. The stratum corneum is effectively a 10–15 μm thick matrix of dehydrated, dead keratinocytes embedded in a lipid matrix. Once the drug crosses the stratum corneum, the next epidermal

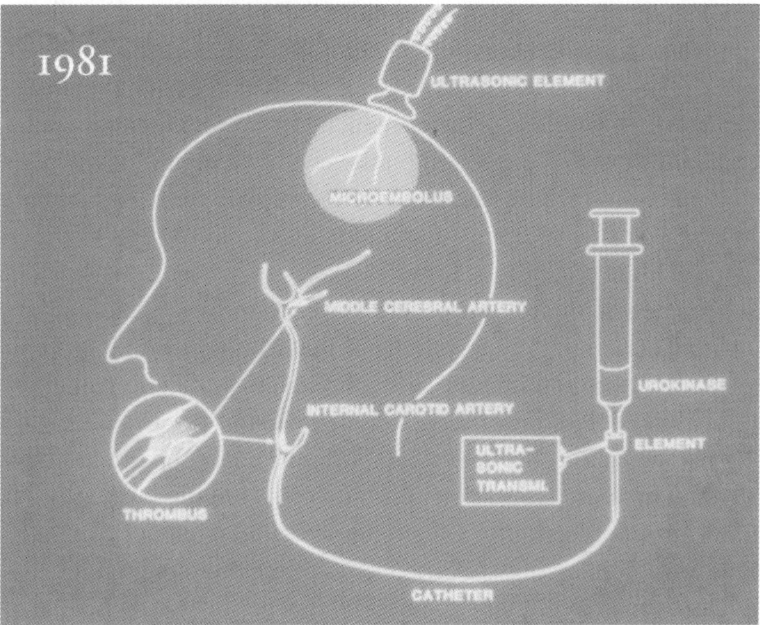

Fig. 3. Early concept drawing of stroke therapy by ultrasound (provided by Shunro Tachibana). Ultrasound was either applied extracorporeally through the skull or by means of miniature ultrasound catheter via the artery. Notice that the catheter also shows ultrasound being generated outside the body and propagating through the tube.

layer is less problematic to traverse, and consequently, the drug can reach the capillary bed to be absorbed. For protein and peptide drugs, the transdermal route has the potential to be an extremely efficient delivery site.

The clinically significant protein in the current delivery literature is that of insulin for controlling the blood glucose level in diabetic patients. Tachibana *et al.* (1991) and Kost *et al.* (1990) in the early 90s first introduced the use of ultrasound for the purpose of delivering insulin through the skin. Transdermal insulin delivery with low-frequency (<1 MHz) ultrasound condition was reported. Diabetic rat and rabbit experiments suggested a very rapid penetration of insulin through the skin, resulting in the reduction of blood glucose concentration. It has been postulated that ultrasound alters the stratum corneum of the skin, which functions as a barrier for most drugs. The disrupted skin surface may contribute to the increased absorption of drug by ultrasound. Acoustic cavitation, which is the production and collapse of countless microbubbles induced by ultrasound, may contribute to increased drug penetration during ultrasound treatment of the skin. Theoretical and experimental results suggested that drug penetration occurred through cavitation-induced keratinocyte intercellular lipid bilayer disordering and depended on the chemical nature of the permeant. Scanning electron microscopic study of the surface of hairless mouse skin revealed that ultrasound energy disrupted the outermost layer of the stratum corneum and induced large, deep crater like clefts where the superficial capillaries became visible. It is suspected that insulin was transported through these artificial openings at the surface of the skin, which induced enhancement of drug absorption into the blood stream. Several companies are now developing small electronic "wearable" ultrasound devices attached to the arm or wrist which may become available in the near future (See Chap. VII).

Genes, which are carried on chromosomes, are the basic physical and functional units of heredity. Genes are specific sequences of bases that encode information on how to produce proteins, fundamental for life functions and majority of cellular structures. Gene therapy is a technique for correcting defective genes responsible for disease development. Researchers are currently developing several approaches for correcting faulty genes to cure various diseases. A normal gene may be inserted into a nonspecific location within the genome to replace a nonfunctional gene or an abnormal gene could be replaced for a normal gene through homologous recombination. Additionally, such methods for regulation (the degree to which a gene is turned on or off) of a particular gene could be altered. The major drawbacks of gene therapy are the short-lived nature of gene expression. The therapeutic DNA introduced into target cells must remain functional and the cells containing the therapeutic DNA must be long-lived and stable to completely cure the patient. The immune response prevents repeated gene therapy. The current system of using viruses as the carrier DNA to the target lesion presents a variety of potential problems to the patient, toxicity, immune and inflammatory responses, and gene control are among them. Certain tissues such as muscle have been reported to take up and express non-viral carried naked plasmid DNA *in vivo*. In general, however, the level of transfection after direct injection of naked plasmid DNA is variable and low. Greenleaf *et al.* (1998) first approached these problems by way of using non-viral plasmid DNA in combination with ultrasound. It was postulated that ultrasound would initiate the delivery of DNA through the celluar membrane to within the cells and would not produce irreversible damage to the cells simultaneously. Bao *et al.* (1997) further added microbubbles to increase the rate of DNA transfer. Ward *et al.* (1999) and Tachibana *et al.* (1999) had earlier theorized that liquid microjets induced in the event of collapse of microbubbles could be the mechanism by which DNA easily penetrates the cell membrane. Scanning electron microscopy and high-speed video imaging technologies have recently revealed images of collapsing microbubbles and ruptured cell membrane surface that supports this theory. Unger (2004) introduced the concept of "tailored made" microbubbles and nanobubbles that target specific tissue lesions to deliver drugs and DNA.

Today, the concept of applying ultrasound as a means for altering the pharmacokinetics in various tissues and drug permeability through cell membranes, has expanded into a whole new field ranging from gene therapy to anti cancer drugs. A new generation of microbubbles and nano-sized bubbles are under development specifically for the purpose of "target and deliver" drug treatment with non-thermal ultrasound.

3. Stroke Therapy

The Stroke is the third most common cause of death in the United States, ranked only after heart disease and cancer. Approximately 700,000 new cases are reported in the US annually and ~160,000 Americans die each year from stroke. Stroke is caused by an interruption of the flow of blood to the brain (*i.e.*, an ischemic stroke) or the rupture of blood vessels in the brain (*i.e.*, a hemorrhagic stroke), which in turn causes brain cells in the affected area to die. The thrombolytic agent, tissue plasminogen activator (t-PA), is the most effective FDA approved drug to treat ischemic stroke; however, most stroke patients are not treated with t-PA because it must be administered within three hours of a stroke to be effective. Even if administrated with this drug, in some cases, there is no response to the drug due to reasons unknown. Large scale clinical trials such as the Pro-urokinase in Acute Cerebral Thromboembolism (PROACT) study (Del Zoppo *et al.*, 1998) have been conducted. In general, higher dosages of lytics increases the treatment success rate but have also resulted in higher incidence of side effects such as unwanted bleeding in the brain and the digestive system.

It is well known that the thrombus structure resembles a fibrin net, with considerable space between the fibrin and red cells. Transport of fibrinolytic drugs into the thrombus is an important determination of the clot lysis rate. However, in the early stages of thrombolytic therapy, only a fraction of therapeutically administered plasmingogen activators can penetrate into the clots by passive diffusion. Investigators have not yet determined the exact mechanisms by which ultrasound accelerates fibrinolysis. To date, it is theorized that non-thermal ultrasound changes the pharmacokinetics of the surface or within the thrombus during fibrinolysis. There have been observations of ultrasound-induced heating in the these experiments, however, researchers have found that temperature increase made little contribution to the enhancement of fibrinolysis. Furthermore, ultrasound itself does not seem to activate the fibrinolytic cascade. Blinc (1993) demonstrated that ultrasound energy did not accelerate the hydrolysis of a peptide substrate by rt-PA, and the rate of plasmin degradation of fibrinogen was not increased. Acceleration of fibrinolysis by ultrasound also required the presence of a fibrin gel and was seen with clots of whole blood, plasma, and purified fibrin. Kimura *et al.* (1994) confirmed the increase of clot lysis and the fibrin degradation product, D-dimer, after ultrasound exposure plus re-PA. These data support the theory that the acceleration of fibrinolysis by ultrasound is primarily due to enhancement of drug transport within the clots through non-thermal ultrasound related mechanisms. The most likely mechanism in which ultrasound provokes drug movement into the thrombus is acoustic cavitation, which can be defined as the formation and collapse of bubbles in liquids. Acoustic cavitation can generate high streaming velocity in liquid and it in turn can assist drug diffusion, especially at locations where acoustic impedance differs. Tachibana *et al.* (1995) reported further acceleration of fibrinolysis by ultrasound in the presence of albumin microbubbles around the clots. These microbubbles were originally used as diagnostic echo contrast agents, however, when they were exposed to more intense ultrasound in this case, it was postulated that this material served as a source for cavitation, thus resulting in more fibrinolysis.

Tachibana *et al.* (1992) demonstrated *in vitro* that relatively low-intensity ultrasound irradiation of clots in the presence of lytic agents can reduce the amount of drug required by a factor of ten, and shorten the lysis duration to one-fifth of the original time. This phenomenon has also been confirmed by other researchers (Francis, 1992; Blinc, 1993). Although the minimum ultrasound intensity needed to induce acceleration of fibrinolysis is currently under discussion, recent reports have shown that ultrasound of mechanical index (MI) ranging from 0.1 to 1.0 can produce enhanced fibrinolytic effects. Nonthermal effects of ultrasound contribute to the penetration of drugs into the thrombus. Experiments under conditions where cavitation is more easily produced have resulted in further enhancement of thrombolysis. Increased thrombolysis may also be associated to the unidirectional motion of a fluid or drug known as acoustic streaming, which originates within close range of the ultrasound transducers. Researchers have studied the driving force of acoustic streaming of microparticles theoretically and experimentally in various fluid conditions. Another possible explanation for the increased thrombolysis may be the temporary effect of ultrasound on the thrombus itself. It was suggested that bubble formation, growth and collapse causes reversible alteration in the fibrin structure that may result in an increased flow of the drug into the thrombus.

Clinical application of this new therapeutic ultrasound method for producing thrombosis has already started since 2001. Clinical trials in Europe and in the USA have been reported using miniature ultrasound transducers at the tip of catheters that approach the clots via arterial vessels (MicroLysUS infusion catheter, EKOS Corp, USA). The lytic drug, urokinase, is released at the distal end of the catheter during ultrasound irradiation (Figs. 4 and 5). The major goal of the catheters used in this study was to apply ultrasound at shorter distances with smaller ultrasound probes, and at the same time minimize damage to the surrounding normal tissues. Mahon (2003) presented early experience with the MicroLysUS infusion catheter for acute embolic stroke treatment in North America. This study was designed to demonstrate the safety of the device and to determine if ultrasound accelerates thrombolysis and improves clinical outcomes. Fourteen patients aged 40–77 years with anterior- or posterior-circulation occlusion, presented with cerebral ischemia 3–13 hours after symptom onset. Patients were treated with the catheter and simultaneous intraarterial thrombolysis. Procedural and clinical information, including time to lysis, degree of recanalization, NIHSS score, and modified Rankin Scale (mRS) score was recorded both before

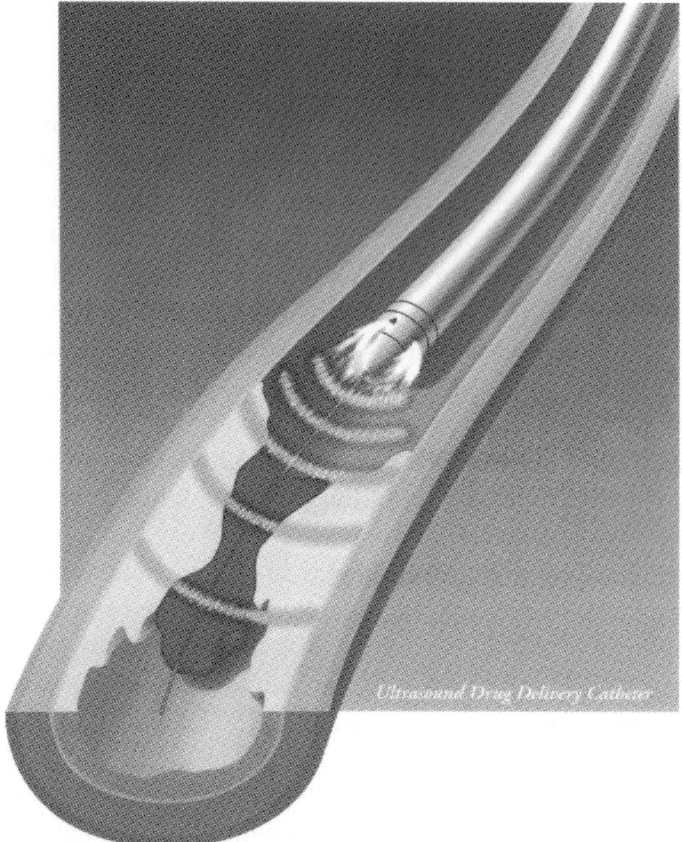

Fig. 4.   Catheter type therapeutic ultrasound device that could be inserted into the artery. Miniature ultrasound generating element was attached to the very tip of catheter. Ultrasound and drug such as urokinase can be delivered at the same time near the target thrombus.

treatment and afterward. The numbers in the study were small, but the trends demonstrated that the rates of recanalization and neurologic outcomes in patients treated with the new ultrasound catheter were equivalent or slightly better than those in patients treated with standard microinfusion. The EKOS catheter for leg peripheral arterial thrombolysis was approved by the FDA in 2004 and will probably be the first drug/ultrasound combination product to be marketed in the cardiovascular field.

Ishibashi *et al.* (2002) have accepted the challenge of sonicating transcranially to accelerate thrombolysis. A noninvasive method was tested

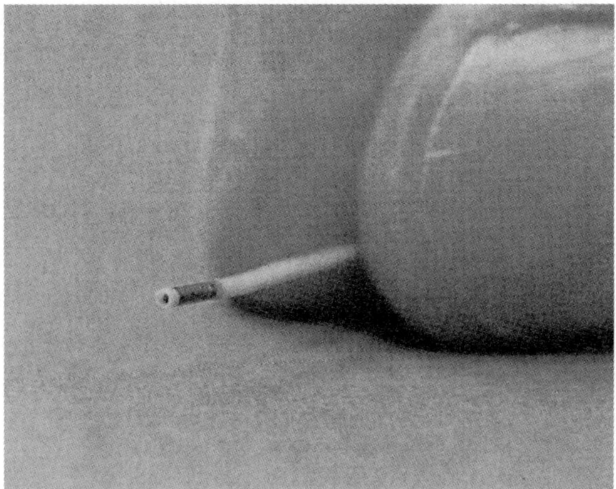

Fig. 5.   EKOS Corporation therapeutic device for strok therapy. A 2.5F (0.7 mm diameter) miniature catheter (MicroLysUS Infusion System) can be inserted deep inside the brain via the artery. Thrombolytic agents can be released at the tip of the catheter while applying ultrasound.

in an occlusion model of rabbit femoral artery, produced with thrombin after constriction of the artery led to stenotic flow and endothelial damage. After stable occlusion was confirmed, monteplase (mtPA) was administered intravenously, and ultrasound (490 kHz, 0.13 W/cm^2) was applied (TUS group). The ultrasound intensity was reduced from a higher value by passage of the ultrasound through a piece of temporal bone to simulate transcranial applications. The recanalization ratio in the TUS group was higher than that in the tPA group. Pfaffenberger *et al.* (2004) modified this experiment to determine if a 1.8-MHz commercial diagnostic ultrasound device would accelerate thrombolysis. Duplex-Doppler, continuous wave-Doppler, and pulsed wave (PW)-Doppler were compared on their impact on recombinant tissue plasminogen activator (rtPA) mediated thrombolysis. Blood clots were transtemporally sonicated in a human stroke model. Furthermore, ultrasound attenuation of 5 temporal bones of different thickness was determined. Results showed only PW-Doppler accelerated rtPA mediated thrombolysis significantly. Without attenuation by temporal bone, PW-Doppler plus rtPA showed a significant enhancement in relative clot weight loss. Measurements made when ultrasound was attenuated by passage through temporal bone revealed decreases of the output intensity of over 85%, depending on temporal bone thickness. Ultrasound attenuation by the bone is a major limiting factor in the case of high frequency transcranial ultrasound application.

Clinical investigations were aggressively carried out by Alexandrov *et al.* (2004) with diagnostic transcranial ultrasound. The initial study included 40 acute stroke patients with occlusions of the middle cerebral artery (MCA), internal carotid artery or basilar artery, which revealed high rates of complete recanalization with dramatic clinical recovering, when continuous transcranial Doppler (TCD) monitoring was used during tissue plasminogen activator (tPA) infusion. Alexandrov *et al.* (2004) reported findings from a large phase II clinical trial entitled "Combined Lysis of Thrombus in Brain Ischemia using Transcranial Ultrasound and Systemic tPA (CLOTBUST). In this trial involving 126 patients, evidence was obtained for the existence of ultrasound-enhanced thrombolysis in the middle cerebral artery thrombus. The CLOTBUST aims were: (1) To compare recanalization and recovery in patients with standard IV tPA therapy and those receiving additional continuous targeted ultrasound monitoring. (2) Compare safety in the two groups. Patients had to meet standard tPA treatment criteria of symptom onset less than 3 hours prior to treatment and also show middle cerebral occlusion on TCD. The primary end point included clinical recovery or TCD recanalization at 2 hours with 24-hour and 3-month follow up. The safety end point was intracranial hemorrhage with clinical worsening. The final results reported revealed symptomatic intracerebral hemorrhage occurrence in three patients in the target group, and three in the control group. Complete recanalization or dramatic clinical recovery within two hours after the administration of a t-PA bolus occurred in 31 patients in the target group (49%), compared with 19 patients in the control group (30%). Twenty-four hours after treatment of the patients eligible for follow-up, 24 in the target group (44%) and 21 in the control group (40%) had dramatic clinical recovery. This large clinical trial concluded that continuous transcranial Doppler augmented t-PA-induced arterial recanalization, with a non significant trend toward an increased rate of recovery from stroke, as compared with placebo. More evaluation is needed to see if diagnostic level ultrasound intensity can truly penetrate the skull and accelerate thrombolysis.

To summarize, the differences between external and internal ultrasound applications are: (1) in external application, relatively higher energy and perhaps lower frequency ultrasound is needed at the surface of the body to sufficiently deliver energy to deeply located thrombus; (2) ultrasound must propagate through the skull, preventing sufficient ultrasound energy from reaching the target accurately; (3) for internal catheter ultrasound, the number of hospitals that can actually conduct this treatment within 3 to 6 hours after onset of stroke is limited. More clinical studies are needed to evaluate the medical significance of accelerated thrombolysis by ultrasound energy. However, this therapeutic ultrasound application for stroke seems to be the most promising among various ultrasound drug delivery clinical trials known to date.

4. Microbubbles

It is well known that microbodies of air or a gas, suspended in a liquid are exceptionally efficient ultrasound scatterers for echography; they are useful as ultrasonic contrast agents. For instance, injecting suspensions of gas microbubbles (in the range of 0.5 to 10 μm in diameter) in a carrier liquid into the bloodstream of living bodies, will strongly reinforce ultrasonic echography imaging, thus aiding the visualization of internal organs, for the detection of cardiovascular and other diseases. Coated microbubbles have the advantage of being stable in the body for a significant period of time, as the shells serve to protect the gases of the microbubbles from diffusion into the bloodstream. There has been a considerable degree of excitement in diagnostic ultrasound imaging regarding improvement, which come from the introduction of these echo contrast agents. Second-generation microbubbles contain perfluorocarbon gas rather than air, which results in an even longer life span of contrast agents within the circulatory system. This permits a longer window time for the echographers to observe patients. Recently, various *in vitro* and *in vivo* experiments have demonstrated that echo contrast agent microbubbles can be intentionally ruptured by diagnostic and therapeutic ultrasound. This acoustically induced destruction and collapse of the microbubbles produces a high amplitude response. Violent liquid jets and microstreaming can be produced during microbubble collapse. Researchers have hypothesized that these microjets or microstreaming could be applied to promote diffusion of drugs into various tissues and lesions. Albumin microbubbles were first used in conjunction with ultrasound to further enhance the effects of thrombolytic agents (Tachibana, 1995).

Porter later (1996) reported that intravenous perfluorocarbon-exposed sonicated dextrose albumin (PESDA) microbubbles in the presence of low frequency ultrasound can lyse very small clots without the help of lytic agents. They developed a method to declot full-size arteriovenous dialysis grafts in animals. In a trial, three declotting techniques were randomly applied during sonication: (1) direct injection of PESDA; (2) direct injection of saline; and (3) intravenous PESDA. Declotting was graded by cine-angiography score. Results showed high mean patency scores for direct PESDA and for IV PESDA, *vs* saline. The frequency and intensity of ultrasound were 1 MHz and 0.6 W/cm^2. Mizushige *et al.* (1999) reported comparison of different types of microbubble ultrasound contrast agent [sonicated albumin (A)-, SH-U508A (SH)- and dodecafluoropentane emulsion (DDFP)] for drug-mediated thrombolysis. A catheter-type transducer capable of US emission (*i.e.*, 10 MHz, spatial peak temporal average intensity 1.02 W/cm^2 and peak negative pressure 0.33 MPa) in the continuous-wave mode was employed during *in vitro* exposure of artificial white thrombi. Serial changes in acoustic properties monitored by echography showed greatest reduction of the thrombus in the DDFP, and indicated that in the sonicated albumin, microbubble was not significantly different from controls. The stability of the microbubbles was an important factor for the difference. Culp (2004) conducted a transcranial ultrasound experiment in swine (1 MHz, 2.0 W/cm^2) in combination with platelet-targeted microbubbles and obtained rapid opening of intracranial thrombotic occlusions. Based on these results, ImaRx Therapeutics, Inc. (Arizona, USA) recently announced initiation of a multicenter Phase II clinical trial with a 40-patient, randomized and blinded study. This will evaluate the safety and effectiveness of thrombolysis with nanosized bubbles and ultrasound for the treatment of acute ischemic stroke, without the use of lytic drugs. Results showing whether microbubble alone in the presence of ultrasound could breakup thrombus in the middle cereberal artery are anticipated from the trial. Other applications in a range of thrombus related conditions, including myocardial infarction, deep vein thrombosis and thrombi in dialysis grafts, are also under consideration.

Another emerging application, which cannot be ignored, comes from the possibility of using microbubbles to carry various drugs to target sites, and rupturing the microbubbles by localized ultrasound energy. At moderately high sound pressure amplitudes, the acoustic pressure waves can cause the shells of coated microbubbles to rupture, freeing the bubbles so that they behave as non coated microbubbles until they diffuse into the bloodstream. Drug-filled or drug-coated microspheres carrying a therapeutic compound may be targeted to specific tissues through the use of sonic energy, which is directed to the target area and causes the microspheres to rupture and release the therapeutic compound. Targeted drug delivery methods are particularly important where the toxicity of the drug is an issue. Specific drug delivery methods potentially serve to minimize toxic side effects, lower the required dosage amounts, and decrease costs for the patient. The most exciting application of this method is probably gene therapy. The methods and materials in the prior technology for the introduction of genetic materials to, *e.g.*, living cells, are limited and ineffective. Better means of delivery for therapeutics such as genetic materials are needed to treat a wide variety of diseases. Great strides have been made in characterizing genetic diseases and in understanding protein transcription, but relatively little progress has been made in delivering genetic material to cells for treatment. To date, several different mechanisms have been developed to deliver genetic material. These delivery mechanisms include techniques such as calcium phosphate precipitation and electroporation, and carriers such as cationic polymers and aqueous-filled liposomes. These methods have all been relatively ineffective *in vivo* and only of limited use for cell culture transfection. None of these methods potentiate local release, delivery and integration of genetic material to the target cell. A principal difficulty has been to deliver the genetic material from the extracellular space to the intracellular space or even to effectively localize genetic material at the surface of selected cell membranes. Viruses such as adenoviruses and retroviruses have been used as vectors to transfer genetic material to cells. However, it has also been difficult to develop a successfully targeted viral-mediated vector for the delivery of genetic material *in vivo*.

Instead of viral vectors as the carrier of genes to targeted locations, pure plasmid DNA can be attached either to the outside or inside of the microbubble capsule wall. Bubbles can be collapsed by extracorporeal ultrasound

Table 1. Comparison of delivery of plasmid DNA by sonoporation or electroporation vs viral vectors.

	Sonoporation (non-viral)	Electroporation (non-viral)	Viral vectors
Tissue invasiveness[1]	(−)	(+)	(−)
Mechanical or physical damage[2]	(−)	(+)	(−)
Extreme localization[3]	(++)	(+)	(−)
Systemic toxicity	(−)	(−)	(+)
Targeted timing of transfection[4]	(+)	(+)	(−)
Homogeneous transfection at target[5]	(−)	(+)	(+)
Monitoring location of DNA in tissue	DNA/microbubbles can be visualized with diagnostic US	(−)	(−)
Clinical experience	(−)	(−)	(+)
Technical difficulty in performing treatment[6]	(−)	(+)	(−)
Treatment for large volume targets	(+)	(−)	(+)
Cost performance	Cost of microbubbles is relative expensive at present	Electrodes are relatively expensive	Viral vectors are expensive to manufacture
Others	Microbubbles have to be combined with DNA		

[1]Sonoporation and viral vectors treatment is basically minimally invasive, whereas electrodes have to be invasively inserted into the target tissue area in the case of electroporation.

[2]Although ultrasound can induce damage to the tissue at high intensities, outcome could be obtained with non-harmful levels. Electroporation could result in burns near the electrodes.

[3]Gene transfection by sonoporation or electroporation can be targeted to an extremely localized area either by local injection of DNA or focused energy.

[4]Gene transfection could be obtained in a matter of seconds with sonoporation or electroporation whereas viral vectors requires hours or days.

[5]Viral vectors and electroporation gene transfection occurs diffusively within tissues whereas some papers suggest "cobble stone" like transfection in the case of sonoporation.

[6]Custom made electrodes are required for each treatment for electroporation whereas ultrasound probes are reusable and could be applied for various situations.

or by intravascular ultrasound catheter, permitting the DNA to penetrate directly into the tissue and cells. Greenleaf *et al.* (1997) demonstrated an increase in the transfection rate of DNA in the presence of albumin microbubbles *in vitro*. Unger *et al.* (1997). demonstrated similar results with microbubble liposomes. Porter *et al.* (2001) succeeded in reducing restenosis by antisense to the c-myc protooncogene bound to perflurocarbon microbubbles in pigs. Ultrasound may become a new, effective and safe means for introducing genetic material into the target cells of tissues. Although the exact mechanism is still unknown, it is believed that microspheres, upon rupture, create a local increase in membrane fluidity, thereby enhancing cellular uptake of the therapeutic compound (Ogawa *et al.*, 2001). There have been reports that differences in the gene transfer rate depended on the type of microbubbles similar to the results from the thrombolysis (Tachibana *et al.*, 2003). However, it is clear that gene delivery phenomenon occurs at a far smaller scale, thus further investigation is needed to understand the exact mechanism involved in ultrasound microbubble gene transfer. Recent observation of the collapse of microbubbles by the newly developed high speed video microscope Brandalis-128 system, which has an average speed of 13 million frames per second, has produced massive information on the dynamic behavior of ultrasound insonified encapsulated microbubbles (Postema, 2004). Understanding more on the physics involved in the event of microjet in the following few years will perhaps solve how genes actually penetrate the cell membrane (Marmottant *et al.*, 2003, 2004).

5. Regenerative Medicine

Today, the concept of applying ultrasound as a means to alter the pharmacokinetics of drugs in various tissue and cell membrane permeability to these drugs has expanded into a whole new field beyond just drug delivery. Application of ultrasound for regenerative medicine is one of them. One example is the delivery of genes into cells. Certain tissues such as muscle have been reported to take up and express naked plasmid DNA *in vivo*. In general, however, the level of transfection after direct injection of naked plasmid DNA is variable and low. Different methods have been devised to improve the transfection efficiency. The use of certain viral vectors leads to more efficient transfection, compared with naked plasmid DNA. However, serious concerns have been voiced regarding the use of viral vectors, especially when clinical trials are involved. Instead of viral vectors as the carrier of genes to targeted locations, pure plasmid DNA can be attached either to the outside or inside of the microbubble capsule wall. Bubbles can be collapsed by extracorporeal ultrasound or by intravascular ultrasound catheter, permitting the DNA to penetrate directly into the tissue and cells. Ultrasound may become a new, effective and safe means for introducing genetic material into the target cells of tissues.

Ultrasound can induce cell-membrane porosity (Tachibana *et al.*, 1999), and enhance the delivery of naked plasmid DNA into cells *in vitro* (Fig. 6). Moreover, recent studies have shown enhanced permeability of naked plasmid DNA into tumors *in vivo* (Manome *et al.*, 2000). Li *et al.* (2003) recently made a comparison of gene transfection using various microbubbles available in the market. Ogawa *et al.* (2002) also made comparison with different dissolved gases and found changes in the extent of gene transfection. Although the exact mechanism is still unknown, it is believed that microspheres, upon rupture, create a local increase in membrane fluidity, thereby enhancing cellular uptake of the therapeutic compound. "Sonoporation" as this phenomenon is frequently named, is a new means to overcome limitations of the other gene transduction methods. Different genes for various purposes are now under intensive investigation for possible use in regenerative medicine. These could be for angiogenesis, antiangiogenesis, apoptosis, bone generation and other future treatments methods.

Anti-sense oligodeoxynucleotides (AS-ODNs) have been recognized as a new generation of putative therapeutic agents, Miura *et al.* (2003) established a delivery technique that could transfect AS-ODNs, which are designed for endothelin type B receptor (ETB), into cultured human coronary endothelial cells (HCECs) by exposure to ultrasound in the presence of echo contrast microbubbles. Taniyama (2002) have successfully transfected genes (HGF) for angiogenesis by ultrasound/microbubbles in skeletal muscles. This could lead to a cure for critical limb ischemia. In addition, Taniyama *et al.* (2003) transfected an anti-oncogene (p53) plasmid into carotid artery after balloon injury, as a model of gene therapy for restenosis. Bone morphogenetic proteins (BMPs) are morphogens implicated both in embryonic and regenerative odontogenic differentiation. Gene

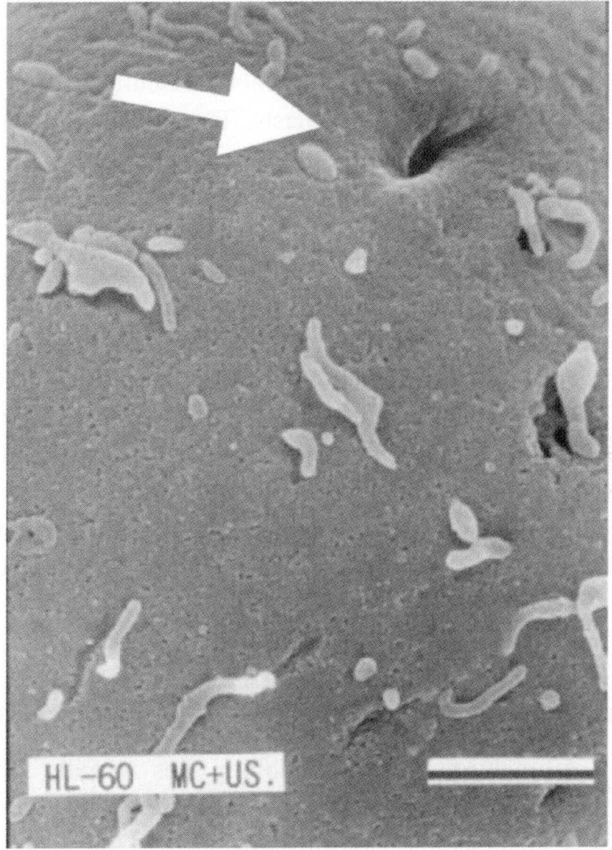

Fig. 6. Scanning electron microscopic image of the surface of cell membrane partially ruptured by microbubble collapse (scale 0.1 μm). The arrow shows where possible disruption of the cell membrane, probably in the event of micro jet impact. Drugs or DNA could easily be delivered into the cells through these openings (cell type: HL-60; 50 kHz; 3 W/cm^2, 2 minutes).

therapy has the potential to improve induction of reparative dentin formation or potent bioactive pulp capping. Nakashima (2003) optimized the gene transfer of Growth/differentiation factor 11 (Gdf11)/Bmp11 plasmid DNA into dental pulp stem cells by sonoporation, *in vivo*. Dental pulp tissue treated with plasmid pEGFP or CMV-LacZ in 5–10% Optison$^\circledR$ and irradiated by ultrasound (1 MHz, 0.5 W/cm^2, 30 sec) showed significant efficiency of gene transfer and high level of protein production selectively in the insonated region, within 300 μm under the amputated site of the pulp tissue. The Gdf11 cDNA plasmid transferred into dental pulp tissue by sonoporation *in vitro*, induced the expression of Dentin sialoprotein (Dsp), a differentiation marker for odontoblasts. The transfection of Gdf11 by sonoporation stimulated the large amount of reparative dentin formation on the amputated dental pulp in canine teeth *in vivo*. These results suggest the possible use of BMPs, employing ultrasound-mediated gene therapy for endodontic dental treatments. It is estimated that genes for regeneration tissues could become a realistic mode of treatment in future. Other genes that have potential function for therapy have been reported to increase tranfection rate by ultrasound and microbubbles (Taniyama *et al.*, 2004, 2005). Manome *et al.* (2005) demonstrated that the use of ultrasound (210.4 kHz, $5.0 \, \mathrm{W/cm^2}$, 5 seconds) most effectively transfected a plasmid DNA into culture slices of mouse brain (147-fold increase compared to controls). The effect was reinforced by combination with echo contrast agent, Levovist. Intracranially injected DNA with Levovist also enhanced gene transfection in newborn mice.

6. Breakthrough in Developmental Research

An unexpected breakthrough in technology was recently reported in a publication on developmental research, using chick and mouse embryo. It is surprising that such a non-invasive method as sonoporation for injecting various genes into cells, can lead to the discovery of understanding the function of genes in the early period of development. Ohta *et al.* (2003) recently succeeded in delivering functional gene into chick embryo. This study is probably the first of a series of discoveries in understanding the early development stages of animals using ultrasound. The gene transduction technique is a useful method to study gene functions that underlie especially in vertebrate embryogenesis. Gene transduction technique was reported using microbubble-enhanced sonoporation to achieve ectopic and transient gene expression for several embryonic organs including embryonic chick limb bud mesenchymes (Fig. 7). The technique has the advantage of (1) relatively simple gene transduction procedures, and (2) efficient exogenous gene transduction and expression with lower damages to embryos. Green fluorescent protein (GFP) or LacZ was

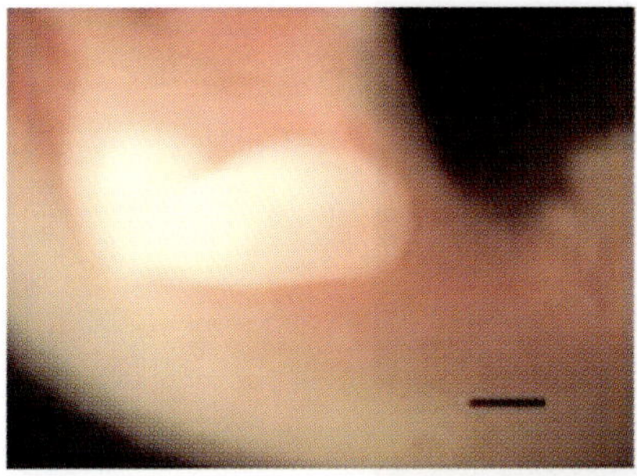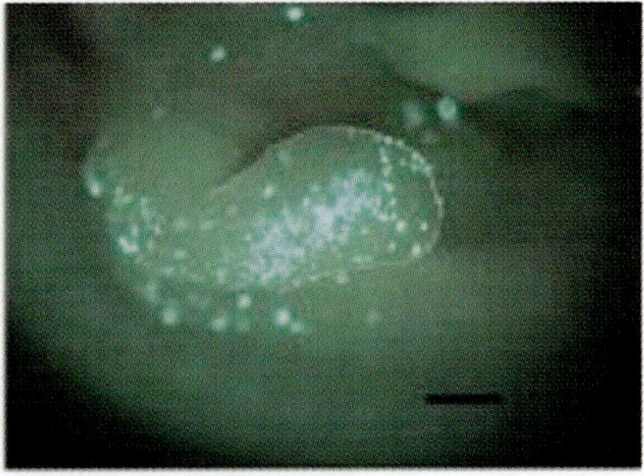

Fig. 7. Limb bud ectoderm of mouse embryo. Induction of GFP was obtained by ultrasound and microbubble collapse. Left photo shows gross view of the limb. Fluorecent microscope was used to visualize localized transfection of GFP genes. Green glow spots were observed around the limb skin (US: 1 MHz, 2 W/cm^2, 1 minute).

misexpressed in limb bud mesenchymes by sonoporation, with the introduced expression transiently detected in the injected sites. Most of the transduced chick embryos survived without showing significant embryonic abnormalities or cell death after sonoporation. To demonstrate its efficacy for assessing the effect of transient gene transduction, the *Shh* (*sonic hedgehog*) was transduced into the developing chick limb bud. The transduced limb bud displayed limb malformations, including partial digit duplication.

Recent research at our lab (unpublished data) has suggested a revolutionary technique in "ultra site specific" drug delivery into honeybee brain. A high molecular weight Rhodamine labeled dextran was selectively injected into several neurons of the brain tissue, without irreversible damage to the cells (microbubble: BR14, Bracco: 750 kHz, 2.0 W/cm^2, SonoPore KTAC-3000). The object was to visualize the axon of the cells in the brain in order to evaluate the neural network involved in basic behavioral functions, such as language or communication among insects. We were able to identify single nerve cells in the brain by using 3-dimensionally reconstructed images by confocal laser microscopy (Fig. 8). This ultra-localized "injection" technology of various substances into single cells, still in the infant stage, may help in understanding the neural network and mechanism of the function of the brain and could be applied for research in artificial intelligence and robot technology in future (Fig. 9).

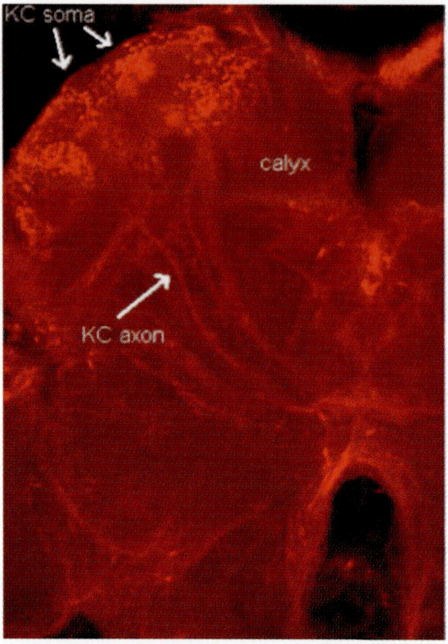

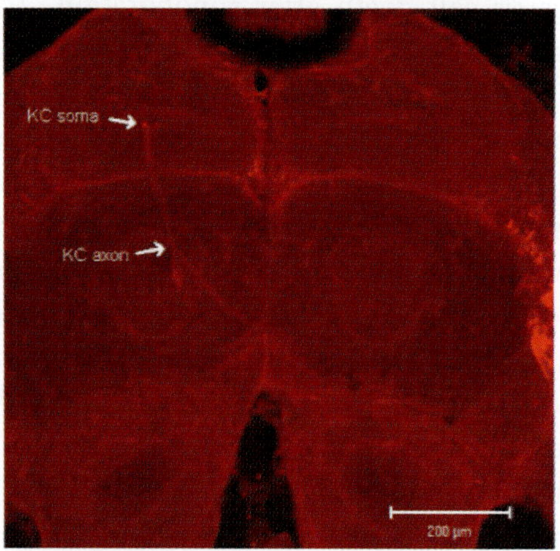

Fig. 8. Staining of single nerve fibers in Honeybee brain by ultrasound (tetra-methylrhodamine-dextran staining). Optison microbubbles were attached to the surface of the brain and irradiated by ultrasound (1 MHz, 2 W/cm^2, 1 minute) in the presence of the stain. Sliced cross section view of the brain shows staining at the surface of the bee brain (above arrows) as well as the axons in the deep layers.

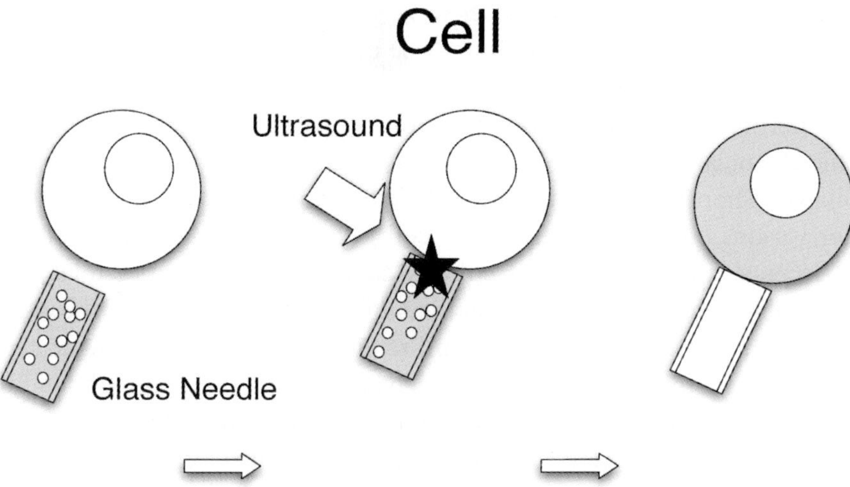

Fig. 9.   Illustraion of possible injection of drug into a single living cell by "ultra" targeted sonoporation method without irreversible damage. Microbubble and the target drug can be carried at high concentrations by a micro glass needle (far left). Ultrasound could be irradiated at a certain intensity of duration (center). Drug can penetrate the cell membrane without irreversible damage to the cell.

7. Sonodynamic Therapy

As physical methods used for the treatment of leukemia and solid cancers, compared with radiotherapy and light irradiation, ultrasonic irradiation is superior in that the applied energy can be focused solely on the cancer tissues to be treated with little effect upon normal tissues, and is better than light irradiation in terms of the degree of penetration. Umemura *et al.* (1990) pioneered the development of non-thermal ultrasound to activate a group of chemicals that were originally used as light activated chemicals for cancer therapy. This new ultrasound therapy has been termed as sonodynamic therapy. Ultrasonic waves are known to cause chemical actions if cavitation occurs; for example, irradiation of water can cause a reaction to generate hydrogen peroxide. It was found that certain drugs, upon ultrasonic irradiation, create active oxygen such as superoxide radicals and singlet oxygen, effectively destroying cancer tissues (Miyoshi *et al.*, 1995). The agents themselves have no anti tumor activity and are very low in toxicity, exhibiting anti tumor activity only by the chemical action caused by ultrasonic irradiation. Thus, there is significantly less risk in causing any systemic disorder. In addition, these drug act exclusively upon tumor tissues when combined with ultrasonic irradiation, with no adverse effect upon normal tissues. An important factor involved in ultrasound irradiation is the chemical reactions induced during the course of violent microbubble collapse. Short lived free radicals can be created by ultrasound that could alter various compounds leading to cell killing (Yumita, 2003). Sonoluminescence (the production of light by cavitation) may also be related to the complex sonochemical or sonodynamic reactions. However, the exact mechanism related to cytotoxicity still remains to be solved. Acoustic cavitation can chemically activate photosensitive drugs specifically bound to malignant cell membrane, which could result in cell surface disruption (Uchida *et al.*, 1997). Recent experiments with Adult T cell leukemia cells were specifically killed by low intensity ultrasound of $0.3\,\text{W/cm}^2$ in the presence of porfimer sodium (Tachibana *et al.*, 1997). Abe *et al.* (2002) developed a strategy for the selective destruction of cancer cells by ultrasonic irradiation in the presence of an antibody-conjugated photosensitizer. A photoimmunoconjugate (PIC) was prepared between ATX-70, a photosensitizer of a gallium-porphyrin analogue, and F11-39, a high affinity monoclonal antibody (MAb) against carcinoembryonic antigen (CEA), which is often overexpressed in various carcinoma cells. The conjugate, designated F39/ATX-70, retained immunoreactivity against purified CEA and CEA-expressing cells as determined by enzyme-linked immunosorbent assay, flow cytometry and immunofluorescence microscopic analysis. The cytotoxicity of F39/ATX-70 against CEA-expressing human gastric carcinoma cells *in vitro* was found to be greater than that of ATX-70, when applied in combination with ultrasound irradiation. *In vivo* anti tumor effects in a mouse xenograft model resulted in a marked growth inhibition of tumor, compared with ultrasound alone or ultrasound after administration of ATX-70. Arakawa *et al.* (2003) demonstrated that PAD-S31, a water-soluble, chlorin-derivative sonochemical sensitizer, can be used for sonodynamic therapy on neointimal hyperplasia in a rabbit stent model. One hour after the intravenous administration of PAD-S31, ultrasound energy (1 MHz, $0.3\,\text{W/cm}^2$) was delivered transdermally to the sonodynamic therapy group. At 28 days, all stent sites were analyzed morphometrically. The ratio of the intimal and medial cross-sectional area was smaller in the sonodynamic therapy group than in the control, ultrasound, and PAD-S31 groups. It was concluded that sonodynamic therapy might be a feasible treatment modality for noninvasively inhibiting neointimal hyperplasia.

Anti-angiogenesis therapy is considered to be a new approach to various human cancers because angiogenesis is crucial for tumor growth (Emoto *et al.*, 2003). Moreover, ultrasound energy has been shown to enhance an anti tumor effect of a chemotherapeutic agent *in vitro* and *in vivo*. Uterine sarcoma is the most malignant neoplasm among the known uterine malignancies, which has a poor response to any chemotherapeutic agent currently used and also to radiotherapy. Our previous study (unpublished) showed anti tumor effect of TNP-470 (an analogue of fumagillin), an angiogenesis inhibitor, for human uterine sarcoma, *in vitro* and *in vivo*. This study firstly examined the therapeutic effect of angiogenesis inhibitor, combined with ultrasound irradiation for human cancer *in vivo*, and evaluated its vascularity real-time using a microbubble ultrasound contrast agent (Optison®). The uterine sarcoma xenografts were treated by 1 MHz ultrasound with an intensity of $2.0\,\text{W/cm}^2$ for 4 minutes three times per week, each after subcutaneous injection of TNP-470 at a dose of 30 mg/kg and this therapy was continued for eight weeks. The reduction of the volume, as well as the weight of the xenografts was significantly shown by this combined therapy, in comparison to a group of drug used alone or in the controls. No major side effect was observed in any mice of the groups. The effect of anti-angiogenesis for this tumor was demonstrated real-time by contrasted color ultrasound, non-invasively. The microvessel density of the tumors was significantly decreased in this combination therapy, compared with other groups. These results suggest that there is an accelerated (boosting) effect of ultrasound for anti-angiogenesis drug therapy for human uterine sarcoma, and this combination therapy might be a potential candidate for new cancer treatment.

Feril *et al.* (2005) recently reported monocytic leukemia cells (U937) killing effect by combining hyperthermia sensitive drug, 2,2′-azobis (2-amidinopropane) dihydrochloride (AAPH) and exposure to nonthermal 1 MHz US for 1 minute at an intensity of $2.0\,\text{W/cm}^2$. Apoptosis measured by flow cytometry and free radical investigation using electron paramagnetic resonance (EPR) spin trapping, showed that US-induced cell lysis and apoptosis were enhanced in the presence of AAPH, regardless of the temperature at the time of sonication. Although free radicals were increased in the combined treatment, this increase did not correlate well with cell killing. The mechanism of enhancement pointed to the increased uptake of the agent during sonication rather than potentiation by AAPH. Although much more research is needed to transfer experimental information to actual clinical cases, rapid advancement of HIFU (high intensity focused ultrasound) will act as an accelerating factor for future therapeutic strategies, combining anti cancer drug and ultrasound in patients (See Chap. VIII).

8. Molecular Imaging and Therapy

Molecular imaging is currently one of the most promising fields in medical research for the noninvasive assessment of physiologic and pathologic processes at the molecular level. Molecular imaging is not just an extension of the traditional process of image formation and interpretation, but is meant to improve diagnostic accuracy by providing an *in vivo* analog of immunocytochemistry or *in situ* hybridization. In this sense, molecular imaging is a revolutionary leap forward to diagnose a disease not just from morphological information, but by obtaining clues of the pathological malfunction of the lesion of interest at the molecular level. The object is to enhance the conspicuity of subtle pathologies by targeting the molecular components or processes that are the causes of disease. Recent advancements in nuclear imaging, ultrasound, MRI have initiated interest in molecular imaging across all modalities and across various medical fields, ranging from cancer to cardivascular areas. This new direction has only become possible because of the rapid progress in biotechnology (*e.g.*, the finalized human genome project, proteomics, and bioinformatics). Intense research and effort is currently being spent on identifying suitable molecular targets and preparing the specific sensitive site-targeted contrast agents. The use of ultrasound is undoubtedly a potential modality for molecular imaging.

The use of ultrasound has several characteristics that distinguishes it from the other molecular imaging modalities: (1) real time imaging is possible; (2) relatively short and efficient imaging protocols, compared with MRI or nuclear imaging; (3) non-invasiveness, minimal patient discomfort; (4) low operating costs; and lastly, (5) complementary therapeutic and imaging capabilities which neither MRI nor nuclear imaging can offer. The last item is by far the most outstanding characteristic. The major areas where diagnostic ultrasound molecular imaging is being evaluated include angiogenesis (both endogenous and therapeutic), thrombus and cancer detection, identification of atherosclerotic plaque at risk for rupture and detection and quantification of markers of inflammation. In fact, therapeutic application is equally being considered in the same field as targeted drug delivery (See Chap. VI) and gene therapy (See Chap. III).

Although there are many strategies for designing microbubbles, there are mainly two types: passive/nonspecific targeting which relies on the properties of the shell and diameter of the bubble for accumulation in the vasculature; and active targeting, also known as specific targeting. The latter relies on adhesion ligands which makes it possible for the micro or nano bubbles to accumulate at a specific site. The current favorite molecular target for ultrasound is the expression of inflammation or immuno-associated molecules which can be visualized with molecular ultrasonography. Targeted contrast ultrasound has previously been utilized to detect vascular disease, including thrombi using fibrinogen targeted microbubbles (Unger *et al.*, 1998), inflammation using MBs targeted to P-selectin (Lindner *et al.*, 2001) or ICAM-1 (Villanueva *et al.*, 1998), and acute cardiac transplant rejection by targeting ICAM-1 (Weller *et al.*, 2003). Newly targeted microbubbles directed to the GPIIb IIIa receptor have been developed. These bioconjugate ligands were inserted into lipid-coated membranes of perfluorocarbon gas microbubbles and binding studies performed on activated platelets immobilized on cell culture plates. Targeted microbubble binding to clots in a flow through chamber was also being assessed. Microbubble binding studies on arteriolar and venular clots in a mouse cremasteric muscle model showed improved binding to vascular thrombi (Schumann *et al.*, 2002). Recent studies have shown the feasibility of using intravenously administered L-selectin ligand-specific polymer-stabilized air-filled microparticles for active targeting of peripheral lymph nodes under normal condition in animal models (Hauff *et al.*, 2004). This visualization technology can be applied as an indirect method of lymphography, thus making accurate identification of lymph nodes for biopsy and therapy possible. Endothelial cells of angiogenic tumor vasculature are characterized by altered expression of molecular markers on their surface. Numerous peptides have been identified that specifically bind tumor angiogenic endothelium, including the tripeptide arginine-arginine-leucine (RRL).

Weller *et al.* (2005) recently hypothesized that ultrasound contrast microbubbles targeted via linkage with RRL would specifically adhere to tumor angiogenic endothelium versus normal myocardium, and that this selective adhesion could be detected ultrasonically. Experimental results showed microbubble binding *in vitro* to tumor-derived cultured endothelium. Furthermore, *in vivo* ultrasonic detection of angiogenic tumor vasculature in a tumor-bearing mouse model demonstrated and showed that this technique could distinguish between normal tissue and tumor tissue.

Great advances have been reported in applying to various targets, including smaller microbubbles in the nanosize range which could function as indicators for ultrasound visualization. Targeted perfluorocarbon nanoparticles were the first reported molecular imaging agent for ultrasound applications and were shown to augment reflectivity from fibrin thrombi (Unger *et al.*, 1998). Additionally, targeting to vascular epitopes such as tissue factor, whose expression is induced in smooth muscle cells is possible, because these particles can penetrate through microfissures into the vascular media (Wickline *et al.*, 2003; Lanza *et al.*, 2003). Reflective microbubbles and liposomes have also been used to specifically target endothelial integrins (Dayton *et al.*, 2004; Leong-Poi *et al.*, 2003).

The ability to incorporate drugs or genes into detectable site-targeted nanosystems represents a new paradigm in therapeutics. Payloads of therapeutic agents, such as genes or radionuclides, can be complexed to the carriers themselves. Drugs can be linked to or dissolved within carrier lipid coatings, deposited in subsurface oil layers, or trapped within the carriers themselves. Drug delivery to specific cells from nanocarriers can occur by diffusion, particle fusion and internalization into cells, component (lipid-lipid) exchange and convective flux, biolistics, or some combination of these mechanisms. Nanoparticles are also useful for the delivery of pharmaceutical agents, after binding to target cellular epitopes by a mechanism known as "contact facilitated drug delivery". Binding and close apposition to the targeted cell membrane permits enhanced lipid-lipid exchange with the lipid monolayer of the nanoparticle, which accelerates convective flux of lipophilic drugs (*e.g.*, paclitaxel) dissolved in the outer lipid membrane of the nanoparticles into the targeted cells. The progress in molecular imaging by micro/nanobubbles will probably initiate further excitement for using this very technology for drug delivery. Ultrasound is technically the most appropriate modality for this purpose, which will introduce new medical fields that are fusions between diagnostic and therapeutic.

9. Conclusions and Outlook

Research on the bioeffects of ultrasound alone and in the presence of various drugs to the patients has only just begun. Most investigations are still highly experimental and are far from being applicable in the clinical situation. However, such applications as HIFU therapy (see, Chap. VIII) for prostate cancer are already beginning to be widely used in patients as alternative non-operative modalities. Additionally, there exists an interesting biological phenomenon that cannot be ignored when non-thermal ultrasound is applied. The interaction between ultrasound and drugs can range from a change in the permeability of biological membrane to the manipulation of DNA into the cells. Recent discoveries have triggered the imagination of researchers in regenerative medicine and developmental research. Understanding the mechanism of micro/nano bubble collapse will eventually result in the optimization of the acoustics and the design of ultrasound devices for wider clinical therapeutic applications and research.

Acknowledgments

This review was supported in part by a Grant-in-Aid for Scientific Research on Priority Areas (15300187, 16500328) from the Ministry of Education, Culture, Sports, Science and Technology, Japan, and from Fukuoka University Central Research Institute.

References

Abe H, Kuroki M, Tachibana K, *et al.* Targeted sonodynamic therapy of cancer using a photosensitizer conjugated with antibody against carcinoembryonic antigen. *Anti Cancer Res* (2002) **22**(3): 1575–1580.

Alexandrov AV, Demchuk AM, Hill MD. CLOTBUST: Phase I data on ultrasound enhanced thrombolysis for stroke. *Stroke* (2002) **33**: 354–355.

Alexandrov AV, Molina CA, Grotta JC, *et al.* Ultrasound-enhanced systemic thrombolysis for acute ischemic stroke. *N Engl J Med* (2004) **351**(21): 2170–2178.

Arakawa K, Hagisawa K, Kusano H, *et al.* Sonodynamic therapy decreased neointimal hyperplasia after stenting in the rabbit iliac artery. *Circulation* (2002) **105**(2): 149–151.

Bao S, Thrall BD, Miller DL. Transfection of a reporter plasmid into cultured cells by sonoporation *in vitro*. *Ultrasound Med Biol* (1997) **23**(6): 953–959.

Blinc A, Francis CW, Trudnowski JL, Carstensen EL. Characterization of ultrasound-potentiated fibrinolysis *in vitro*. *Blood* (1993) **81**(10): 2636–2643

Culp WC, Porter TR, Lowery J, *et al.* Intracranial clot lysis with intravenous microbubbles and transcranial ultrasound in swine. *Stroke* (2004) **35**(10): 2407–2411.

Daffertshofer M, Fatar M. Therapeutic ultrasound in ischemic stroke treatment: Experimental evidence. *Eur J Ultrasound* (2002) **16**(1–2): 121–130.

Daffertshofer M, Hennerici M. Ultrasound in the treatment of ischaemic stroke. *Lancet Neurol* (2003) **2**(5): 283–290.

Dayton PA, Pearson D, Clark J, *et al.* Ultrasonic analysis of peptide- and antibody-targeted microbubble contrast agents for molecular imaging of alphavbeta3-expressing cells. *Mol Imag* (2004) **3**(2): 125–134.

del Zoppo GJ, Higashida RT, Furlan AJ, *et al.* PROACT: A phase II randomized trial of recombinant pro-urokinase by direct arterial delivery in acute middle cerebral artery stroke. *Stroke* (1998) **29**(1): 4–11.

Emoto M, Ishiguro M, Iwasaki H, Kikuchi M, Kawarabayashi T. Effect of angiogenesis inhibitor TNP-470 on the growth, blood flow, and microvessel density in xenografts of human uterine carcinosarcoma in nude mice. *Gynecol Oncol* (2003) **89**(1): 88–94.

Feril LB Jr, Kondo T, Zhao QL, *et al.* Enhancement of ultrasound-induced apoptosis and cell lysis by echo-contrast agents. *Ultrasound Med Biol* (2003) **29**(2): 331–337.

Feril LB Jr, Ogawa R, Kobayashi H, Kikuchi H, Kondo T. Ultrasound enhances liposome-mediated gene transfection. *Ultrason Sonochem* (2005) **12**(6): 489–493.

Furuhata H, Kudo S. Thrombolysis with ultrasound effect. *Tokyo Jikeikai Med J* (1989) **104**: 1005–1012.

Francis CW, Onundarson PT, Carstensen EL, *et al.* Enhancement of fibrinolysis *in vitro* by ultrasound. *J Clin Invest* (1992) **90**(5): 2063–2068.

Greenleaf WJ, Bolander ME, Sarkar G, Goldring MB, Greenleaf JF. Artificial cavitation nuclei significantly enhance acoustically induced cell transfection. *Ultrasound Med Biol* (1998) **24**(4): 587–595.

Harrison GH, Balcer-Kubiczek EK, Eddy HA. Potentiation of chemotherapy by low-level ultrasound. *Int J Radiat Biol* (1991) **59**(6): 1453–1466.

Hashiya N, Aoki M, Tachibana K, *et al.* Local delivery of E2F decoy oligodeoxynucleotides using ultrasound with microbubble agent (Optison) inhibits intimal hyperplasia after balloon injury in rat carotid artery model. *Biochem Biophys Res Commun* (2004) **317**(2): 508–514.

Hauff P, Reinhardt M, Briel A, Debus N, Schirner M. Molecular targeting of lymph nodes with L-selectin ligand-specific US contrast agent: A feasibility study in mice and dogs. *Radiology* (2004) **231**(3): 667–673.

Ishibashi T, Akiyama M, Onoue H, Abe T, Furuhata H. Can transcranial ultrasonication increase recanalization flow with tissue plasminogen activator? *Stroke* (2002) **33**(5): 1399–1404.

Kimura M, Iijima S, Kobayashi K, Furuhata H. Evaluation of the thrombolytic effect of tissue-type plasminogen activator with ultrasonic irradiation: *In vitro* experiment involving assay of the fibrin degradation products from the clot. *Biol Pharm Bull* (1994) **17**(1): 126–130.

Koike H, Tomita N, Azuma H, *et al.* An efficient gene transfer method mediated by ultrasound and microbubbles into the kidney. *J Gene Med* (2005) **7**(1): 108–116.

Kremkau FW, Kaufmann JS, Walker MM, Burch PG, Spurr CL. Ultrasonic enhancement of nitrogen mustard cytotoxicity in mouse leukemia. *Cancer* (1976) **37**(4): 1643–1647.

Lanza GM, Wickline SA. Targeted ultrasonic contrast agents for molecular imaging and therapy. *Curr Probl Cardiol* (2003) **28**(12): 625–653.

Leong-Poi H, Christiansen J, Klibanov AL, Kaul S, Lindner JR. Noninvasive assessment of angiogenesis by ultrasound and microbubbles targeted to alpha(v)-integrins. *Circulation* (2003) **107**(3): 455–460.

Li T, Tachibana K, Kuroki M, Kuroki M. Gene transfer with echo-enhanced contrast agents: Comparison between Albunex, Optison, and Levovist in mice–initial results. *Radiology* (2003) **229**(2): 423–428.

Lindner JR, Song J, Christiansen J, *et al.* Ultrasound assessment of inflammation and renal tissue injury with microbubbles targeted to P-selectin. *Circulation* (2001) **104**(17): 2107–2112.

Mahon BR, Nesbit GM, Barnwell SL, *et al.* North American clinical experience with the EKOS MicroLysUS infusion catheter for the treatment of embolic stroke. *AJNR Am J Neuroradiol* (2003) **24**(3): 534–538.

Manome Y, Nakamura M, Ohno T, Furuhata H. Ultrasound facilitates transduction of naked plasmid DNA into colon carcinoma cells *in vitro* and *in vivo*. *Hum Gene Ther* (2000) 20;**11**(11): 1521–1528.

Manome Y, Nakayama N, Nakayama K, Furuhata H. Insonation facilitates plasmid DNA transfection into the central nervous system and microbubbles enhance the effect. *Ultrasound Med Biol* (2005) **31**(5): 693–702.

Marmottant P, Hilgenfeldt S. Controlled vesicle deformation and lysis by single oscillating bubbles. *Nature* (2003) 8;**423**(6936): 153–156.

Marmottant P, Hilgenfeldt S. A bubble-driven microfluidic transport element for bioengineering. *Proc Natl Acad Sci USA* (2004) **101**(26): 9523–9527.

Miura S, Tachibana K, Okamoto T, Saku K. *In vitro* transfer of antisense oligodeoxynucleotides into coronary endothelial cells by ultrasound. *Biochem Biophys Res Commun* (2002) **298**(4): 587–590.

Mitragotri S. Healing sound: The use of ultrasound in drug delivery and other therapeutic applications. *Nat Rev Drug Discov* (2005) **4**(3): 255–260.

Miyoshi N, Misik V, Fukuda M, Riesz P. Effect of gallium-porphyrin analogue ATX-70 on nitroxide formation from a cyclic secondary amine by ultrasound: On the mechanism of sonodynamic activation. *Radiat Res* (1995) **143**(2): 194–202.

Mizushige K, Kondo I, Ohmori K, Hirao K, Matsuo H. Enhancement of ultrasound-accelerated thrombolysis by echo contrast agents: Dependence on microbubble structure. *Ultrasound Med Biol* (1999) **25**(9): 1431–1437.

Nakashima M, Tachibana K, Iohara K, *et al.* Induction of reparative dentin formation by ultrasound-mediated gene delivery of growth/differentiation factor 11. *Hum Gene Ther* (2003) **14**(6): 591–597.

Ogawa K, Tachibana K, Uchida T, *et al.* High-resolution scanning electron microscopic evaluation of cell-membrane porosity by ultrasound. *Med Electron Microsc* (2001) **34**(4): 249–253.

Ogawa R, Kondo T, Honda H, *et al.* Effects of dissolved gases and an echo contrast agent on ultrasound mediated *in vitro* gene transfection. *Ultrason Sonochem* (2002) **9**(4): 197–203.

Ohta S, Suzuki K, Tachibana K, Yamada G. Microbubble-enhanced sonoporation: Efficient gene transduction technique for chick embryos. *Genesis* (2003) **37**(2): 91–101.

Porter TR, LeVeen RF, Fox R, Kricsfeld A, Xie F. Thrombolytic enhancement with perfluorocarbon-exposed sonicated dextrose albumin microbubbles. *Am Heart J* (1996) **132**(5): 964–968.

Porter TR, Hiser WL, Kricsfeld D, *et al.* Inhibition of carotid artery neointimal formation with intravenous microbubbles. *Ultrasound Med Biol* (2001) **27**(2): 259–265.

Postema M, van Wamel A, Lancee CT, de Jong N. Ultrasound-induced encapsulated microbubble phenomena. *Ultrasound Med Biol* (2004) **30**(6): 827–840.

Pfaffenberger S, Devcic-Kuhar B, Kollmann C, *et al.* Can a commercial diagnostic ultrasound device accelerate thrombolysis? An *in vitro* skull model. *Stroke* (2005) **36**(1): 124–128.

Saad AH, Hahn GM. Ultrasound enhanced drug toxicity on Chinese hamster ovary cells *in vitro*. *Cancer Res* (1989) **49**(21): 5931–5934.

Schumann PA, Christiansen JP, Quigley RM, *et al.* Targeted-microbubble binding selectively to GPIIb IIIa receptors of platelet thrombi. *Invest Radiol* (2002) **37**(11): 587–593.

Tachibana S, Koga E. Ultrasonic vibration for boosting fibrinolytic effect of urokinase. *Blood and Vessel* (1981) **12**: 450–453.

Tachibana K, Tachibana S. Transdermal delivery of insulin by ultrasonic vibration. *J Pharm Pharmacol* (1991) **43**(4): 270–271.

Tachibana K. Enhancement of fibrinolysis with ultrasound energy. *J Vasc Interv Radiol* (1992) **3**(2): 299–303.

Tachibana K. Transdermal delivery of insulin to alloxan-diabetic rabbits by ultrasound exposure. *Pharm Res* (1992) **9**(7): 952–954.

Tachibana K, Tachibana S. Albumin microbubble echo-contrast material as an enhancer for ultrasound accelerated thrombolysis. *Circulation* (1995) **92**: 1148–1150.

Tachibana K, Uchida T, Hisano S, Morioka E. Eliminating adult T-cell leukaemia cells with ultrasound. *Lancet* (1997) **349**(9048): 325.

Tachibana K, Uchida T, Ogawa K, Yamashita N, Tamura K. Induction of cell-membrane porosity by ultrasound. *Lancet* (1999) **353**(9162): 1409.

Taniyama Y, Tachibana K, Hiraoka K, *et al.* Development of safe and efficient novel nonviral gene transfer using ultrasound: Enhancement of transfection efficiency of naked plasmid DNA in skeletal muscle. *Gene Ther* (2002) **9**(6): 372–380.

Taniyama Y, Tachibana K, Hiraoka K, *et al.* Local delivery of plasmid DNA into rat carotid artery using ultrasound. *Circulation* (2002) **105**(10): 1233–1239.

Uchida T, Tachibana K, Hisano S, Morioka E. Elimination of adult T cell leukemia cells by ultrasound in the presence of porfimer sodium. *Anti cancer Drugs* (1997) **8**(4): 329–335.

Unger EC, McCreery TP, Sweitzer RH. Ultrasound enhances gene expression of liposomal transfection. *Invest Radiol* (1997) **32**(12): 723–727.

Unger EC, McCreery TP, Sweitzer RH, Shen D, Wu G. *In vitro* studies of a new thrombus-specific ultrasound contrast agent. *Am J Cardiol* (1998) **81**(12A): 58G–61G.

Unger EC, Porter T, Culp W, *et al.* Therapeutic applications of lipid-coated microbubbles. *Adv Drug Deliv Rev* (2004) **56**(9): 1291–1314.

 K. Tachibana & S. Tachibana

Umemura S, Yumita N, Nishigaki R, Umemura K. Mechanism of cell damage by ultrasound in combination with hematoporphyrin. *Jpn J Cancer Res* (1990) **81**(9): 962–966.

Villanueva FS, Jankowski RJ, Klibanov S, *et al.* Microbubbles targeted to intercellular adhesion molecule-1 bind to activated coronary artery endothelial cells. *Circulation* (1998) **98**(1): 1–5.

Ward M, Wu J, Chiu JF. Ultrasound-induced cell lysis and sonoporation enhanced by contrast agents. *J Acoust Soc Am* (1999) **105**(5): 2951–2957.

Weller GE, Lu E, Csikari MM, *et al.* Ultrasound imaging of acute cardiac transplant rejection with microbubbles targeted to intercellular adhesion molecule-1. *Circulation* (2003) **108**(2): 218–224.

Weller GE, Wong MK, Modzelewski RA, Lu E, Klibanov AL, Wagner WR, Villanueva FS. Ultrasonic imaging of tumor angiogenesis using contrast microbubbles targeted via the tumor-binding peptide arginine-arginine-leucine. *Cancer Res* (2005) **65**(2): 533–539.

Wickline SA, Lanza GM. Nanotechnology for molecular imaging and targeted therapy. *Circulation* (2003) **107**(8): 1092–1095.

Yumita N, Sakata I, Nakajima S, Umemura S. Ultrasonically induced cell damage and active oxygen generation by 4-formyloximeetylidene-3-hydroxyl-2-vinyl-deuterio-porphynyl(IX)-6-7-diaspartic acid: On the mechanism of sonodynamic activation. *Biochim Biophys Acta* (2003) **1620**(1–3): 179–184.

V

MRI-GUIDED FOCUSED ULTRASOUND FOR LOCAL TISSUE ABLATION AND OTHER IMAGE-GUIDED INTERVENTIONS

Kullervo Hynynen and Nathan McDannold

The power of being able to focus acoustic energy deep in the body can be largely enhanced by using magnetic resonance imaging (MRI). In addition to providing good soft tissue contrast, MRI offers temperature monitoring and exposure control that has been shown to be important for clinical interventions. This chapter reviews the current clinical and research experience with MRI-guided focused ultrasound devices and their potential for other image-guided interventions such as targeted drug delivery, vascular occlusion and thrombolysis.

1. Introduction

Of all the advantages of ultrasound over other interventional methods, perhaps the greatest is its ability to noninvasively concentrate energy into a controlable focal volume deep in tissue. The ability to focus ultrasound beams was first experimentally explored for therapy by Lynn *et al.* (1942), who demonstrated the feasibility of focal noninvasive ablation of tissue. This research was continued by William and Francis Fry *et al.* (1955a, b) and Lele (1962), resulting in the testing of focused ultrasound beams for the destruction of small tissue volumes in the central nervous system in animals and in humans. The early history of therapeutic ultrasound is reviewed in detail by Kremkau (1979). Most notably, focused ultrasound was used in spinal commissurotomy (Richards *et al.*, 1966), in the treatment of glaucoma

(Coleman *et al.*, 1985) and in the treatment of human malignant melanomas (Burov, 1956; Burov and Adreevskaya, 1956), breast cancer (Oka, 1960), and brain tumors (Oka, 1960).

Focused ultrasound (FUS) surgery has not been widely used, despite some promising results in a large, clinical multi-center eye surgery study (Coleman *et al.*, 1985). Indeed, the medical community has been slow in accepting FUS surgery as a mainstream treatment modality, largely due to the size of the destroyed tissue volume being dependent on the applied power, on the duration of the sonication (Lele, 1962), and on the tissue type (Frizzell *et al.*, 1977). Similarly, the overlying tissues may affect the quality of focusing (Mahoney *et al.*, 2001), (Liu *et al.*, 2005), and likewise, our ability to pinpoint the focal spot location. These factors, taken separately and in combination, have made it difficult to predict the focal tissue coagulation based only on the output parameters of the ultrasound source. During the 1990s, several commercial companies developed clinically focused ultrasound surgery devices that are currently in trials or at the early stages of clinical practice. These prototypes utilized single element transducers or arrays that were mechanically manipulated to aim the beam based on ultrasound images (Gelet *et al.*, 1993; Foster *et al.*, 1993; Vallancien *et al.*, 1992; Wu *et al.*, 2001a). Although ultrasound allows the anatomy to be imaged with reasonable certainty, especially in the eye and prostate, soft tissue contrast is not always adequate for tumor treatments (Hynynen *et al.*, 1990); moreover, it does not allow the ultrasound exposure or tissue damage to be quantified. We have explored the use of Magnetic Resonance Imaging (MRI) to address these problems. MRI offers good soft tissue contrast, the ability to image temperature elevations, and the ability to detect the resulting tissue changes. It is thus well suited for the guidance, monitoring and control of focused ultrasound exposures. Following the first feasibility experiments conducted by our group (Hynynen, 1992; Hynynen *et al.*, 1992; Hynynen *et al.*, 1993b), multiple studies [for example (Hynynen *et al.*, 1993b; Darkazanli *et al.*, 1993; Hynynen *et al.*, 1994; Hynynen *et al.*, 1995b; Hynynen *et al.*, 1996d; Cline *et al.*, 1993; Cline *et al.*, 1995b; Suzuki *et al.*, 1995; Stepanow *et al.*, 1995; Smith *et al.*, 1995; Stafford *et al.*, 2000; Moonen *et al.*, 1997; Palussiere *et al.*, 2003b; Sommer *et al.*, 1997; Chen *et al.*, 1999; Graham *et al.*, 1999)] have demonstrated the benefits of using MRI to guide and monitor the FUS exposures.

In this chapter, we will review the use of MRI-guided FUS for noninvasive thermal surgery, focusing mainly on our experience with this technology. We will describe the progress in high power ultrasound phased array technology that is allowing more control over the energy deposition, and as a result, is permitting procedures such as transcranial treatment of the brain, believed to be impossible in the past, until recently. In addition, we will describe some of our animal results from experiments testing FUS for other interventions, including some that exploit non-thermal bioeffects. Since some of these studies have not yet been published, we invite the reader to evaluate the merits of the research in the relatively detailed accounts offered here.

2. MRI for Guidance, Monitoring and Control of FUS

For most of the 80s, our laboratory was involved in developing and using ultrasound-guided hyperthermia devices (Hynynen *et al.*, 1987). In parallel, we were exploring the potential of short, high power FUS exposures that could be used for thermal surgery (Billard *et al.*, 1990; Dorr and Hynynen, 1992; Damianou and Hynynen, 1993). When this research reached the point where clinical testing appeared feasible, the need for accurate targeting became evident. Ultrasound imaging, however, due to its relatively poor soft tissue contrast, was clearly not the optimal method for achieving this. At the same time, General Electric Medical Systems (GEMS), now GE Healthcare, was developing an interventional MRI scanner (Schenck *et al.*, 1995) and was actively seeking minimally invasive and noninvasive methods for various therapeutic interventions. It was introduced to our ultrasound research at the University of Arizona, and we jointly decided to explore the feasibility of performing sonications in the magnet. Since our laboratory is capable of constructing ultrasound transducers "in-house", we quickly demonstrated that non-magnetic high power ultrasound transducers can be built and that sonications can be performed during MR (Magnetic Resonance) imaging (Hynynen, 1992; Hynynen *et al.*, 1992; Hynynen *et al.*, 1993b). These initial results convinced GEMS to collaborate with our laboratory in developing this technology for clinical use (Cline *et al.*, 1995b; Hynynen *et al.*, 1996d). Since MRI gives good soft tissue contrast and allows the ultrasound beam to be safely aimed, we were most interested in pursuing this line of research. Even more compeling, some MRI parameters are temperature sensitive (Parker 1984; Kuroda *et al.*, 1996; Quesson *et al.*, 2000), making it possible to detect the focal spot location, perhaps even at power levels low enough to assure precise targeting before thermal ablation begins. However, since the MRI parameters for thermometry in use at that time, based on the sensitivity of T1 (the spin-lattice relaxation time) or the diffusion coefficient, are dependent on other tissue changes beside temperature change, actual tissue temperature quantification was not feasible over the temperature range used for FUS thermal ablation (Young *et al.*, 1994; Hynynen *et al.*, 1996d). Fortunately, new MRI thermometry methods that allow temperature elevations to be quantified during short ultrasound exposures were developed, after the initial deployment of MRI guided FUS.

To date, the most promising results for temperature monitoring with MRI have been obtained by exploiting the temperature sensitivity of the water proton resonance frequency (PRF) shift (Hindman, 1966). Changes in the PRF are linearly related to temperature and can be mapped rapidly with standard MR imaging sequences, using changes in phase images (Cline *et al.*, 1996; Chung *et al.*, 1996a; Cline *et al.*, 1995a). The major disadvantages of the frequency shift technique, however, are its insensitivity to temperature changes in fat (Kuroda *et al.*, 1995) and its motion sensitivity due to the need for image subtractions (Ishihara *et al.*, 1995). Based on *ex vivo* (Kuroda *et al.*, 1995; Peters *et al.*, 1998) and *in vivo* (Kuroda *et al.*, 1998) studies with different soft tissues, it has been shown that the temperature sensitivity of the water PRF is mostly insensitive to tissue type and to temperature-induced changes to the tissue (*i.e.*, coagulation). The temperature-time history can therefore be used to estimate the biological effect or thermal dose induced by FUS exposure (Chung *et al.*, 1996b; Chung *et al.*, 1999). The thermal dose is a nonlinear function of the temperature and time that converts an arbitrary temperature trajectory to an equivalent exposure at 43°C (Sapareto and Dewey, 1984). These studies have demonstrated that the temperature sensitive MRI sequences can be used to detect small temperature elevations to localize the focal spot at levels that do not induce any observable tissue damage (Hynynen *et al.*, 1997) (Fig. 1). Thus, the targeting can be verified *prior* to inducing irreversible changes. Temperature sensitive sequences allow estimates of the achieved focal temperature, which, in turn, assure the target volume is adequately covered and

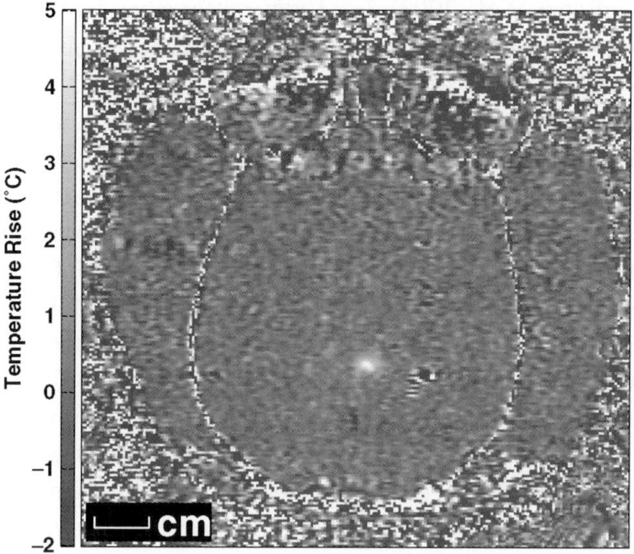

Fig. 1. A MRI thermometry image in the focal plane of a low power test sonication in the brain of a rhesus monkey *in vivo* demonstrating the visibility of the focal spot location at sub-threshold power levels (McDannold *et al.*, 2003). The peak temperature rise in this case was about 5°C during a 10 s sonication.

the critical structures are spared. Numerous studies have recently shown that MRI-based temperature or thermal dose predictions correlate well with both the onset and the spatial extent of the resulting thermal damage (McDannold *et al.*, 1998; McDannold *et al.*, 1999; McDannold *et al.*, 2000; Hazle *et al.*, 2002). It has also been shown that tissue swelling can distort the temperature maps if the heating times are longer than $\sim$1 min, so caution must be exercised when long exposure times are used (McDannold *et al.*, 2001).

Finally, tissue changes induced by the sonications can be detected with MRI. Signal intensities in T1 and T2 (spin-spin relaxation time)-weighted images are affected by thermal tissue damage and by the accompanying reactive response. Similarly, areas with coagulated capillaries, induced by thermal ablation, can be detected by a lack of contrast agent uptake (Hynynen *et al.*, 1994; Tempany *et al.*, 2003). However, in some cases, it is difficult to distinguish changes due to thermal ablation from other pathologies, such as tumors (Hynynen *et al.*, 1993a). Recent work has suggested that these might be distinguished using dynamic contrast uptake curves (Gianfelice *et al.*, 2003). For further references for the MRI aspects of monitoring thermal ablations see reviews by McDannold (McDannold 2005) or Quesson *et al.* (2000).

The ability to quantify the temperature rise and accumulated thermal dose during thermal ablation allows for online feedback control. In most cases, this control has been performed with human feedback, *i.e.*, the operator either controls the power level while watching the progression of the temperature or thermal dose isocontour; or in the case of focused ultrasound exposures, the isocontours are observed after each sonication, and the power, focal pattern, and position are modified until the target volume achieves full coverage.

In simulations (Hutchinson *et al.*, 1998) and in animal models, the feasibility of employing fully automated closed-loop feedback control during thermal therapy has been established. In this method, the power and sometimes the spatial distribution of the heat source is automatically controlled based on the MRI-based temperature measurements. This was first demonstrated using simple methods, such as PID (Proportional Integral and Derivative) controllers, that force the temperature at a single point to follow a predetermined trajectory during long-duration heating with ultrasound (Vimeux *et al.*, 1999; Smith *et al.*, 2001) — an approach similar to what was done earlier with invasive temperature measurements (Lin *et al.*, 1990). Advances in this method, where a physical model of the energy deposition and thermal conduction were taken into account, were next reported (Salomir *et al.*, 2000). Others have suggested methods for automatic control during short-duration focused ultrasound exposures (Vanne and Hynynen, 2003). Automatic feedback has also been shown to be effective in controlling interstitial laser ablation (McNichols *et al.*, 2004a), and in controling hyperthermia with a microwave phased array (Behnia *et al.*, 2002; Kowalski *et al.*, 2002).

Two-dimensional MR thermometry-based control of ultrasound hyperthermia using phased arrays has also been proposed (Hutchinson *et al.*, 1998). Control over two-dimensional heating patterns produced during heating with a microwave phased array has been demonstrated as well (Behnia *et al.*, 2002; Kowalski *et al.*, 2002). The most advanced example of automatic, two-dimensional control to date has been shown in papers by Salomir *et al.*, Palussiere *et al.*, and Mougenot *et al.*, who used real-time

MRI-based temperature feedback to control both the temperature trajectory and the spatial thermal distribution during long-duration focused ultrasound heating in animal tissues (Salomir *et al.*, 2000; Palussiere *et al.*, 2003a; Mougenot *et al.*, 2004). With this method, the ultrasound transducer is moved in such a way that the focal coordinate travels in a double spiral trajectory. Temperature measurements acquired during the first spiral are used to modify the velocity of the transducer during the second spiral. In this way, uniform heating over the target volume is achieved. This method has worked well in animal tumor experiments where the imaging plane is positioned across the scan plane. However, the authors did not demonstrate how the temperature would be controled in the depth direction — a task that has been historically difficult (Lin *et al.*, 1990). Similarly, the sensitivity of the MRI thermometry to motion may introduce additional challenges for the clinical implementation of any closed loop feedback control method.

3. Clinical MRI-guided Focused Ultrasound Surgery Devices

3.1. *Fixed focus devices*

The first prototype MR-guided ultrasound device for breast tumor surgery was manufactured by General Electric Medical Systems and CRD, in collaboration with researchers from the Brigham and Women's Hospital. The ultrasound fields were generated by a single element, spherically focused transducer mounted in a standard MRI table. Adjusted by a computer-controled positioning device in the x, y, and z directions, the transducer was submerged in a water bath that acted as a coupling medium. In the initial prototype device, the positioning was accomplished with a hydraulic system that was found unreliable in early trials; hence, subsequent versions utilized piezoelectric servo-motors mounted at the end of the scanner table, and later at the end of the positioner (Fig. 2). A workstation, programed to aim the ultrasound beam at a location defined on an MR image, controled the transducer motion (Cline *et al.*, 1995b; Hynynen *et al.*, 1996d). Once this system was in place, temperature-sensitive images could be reconstructed and visualized, effectively yielding temperature measurements at single time points.

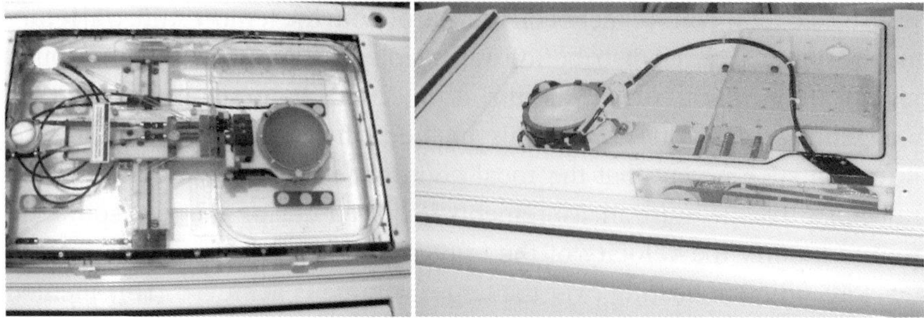

Fig. 2. Two mechanical prototype devices designed to move a focused ultrasound transducer under MRI guidance. The systems were built by General Electric CRD (left), and TxSonics Inc. (currently InSightec Inc.) (right).

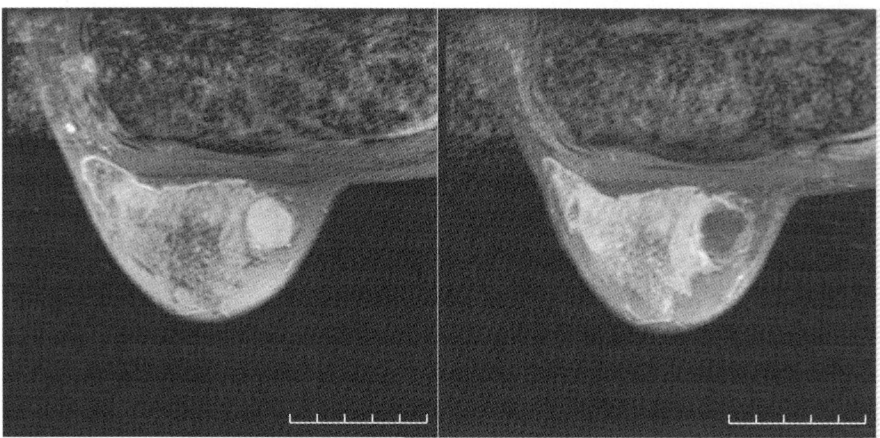

Fig. 3. Breast fibroadenoma treatment (Hynynen *et al.*, 2001b). Left: Contrast enhanced MRI scan before the treatment showing enhancing tumor. Right: The same MRI scan after the treatment showing non-enhancing treated tumor region indicating that the tissue is coagulated and the blood vessels are occluded.

The feasibility of using this method for *in vivo* thermal ablation was demonstrated by treating normal tissues (Hynynen *et al.*, 1996d; Hynynen *et al.*, 1995b) and implanted tumors in rabbits (McDannold *et al.*, 1998; Hazle *et al.*, 2002). Tests of this system in breast fibroadenomas demonstrated the clinical feasibility (Fig. 3). The method was promising in the treatment of breast cancer (Gianfelice *et al.*, 2003a, b; Gianfelice *et al.*, 1999). This result was further supported by a case report involving another clinical prototype utilizing a single transducer, MRI-guided system developed by Siemens and other collaborators from Heidelberg, Germany (Huber *et al.*, 2001).

3.2. *A phased array system for uterine fibroid and breast cancer treatments*

Based on computer simulation (Cain and Umemura, 1986; Ebbini and Cain, 1989; McGough *et al.*, 1992; Wan *et al.*, 1996; Fan and Hynynen, 1995; Fan and Hynynen, 1996b; Fjield *et al.*, 1996a, b; Fan and Hynynen, 1996a; Daum *et al.*, 1998; Daum and Hynynen, 1997; Daum and Hynynen, 1999b; Hutchinson and Hynynen, 1996; Hutchinson *et al.*, 1996; Sun and Hynynen, 1998b; Sun and Hynynen, 1998a) and experimental studies (Hynynen *et al.*, 1996b; Daum *et al.*, 1999; Daum and Hynynen, 1999a; Hutchinson *et al.*, 1995; Hynynen and Jolesz 1998; Clement *et al.*, Clement *et al.*, Hynynen *et al.*, 2004; Lin *et al.*, 1997), ultrasound phased arrays will offer significant advantages over single focused transducers for the thermal ablation of tissues. We have extensively explored the phased array construction methods and have developed multi-channel driving hardware (Buchanan and Hynynen 1994b; Daum *et al.*, 1998) to take advantage of this technology, while monitoring the thermal exposures in MRI. InSightec, Inc. (Haifa, Israel), in collaboration with the investigators at Brigham and Women's Hospital in Boston, have utilized this experience along with information collected from the clinical first generation clinical prototype systems and many simulation and animal studies [*e.g.* (Damianou and Hynynen, 1993; Chung *et al.*, 1999; Damianou *et al.*, 1995; Daum and Hynynen, 1999a; Daum and Hynynen, 1998; Daum and Hynynen 1999b; Fan and Hynynen, 1996a, b; Fjield and Hynynen, 1997; McDannold *et al.*, 1998; McDannold *et al.*, 1999)] to develop a clinical MRI-compatible FUS surgery system (ExAblate2000) (Fig. 4). The main features of the system have been described elsewhere (Hynynen and McDannold, 2004). Briefly, the system focuses ultrasound energy using an ultrasound phased array with approximately 200 elements, a 120-mm diameter, and a 160-mm radius of curvature. The frequency can be chosen by the operator ranging approximately from 0.9 to 1.3 MHz. The array allows the focal depth to be electronically moved between 5 cm and 20 cm

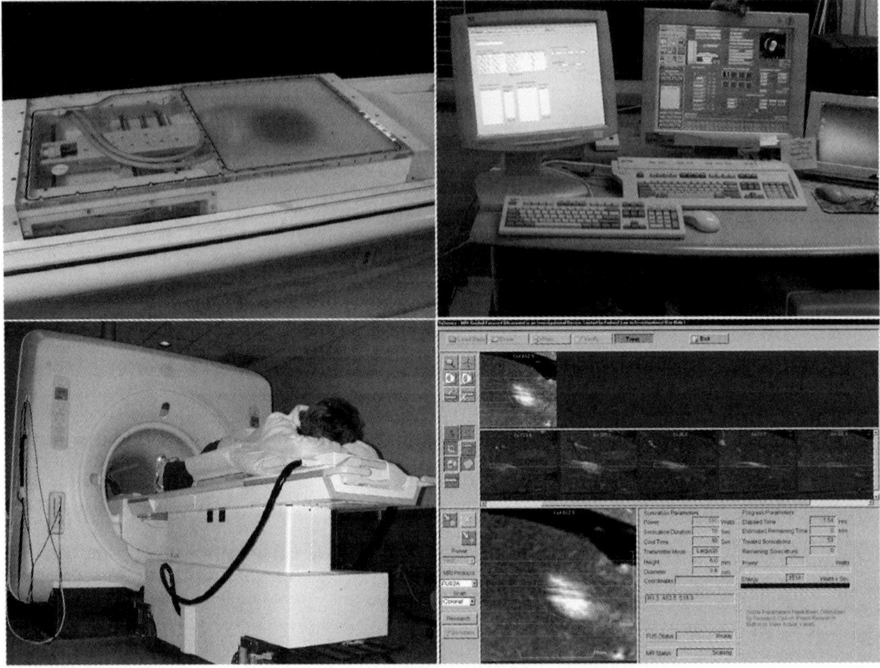

Fig. 4.   Clinical MRI guided focused ultrasound system (Exablate 2000, InSightec, Inc.).

(Fig. 5), and the focal spot size to be controled. The transducer array is mounted in a standard, MR-imaging table in a sealed plastic chamber filled with degassed deionized water. The ultrasound beam propagates up, out of the table through a thin plastic window. For pelvic treatments, the patient lies prone on a gel pad that is placed on top of this window. The transducer is moved and tilted with a computer-controled mechanical positioning device that allows the beam to be targeted based on the MR images obtained at the beginning of and during the treatment session. During the planning, the user interface displays the outline of the beam path to aid the operator in avoiding bone or gas in the field (Hynynen, 1990; Hynynen and DeYoung, 1988) (Fig. 6). The planning software determines the initial value for the power and the pattern of the sonications. These values are used as guides for the initial sonications, after which the operator controls the sonication parameters and the sonication location based on the temperature and thermal dose maps derived from the MRI thermometry and displayed on the

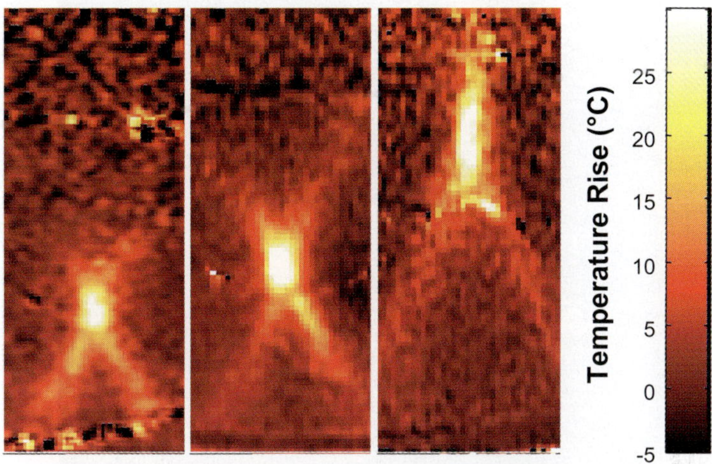

Fig. 5. Three MR thermometry images showing the temperature elevation along the beam path in pig thigh muscle induced *in vivo* by the Exablate 2000. The beam is focused at three different depths using electronic beam steering. The focus is also made wider using electronic phase control of the driving signals of the elements in the phased array (left and in the middle).

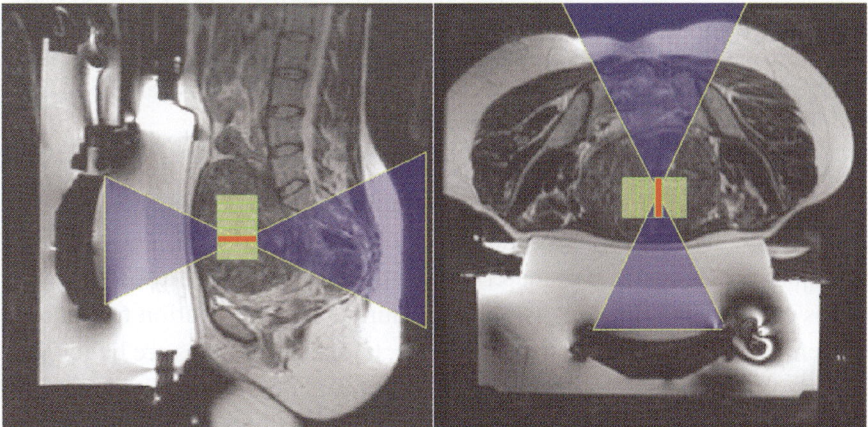

Fig. 6. Treatment planning for a uterine fibroid treatment using the Exablate 2000 system. The treatment consists of sonications at multiple overlapping locations, which are indicated by the boxes. During treatment planning, the location and angle of each spot can be manipulated to ensure that it is safely targeted. The beam path traversed with one sonication is also shown. Displaying the ultrasound beam path during treatment planning ensures that it does not pass through any critical structures.

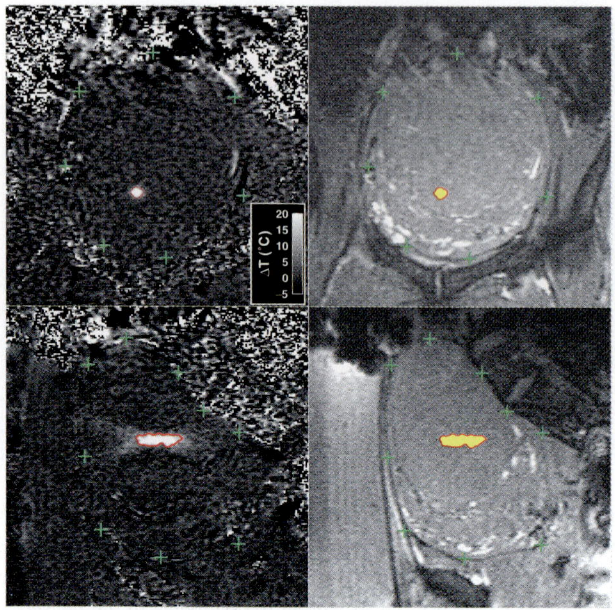

Fig. 7. Temperature images (left) and magnitude images (anatomy) (right) across the focus (top) and along the beam (bottom) obtained during two sonications in a clinical treatment of a uterine fibroid patient with Exablate 2000 system. A time series of these images is acquired during each sonication and are used to ensure that the heating is correctly localized and to estimate online what tissue has reached a lethal thermal dose. Thermal dose contours at 240 equivalent minutes at 43°C are shown for these sonications.

planning images by the system. In addition, feedback from the patients themselves, who are awake and under conscious sedation, is often used to adjust the acoustic parameters if the sonications cause discomfort. A series of temperature maps is obtained during each sonication to evaluate the temperature history. At the same time, temperature maps are being generated, a regular gradient echo image of the anatomy is obtained (Fig. 7). This allows real-time verification of the treatment geometry, ensures that no patient or tumor motion occurs, and that the focal spot is targeted at the desired location.

This system was extensively tested for the treatment of uterine fibroids (Stewart *et al.*, 2003; Tempany *et al.*, 2003; Hindley *et al.*, 2004) and is now FDA-approved for this condition. To our knowledge, this system was the first FDA- approved device that employs the MRI-based thermometry.

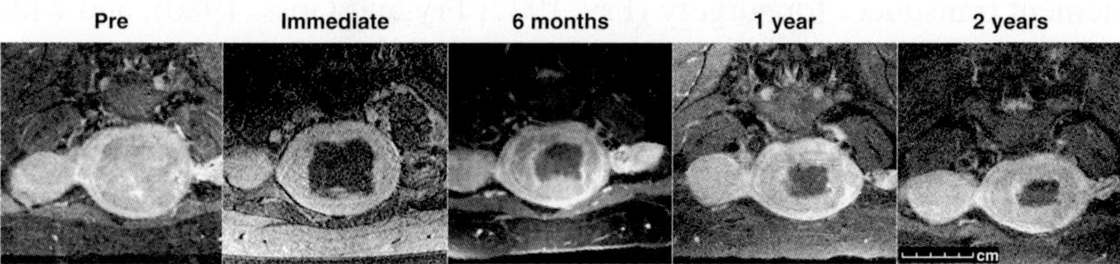

Fig. 8. A uterine fibroid volume before treatment and its shrinkage as a function of time after the ultrasound treatment shown by T1-weighted contrast enhanced MRI. The treated volume does not enhance due to thermal coagulation of the blood vessels and slowly shrinks as a function of time.

A successful treatment results in a coagulated tissue volume that is seen as non-enhancing in the post-treatment, contrast enhanced imaging. The coagulated tissue volume is slowly absorbed by the body, resulting in reduced tumor volume (Fig. 8), and in an improvement in patients' symptoms (Hindley *et al.*, 2004). The system appears promising in the treatment of breast cancer, though it should be noted that the patient population has been small, compared with that of fibroid treatments (Gianfelice *et al.*, 2003a, b).

3.3. *Brain treatments*

Brain tumors are the ideal target for noninvasive surgery since disturbances of overlying or surrounding brain tissue can produce severe complications. For this reason, focused ultrasound was first developed for brain treatments (Lynn and Putnam, 1944; Lynn *et al.*, 1942). However, excessive temperature elevations occur in the skull bone when it is sonicated due to its high ultrasound attenuation and acoustic impedance. Approximately 90% of the propagating beam is lost while propagating through a human skull (Fry and Barger, 1978; Clement and Hynynen, 2002a). Skull also has a high sound speed compared with soft tissue, and has a variable thickness that distorts the wave propagation and destroys the focus of a beam. Thus, early treatments had to be delivered through a craniotomy that made the surgery expensive, and consequently, clinicians were reluctant to adopt the procedure (Fry *et al.*, 1955b; Fry and Fry, 1960; Heimburger, 1985; Guthkelch *et al.*, 1991). Although some experimental attempts were made to deliver ultrasound through an *ex vivo* skull bone with a single element transducer for surgery (Fry, 1977; Fry and Goss, 1980), and with small, one-dimensional arrays for imaging (Smith *et al.*, 1977; Thomas and Fink, 1996) and hyperthermia (Thomas and Fink, 1996), it was commonly believed that noninvasive focused ultrasound brain surgery was not possible until recent demonstrations that have proven otherwise (Hynynen and Jolesz, 1998).

In an effort to overcome the problem of skull heating, we have designed a transducer that maximizes the area of skull through which the beam propagates and converges the energy into a small focal spot. Further cooling can be achieved by actively cooling the scalp. Such area coverage has been achieved by designing and constructing a hemispherical phased array that surrounds the head (Sun and Hynynen, 1998a, b; Clement *et al.*, 2000). We have achieved focusing by using a phased array that compensates for skull-induced distortions, based on either phase corrections determined by a hydrophone probe that must be introduced invasively (Clement and Hynynen, 2002c); or by acoustic simulations of the ultrasound wave that use image-derived information of the skull — a completely noninvasive procedure (Hynynen and Sun, 1998). To mathematically predict the wave propagation through the skull, however, its properties must be accurately known. For this purpose, the speed of sound and ultrasound attenuation as a function of CT-derived bone density were studied (Clement and Hynynen, 2002b) (Fig. 9). Methods utilizing the thickness and density information were developed and were shown to work well with *ex vivo* human skulls (Fig. 10) (Clement and Hynynen, 2002a). The temperature elevations in pig and monkey skulls were also measured to determine the maximum power available for human use (McDannold *et al.*, 2004; Hynynen *et al.*, 2006). This research has resulted in an advanced ultrasound phased array system with 500 phased array elements that may be able to ablate deep tumors in the brain through the intact skull (Clement and Hynynen, 2002a) (Fig. 11). InSightec, Inc. has recently developed a clinical prototype with these capabilities, currently undergoing clinical testing at our institution (Hynynen *et al.*, 2004).

Parallel efforts using time-reversal modeling methods (Aubry *et al.*, 2003) or invasive hydrophone based corrections (Aubry *et al.*, 2001) have been explored by others, demonstrating the ability to focus through animal and human skulls. These methods have been based, thus far, on ultrasound imaging guidance, without real time temperature monitoring.

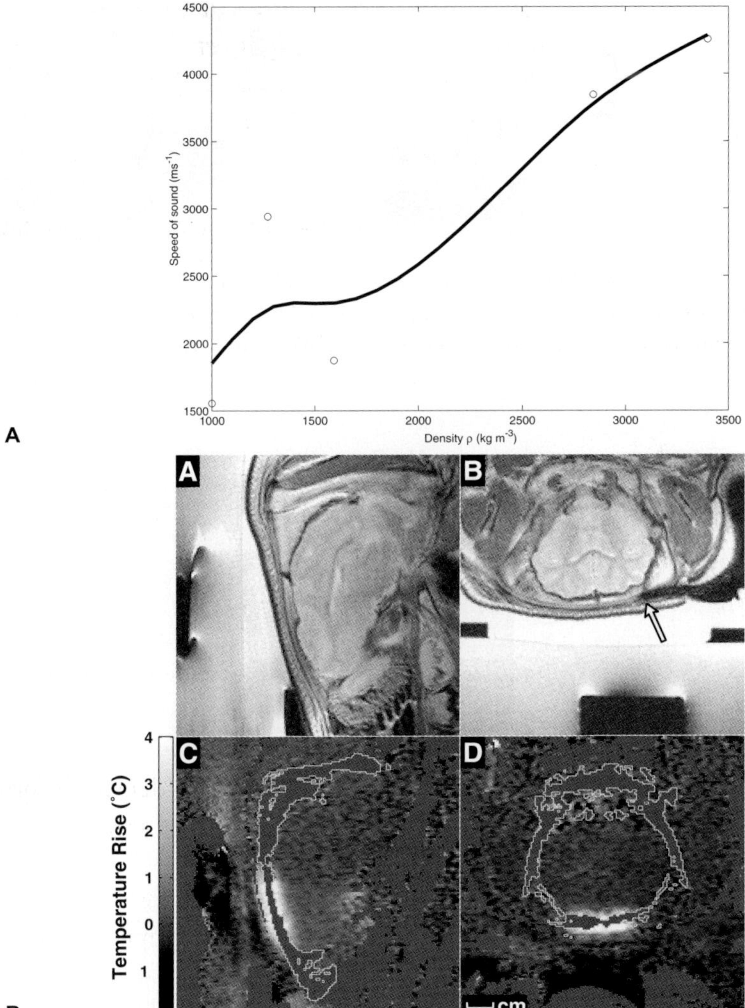

Fig. 9. A: Speed of sound as a function of the bone density as determined by CT scans (Connor *et al.*, 2002); B: Ultrasound induced skull heating as shown by MRI thermometry around a pig skull *in vivo* (bottom). The anatomy is shown in the T2 weighted images on the top (McDannold *et al.*, 2004). The arrow shows the location of an invasive thermocouple probe on the bone surface that was used to verify the MRI thermometry.

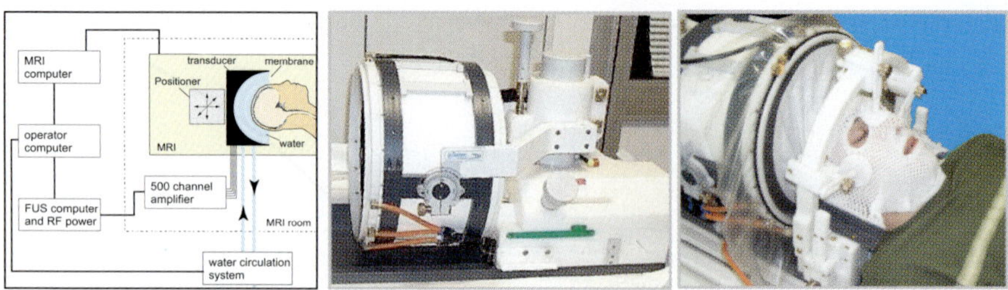

Fig. 10. A prototype clinical phased array system designed for MRI guided transcranial brain surgery. Left a diagram of the complete system. Middle a picture of the hemispherical array. Right the patient immobilization system shown with a volunteer (Hynynen *et al.*, 2004).

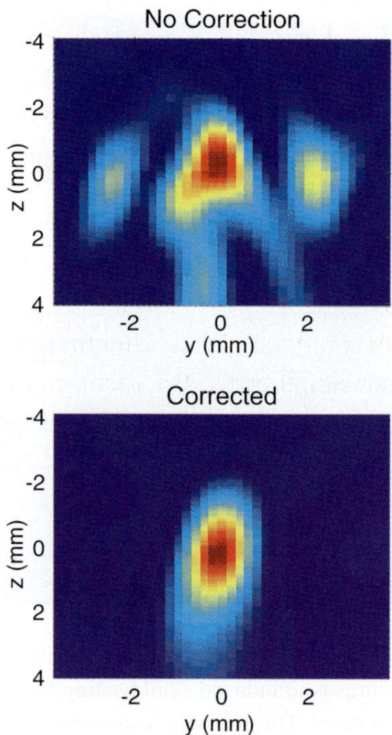

Fig. 11. The ultrasound field distribution of a hemispherical 500 element array (320 elements used) at the focus after the field has propagated through an *ex vivo* human skull. The top figure shows the distortion induced by the skull; the bottom figure shows the focal pattern when the bone induced distortion is compensated for based on an algorithm that derives the bone thickness and density from an CT scan (Clement and Hynynen, 2002a).

4. Pre-clinical Research of MRI-guided Interventions

4.1. *Intracavitary applicators*

4.1.1. *Prostate treatments*

For the past several years, our group has been developing MRI-compatible, intracavitary ultrasound phased array applicators for the treatment of prostate tumors. This research has been driven by earlier array development for hyperthermia treatments (Diederich and Hynynen, 1989; Diederich and Hynynen, 1990; Diederich and Hynynen, 1991; Buchanan and Hynynen, 1994a; Fosmire *et al.*, 1993; Smith *et al.*, 1998), and then by clinical success with single focused transducers (Sanghvi *et al.*, 1996; Chapelon *et al.*, 1999; Chaussy and Thuroff, 2003; Uchida *et al.*, 2002). All of the current clinical treatments using intracavitary ultrasound applicators have been performed under diagnostic ultrasound guidance, without monitoring of the thermal exposure. We have further applied our intracavitary phased array technology to potential applications in MRI-guided prostate surgery. Based on aperiodic design simulations and the empirical width-to-thickness correlation with element efficiency, a 62-element phased array was constructed in an intracavitary applicator (Fig. 12.), effectively making it suitable for transrectal use (Hutchinson *et al.*, 1996; Hutchinson and Hynynen, 1998). Utilizing this one-dimensional array, the focus can be moved only in one plane; at the same time, an ultrasound motor enables control of the focus in the 3D by rotating the array, and thus the focusing plane (Sokka and Hynynen, 2000).

Imasonic, Inc. (Besancon, France), has recently produced for us a linear phased array with slight focusing in the elevation direction. This array, designed by our group, has 128 elements and a half-wavelength, center-to-center spacing that allows full electronic control of the focal spot location. The array was measured to generate a spatial average intensity up to $4\,W/cm^2$ over the array surface. The array has dimensions (width of 25 mm, height approximately 8 mm) similar to those used in the clinical non-focused arrays (Hurwitz *et al.*, 2001), and is thus a good candidate for a prototype clinical prostate applicator for MRI guided surgery.

Promising results with a 1.5 D arrays were recently reported by Seip *et al.* (2005). This approach will allow the beam to be focused in the beam

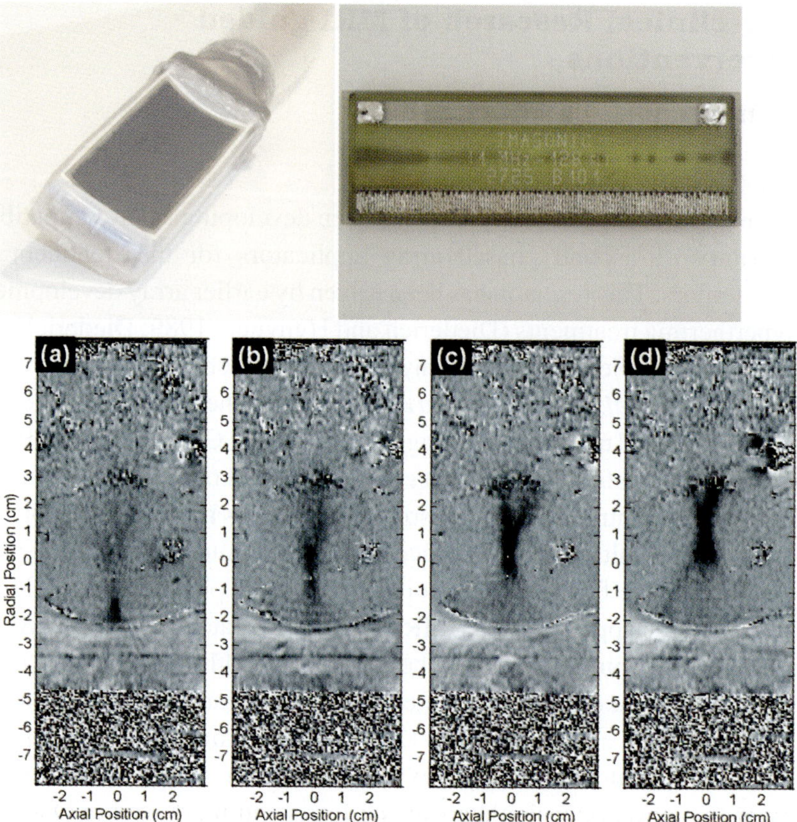

Fig. 12.   A 120 element intracavitary array (in-house assembled) (top, left) and the back side of the piezoelectric transducer head manufactured by Imasonic Inc (top, right). The bottom images show MRI derived temperature maps *in vivo* rabbit muscle tissue along the beam path induced by a 62 element linear array when the focus was electronically steered at different depths (Hutchinson and Hynynen, 1998).

thickness direction. Full 3D electronic control of the focus will require two-dimensional arrays with half-wavelength center-to-center spacing between the transducer elements, resulting in an array with at least 1000 elements. Although arrays with such large numbers of elements have not yet been constructed, current electronics technology could conceivably drive such a system.

4.1.2. *Trans-esophageal focused ultrasound ablation*

RF-catheter ablation of the myocardium has become a treatment of choice for many patients suffering from cardiac arrhythmias, despite the fact that this technique has serious limitations related to the invasiveness of the procedure. All of the access and intracardiac catheter placement-related complications could be eliminated by delivering the energy for tissue heating from a device located outside of the heart. Strickberger *et al.* (1999) have proposed the use of an external ultrasound source for cardiac ablation and have demonstrated the ability to ablate cardiac tissue in open chest experiments, with the eventual goal of using ultrasound targeting through limited access between the ribs. Although this approach will ultimately be the best solution, it will require significant advances in engineering and hardware development. As a result of these challenges, we propose to use focused ultrasound to deliver the energy from the esophagus. Intracavitary ultrasound transducers have been extensively used for the imaging of the heart and a good ultrasound window has already been established. Feasibility of trans-esophageal applicators has also been shown with devices aiming to ablate esophageal cancer (Melodelima *et al.*, 2003; Melodelima *et al.*, 2004). The targeting of the anatomically specific regions can be performed based on online MRI (or diagnostic ultrasound imaging) (Lardo *et al.*, 2000), so there would be no need to insert a catheter to map the conduction pathways in the heart muscle, as is currently done. Our simulation study indicates that such ablation should be possible with a fully two-dimensional array (Yin *et al.*, 2004). We are currently exploring the feasibility of developing such arrays.

4.2. *Utilization of cavitation effects*

Ultrasound can produce both thermal and non-thermal effects in tissue. Thermal effects have several advantages for therapeutic ultrasound, most notably due to the linearity of the temperature rise with the applied acoustic power over the range often used for FUS thermal ablation (Hynynen, 1987) as well as well-established models for predicting when the thermal tissue damage occurs. Thermal ablation with FUS is thus rendered a relatively well-controled procedure that allows straightforward methods for modeling and applying temperature monitoring.

The most potent way to influence tissues by ultrasound is to utilize cavitation, which is the formation and interaction of microbubbles in the ultrasound field. These bubbles strongly interact with the sound field, even at low pressure amplitudes (Coakley, 1971; Lele, 1978; Crum and Fowlkes, 1986; Young, 1989). The severity of these interactions, however, depends on the ultrasound pressure amplitude and frequency, the duration of the sonication, as well as the size and content of the gas bubble, and its location. The ultrasound wave causes the bubbles to contract and expand during compression and rarefaction. The pulsating bubble re-radiates the ultrasound around it, thus removing the energy from the driving wave. It also increases the energy absorption due to viscous and thermal damping mechanisms. Hence, even a small concentration of bubbles can significantly increase the temperature elevation induced by ultrasound (Hynynen, 1991; Lele, 1978; Watmough *et al.*, 1993). The pulsating bubbles cause streaming and shear forces around them. At higher pressure amplitudes, the bubbles collapse due to the incoming momentum of the surrounding fluid (inertial cavitation). This collapse is very violent and is associated with high pressures, temperatures and shear forces (Apfel, 1995; Apfel, 1986; Holland and Apfel, 1990; Young, 1989). Inertial cavitation can be used to completely disintegrate the tissue (Vykhodtseva *et al.*, 1994; Vykhodtseva *et al.*, 1995; Smith and Hynynen, 1998; Tran *et al.*, 2003; Xu *et al.*, 2004). Moreover, the gas bubbles can be introduced or "seeded" via the blood stream or generated by large pressure amplitude sonications in the body.

4.2.1. *Bubble enhanced heating*

Since the first experimental demonstration (Lele, 1978) and the systematic *in vivo* study involving inertial cavitation (Hynynen, 1991), it has been known that enhanced energy absorption and temperature elevation in the tissue is associated with this process. Since this enhancement only happens where cavitation is occurring, the utilization of cavitation could reduce the required time-averaged power needed for thermal ablation, by preferentially depositing the energy in the focal zone. This technique would be especially useful in reducing skull heating during trans-cranial FUS of brain tumors, as discussed in Hynynen and Jolesz (1998). Although cavitation-enhanced heating has most likely been a long-standing part of clinical treatments based on the high intensities reported (Vallancien *et al.*,

1992; Gelet *et al.*, 1996; Wu *et al.*, 2001b), basic theoretical (Chavrier *et al.*, 2000; Holt and Roy, 2001) and experimental (Holt and Roy, 2001; Sokka *et al.*, 2003) studies have only been recently performed, attempting to quantify and optimize it. Our studies have shown that by using a short burst above the cavitation threshold, and then following it with a longer lower power sonication one can achieve a factor of 2–4 gain in the ablated tissue volume, compared with the same temporal average constant power sonication *without* cavitation (Sokka *et al.*, 2003). The tissue damage appeared to be thermal in nature and the tissue damage was predictable by MRI-based thermal dose contours (Fig. 13). This method may offer a way to increase the rate of tissue coagulation, thus allowing larger tumors to be treated.

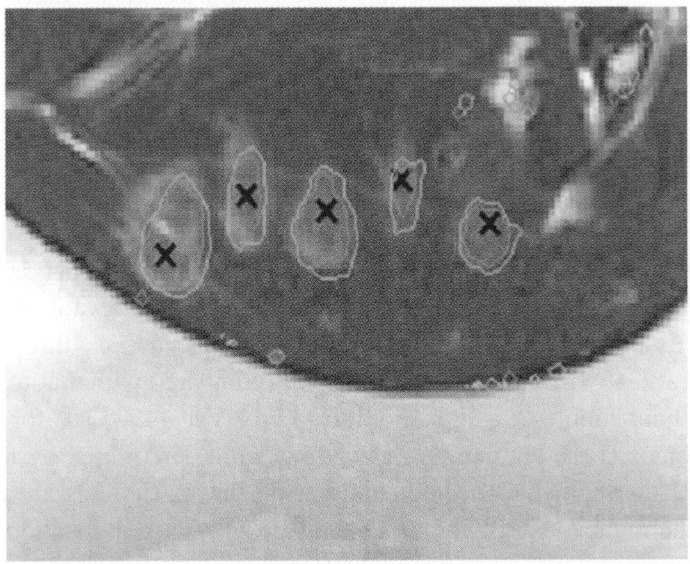

Fig. 13. The thermal lesions shown by a T2-weighted MR image induced in rabbit thigh muscle *in vivo* by five sonications. Each case had the same time-averaged power during the 20 s sonication. Three of these sonications (left, middle, right) consisted of a high power 0.5 s burst followed by a lower power continuous wave exposure. The short burst induced cavitation bubbles that enhanced the ultrasound absorption and increased the lesion size. The other two sonications were performed with constant power. The figure shows the thermal dose contour lines for 30 and 240 equivalent minute exposure at 43°C derived from the MRI thermometry maps (Sokka *et al.*, 2003).

    K. Hynynen & N. McDannold

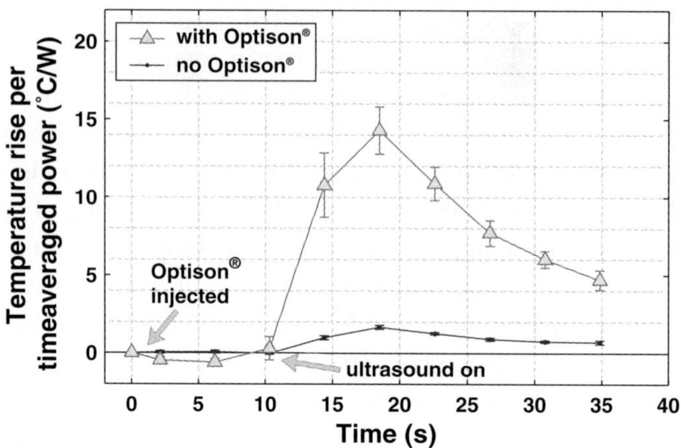

Fig. 14. The temperature elevation/applied acoustic power as a function of time in an *in vivo* rabbit brain sonicated through a craniotomy with a 1.5 MHz focused transducer. The temperature during two different sonications in separate locations are shown with and without intravascular injection of ultrasound contrast agent containing micro-bubbles (Optison®). The presence of the agent greatly enhanced the heating in this case.

Similar temperature gains are expected when ultrasound contrast agents with micro-bubbles are injected in the blood stream during sonication (Simon *et al.*, 1993; Sanghvi *et al.*, 1995). In our studies (McDannold *et al.*, 2006) involving a microbubble-based ultrasound contrast agent (Optison®) in the rabbit brain, we did observe enhanced temperature elevation (Fig. 14), but the tissue damage threshold was much reduced (*i.e.*, threshold for necrosis at ∼43°C for 10–20 s sonications), compared with that of sonications without bubbles (*i.e.*, threshold for necrosis at ∼49–53°C for 10–30 s sonications). These temperature elevations were determined by noninvasive MRI thermometry and indicate that mechanical effects are enhancing the thermal exposure. The tissue damage was noted at locations where the temperature elevation occurred. MRI thermometry-generated isotherms (although at a lower level than without bubbles) were found to be a good predictor of the extent of tissue damage (Fig. 15). This renders MRI thermometry useful in the monitoring and control of this approach. Moreover, because the transducer system does not need to generate such high pressure amplitudes to initiate cavitation, preformed gas bubbles injected into the blood stream offer a considerable advantage over the use of high pressure amplitudes. However, the bubble distribution is dependent on the blood

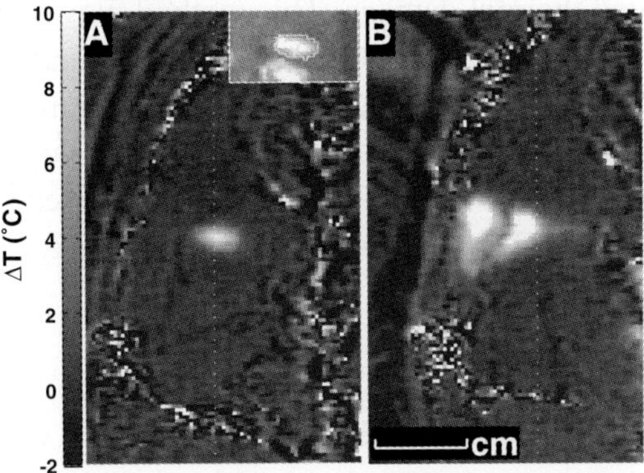

Fig. 15. Two MRI thermometry derived temperature maps along the ultrasound beam during sonications of rabbit brain *in vivo* (bone removed) after an injection of an ultrasound contrast agent (Optison®). Left: low power burst sonication induced a temperature elevation that was localized in the focal zone. The inset shows isotherms drawn from the MRI-based thermometry at 3°C and 4°C, which agree well with imaging of the induced lesion. This low temperature threshold indicates that the lesions were not formed due to heating alone. Right: Higher power continuous wave sonication, which induced heating in front of the focal zone along the ultrasound beam path.

flow and the vasculature, and the necessary contrast agent must still be approved by the FDA. Furthermore, to optimize this sonication strategy and to fully understand its impact upon treatment, more work is needed. In several cases in our study, for example, heating and lesions were produced in the ultrasound beam path away from the focus (Fig. 15).

There are several studies that have utilized two superimposed beams at different frequencies to enhance the cavitation and increase the temperature elevations (Umemura *et al.*, 1996; Umemura *et al.*, 1997; Deng *et al.*, 2000). It may even be possible to reduce the cavitation threshold at the focus and increase it outside the focus, as proposed by Sokka *et al.* (2005). Clearly, to determine the optimal use of cavitation in therapy, additional research is needed. Further study notwithstanding, cavitation offers several extremely promising enhancements over the use of thermal tissue coagulation alone.

4.2.2. *Mechanical destruction of tissue*

There is experimental evidence that high pressure amplitudes associated with strong cavitation can completely disintegrate the exposed tissue without associated thermal damage. This method may be useful in generating holes in the heart for revascularization (Smith and Hynynen, 1998), or for creating a hole through the neonatal atrial septum as a treatment of the hypoplastic left heart syndrome (Xu *et al.*, 2004; Xu *et al.*, 2005). This use of cavitation for removing the tissue has been extensively studied by others (Tran *et al.*, 2003) and offers significant promise.

4.3. *Vascular effects*

Ultrasound can have therapeutically useful interactions with blood vessels. In the following sections, our experience with using ultrasound for vascular interventions will be reviewed.

4.3.1. *Blood vessel occlusion*

Blood vessel occlusion can be effective in controling abdominal, peritoneal, and pelvic hemorrhage, for treating arteriovenous malformations (AVM), and for treating tumors with an identifiable blood supply (Wallance *et al.*, 1981). Such vessel occlusion is usually performed surgically or by using transvascular embolization, radiosurgery or laser induced photothrombosis (Crotty *et al.*, 1993; Watson *et al.*, 1987; Carr *et al.*, 1994). For superficial vascular malformations, the laser technique offers a noninvasive way to occlude the target vessels (Wallance *et al.*, 1976; Wallance *et al.*, 1981), but deep vessels require a transvascular catheter to be positioned within the vessel followed by embolization. For certain small, mostly intracranial AVMs, radiosurgery offers a noninvasive treatment, even though, the delivered radiation dose limits it for a single use and exposes the surrounding tissues to some radiation injury. Therefore, a significant number of patients could benefit from a noninvasive method for vessel occlusion.

Histology studies evaluating ultrasound effects on tissue provided the first evidence that ultrasound can stop blood flow in small blood vessels (for example, Vykhodtseva *et al.*, 1994), and contrast enhanced imaging studies demonstrated that the microcirculation of coagulated tissue volumes was similarly occluded (Hynynen *et al.*, 1994). The first study investigated the feasibility of occluding large blood vessels for treatment purposes and demonstrated that surgically exposed veins can be successfully occluded by ultrasound pulses (Delon-Martin *et al.*, 1995). Following this study, it

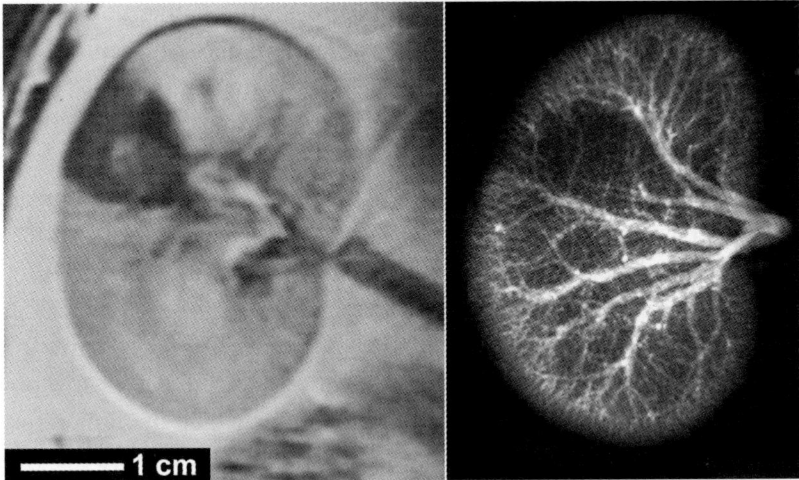

Fig. 16. MRI-guided vessel occlusion *in vivo* in rabbit kidney using focused ultrasound. Left: a contrast enhanced MR image of the kidney after the sonication demonstrating a non-enhancing zone correlating with the area that the targeted artery branch was feeding. Right: a post mortem angiogram of a rabbit kidney showing a sonication induced arterial occlusion.

was shown that temporary constriction of blood vessels can be induced noninvasively by ultrasound exposures deep in the body (Hynynen *et al.*, 1996a; Hynynen *et al.*, 1996c), and that MRI-guided focused ultrasound can be used to occlude relatively large and high flow arteries permanently *in vivo* (Fig. 16). Similar results were obtained later by using ultrasound guidance (Rivens *et al.*, 1999). In addition, ultrasound has been shown to reduce the hemostasis time of punctured large arteries (Vaezy *et al.*, 1998) and to stop bleeding, following liver or spleen incisions (Vaezy *et al.*, 1997; Vaezy *et al.*, 1999b). The results suggest that this hemostatic ability may be useful in controling bleeding during surgery (Vaezy *et al.*, 1999a).

We continued to explore the usefulness of focused ultrasound in occluding large blood vessels by using a rabbit ear model. To investigate the hypothesis that vessel rupture seen in the earlier experiments (Hynynen *et al.*, 1995a) can be eliminated by using higher frequencies (by reducing the resonant size of the bubbles produced during sonication), we sonicated rabbit ear veins and arteries under visual guidance with a sharply focused transducer at 2.02 MHz. The ears having superficial blood vessels allowed us to accurately aim the beam, thereby eliminating uncertainty in the exposure location. In addition, the effects of the intervening tissues were minimized to provide well-controled exposure conditions. A surgical microscope with a video camera aided in aiming the beam, and in visually inspecting the sonication effects. The video signal was recorded for further evaluation. The main artery and vein were targeted in both rabbit ears. Between 1 and 4 locations were sonicated in each vessel at different acoustic power levels between 30 and 210 W for 1s to observe different degrees of tissue damage. This was done in 12 animals.

The 1s sonications caused a varying degree of vessel constriction in both the veins and the arteries. Visual inspection showed that the low power sonications caused a temporary constriction, after which the flow returned slowly. Higher power sonications caused tissue damage around the vessel. Power levels above 117 W caused severe skin damage with little effect on the vessel. In many instances, while the vessel was judged to be occluded based on visual inspection, the X-ray angiograms showed some contrast agent in the lumen of the vessel (Fig. 17). The degree of constriction was power-dependent (Fig. 18). At the highest power reached without causing

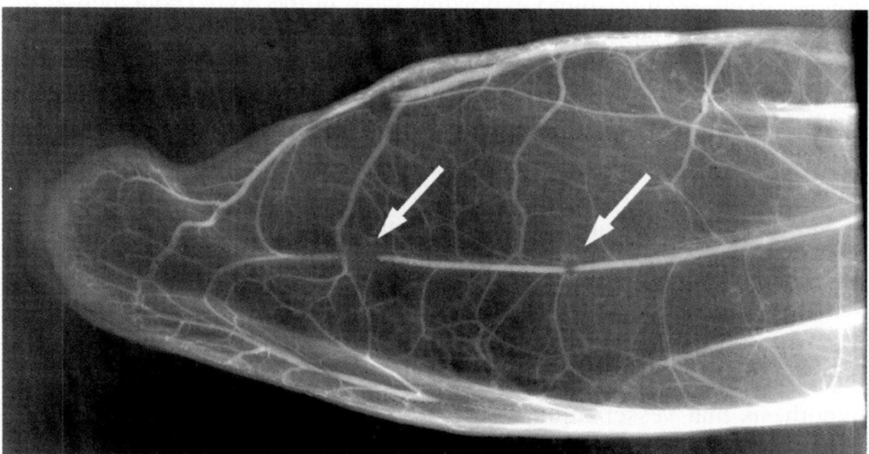

Fig. 17. Post mortem angiography of a rabbit ear after *in vivo* sonication of the central artery and the marginal vein at several locations. The angiogram shows both completed (left arrow) and partial (right arrow) occlusion of the vessels.

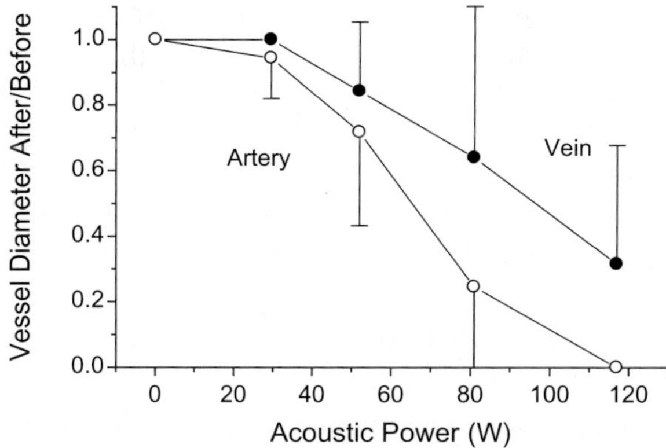

Fig. 18. The normalized vessel diameter vs. applied acoustic power of arteries and veins *in vivo* rabbit ear after 1s sonications at a frequency of 2.02 MHz.

skin damage (117 W), all of the arteries were closed. However, most of the veins remained open, with an average lumen diameter of 30% from the original vessel diameter following sonication.

To determine whether more permanent occlusion could be achieved, the 1s 117 W sonications were followed by a 28 W/10 s sonication, aimed at coagulating the vessel and its surrounding tissue. Only a single sonication was delivered to each artery and vein in both ears. After a 4–6 hr survival, the X-ray angiograms showed complete occlusion in 5/11 arteries. The average lumen diameter of the open vessels was approximately 30% of its original value. The vein sonications produced 5/9 occlusions in the veins and the open vessels had a lumen diameter on average of ∼68% from the initial value. The sonications produced tissue coagulation around the blood vessels and no bleeding was evident in any of the sonications.

These experiments have shown that brief, high power sonications can be used to induce temporary stasis in large arteries and in most veins. This temporary occlusion may be ideal for stabilizing trauma patients, until they can be transported and prepared for surgical interventions. Temporary occlusion also reduces the effects of cooling and allows the tissues around the vessel to coagulate. This, in turn, leads to a permanent occlusion in approximately half of the sonicated vessels. Moreover, we predict, that if longer, low power sonications covering a longer distance of the vessel are successfully delivered, then more vessels may be permanently occluded.

4.3.2. *Thrombolysis*

Several studies over the years have shown that ultrasound can aid in thrombolysis (Rosenschein *et al.*, 1994, Tachibana and Tachibana, 1997; Atar *et al.*, 2001). In particular, several experiments have demonstrated that the effectiveness of thrombolytic agents has increased with the use of intravascular ultrasound devices. A recent study has shown that even exposure to transcranial Doppler imaging, while infusing thrombolytic agents, can result in increased thrombolysis in a clinical setting (Alexandrov *et al.*, 2004).

We have conducted an experimental series investigating the use of high power ultrasound pulses, without any thrombolytic agent in the induction of thrombolysis. The ultrasound fields were generated by single, focused, air backed transducers with 100-mm diameters, 80-mm radius of curvatures and resonant frequencies of 0.68 MHz and 2.0 MHz. In this study, 18 New Zealand white rabbits were anesthetized and the femoral artery and vein were surgically exposed. A stenosis was induced distally by constricting the artery with a silk suture to reduce the flow. A 1 cm segment of the femoral artery was then clamped distally and proximally. Fifty units of bovine thrombi were injected into the artery. The thrombi was dissolved to saline and injected into the vessel. Ten minutes later, the proximal and the distal clamps were released, leaving the vessel occluded by the formed thrombi (Helft *et al.*, 1998). The occluded artery was adjacent to a vein that is also exposed to the ultrasound.

The ultrasound beam was aimed at the occluded segment with the aid of laser pointers that were positioned above the animal. The ultrasound beam propagated through the thigh muscle into the occluded vessel, and then into a layer of acoustic gel (1–2 cm thick) that was placed on the vessel to allow the ultrasound beam to exit the tissue. The sonication was performed by aiming the beam 15 mm upstream from the distal end of the vessel segment. The sonication was performed at that location and then repeated with the interval of 3 mm so that the whole vessel segment was covered. After the sonication, the tissue around the vessel was visually inspected to detect any bleeding or thermal damage. At the conclusion of the sonications, the artery was cut at the distal end of the occluded segment and the blood flow through the vessel was recorded. The animal was sacrificed at the end of the experiment.

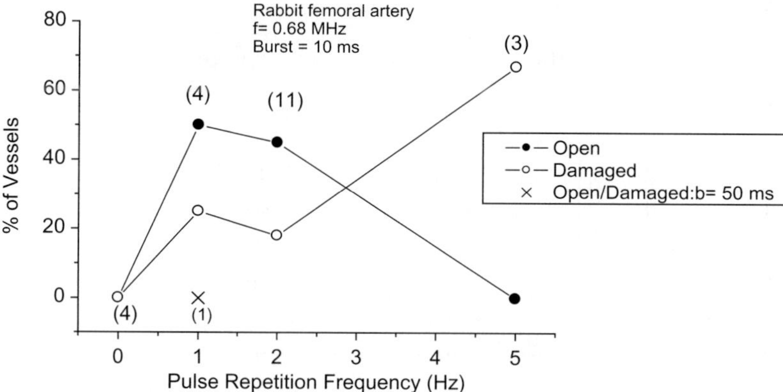

Fig. 19. The percentage of thrombolytic rabbit femoral arteries that were opened or damaged after sonications at a frequency of 0.69 MHz and a burst length of 10 ms as a function of the pulse repletion frequency.

We selected 10 ms sonication bursts at variable pulse repetition frequency. The acoustic power was set at 410 W and the duration of each sonication was 60 s in most of the experiments. Figure 19 plots the percentage of open vessels as a function of the pulse repetition frequency (PRF) of the 60 s sonications and establishes whether vessel damage (bleeding) was induced. It is obvious from the graph that at a frequency of 0.8 MHz, the exposures that caused thrombolysis were overlapping with those that caused the vessel damage. From this we conclude that the cavitation event associated with this frequency is too violent for these small vessels of ∼1 mm in diameter; better results may be obtained by using a higher frequency. The next set of experiments was performed with a frequency of 2 MHz, and in preliminary experiments, the sonication parameters were designated at 270 W acoustic power and a PRF of 1 Hz. From those experiments, it appeared that the vessels could be opened only by 60 s sonications. We also found that no major vessel damage was observed with these sonications. At the PRF of 2 Hz, the vessel was open at 60 s, but these sonications, by contrast, caused tissue damage around the vessel. Finally, the PRF 1 Hz and 60 s sonications were repeated at different power levels. The results, depicted in Fig. 20, demonstrate that the vessels could be opened at power levels as low as about 47 W; further, sonications as high as 270 W did not produce vessel damage. Moreover, these results show that pulsed focused ultrasound has

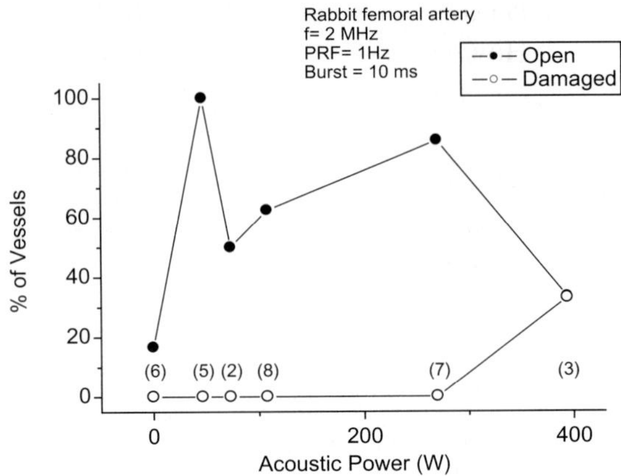

Fig. 20.   The percentage of thrombolytic rabbit femoral arteries that were open or damaged after sonications at a frequency of 2.02 MHz, a burst length of 10 ms, and a repetition frequency of 1 Hz as a function of the applied acoustic power.

definite potential in thrombolysis. However, much more work is needed before this technique can be clinically utilized.

4.3.3. *Blood-brain barrier disruption*

Advances in neuroscience have resulted in the development of new therapeutic and diagnostic agents and genes that may be used to study and treat many central nervous system (CNS) diseases (Pardridge, 2002). However, the use of many potent agents is often limited by their access to the CNS via the blood supply, because the blood-brain barrier (BBB) protects the brain from foreign molecules (Abbott and Romero, 1996; Kroll and Neuwelt, 1998; Pardridge, 2002; Nag, 2003). In addition to a physiological barrier at the level of basal lamina (Muldoon *et al.*, 1999), the BBB is formed by the endothelial cells of the cerebral vessels that connect to each other by intracellular attachments known as "tight junctions" (Abbott and Romero, 1996; Kroll and Neuwelt, 1998). The BBB prevents penetration of ionized, water-soluble drugs, with molecular weights greater than 180 (Kroll and Neuwelt, 1998). By chemically modifying these drugs to make them lipophilic, or by deploying other carriers such as amino acid and peptide carriers, propagation through the barrier might be achieved. Another option is to diffusely alter the function of BBB by temporarily opening the tight junctions, which is now possible with an increasing number of chemicals (Doolittle *et al.*). However, such osmotic method requires an invasive, intra-arterial catheterization that will produce diffuse, non-focal, transient BBB opening within the entire tissue volume supplied by the injected artery branch (Abbott and Romero, 1996; Kroll and Neuwelt, 1998).

A more local and less invasive method for the opening of the BBB for drug delivery would allow the BBB to aid in targeted therapy in the following manner: Agents delivered into the brain via the blood stream are often limited by having a desired therapeutic effect in one brain location, but an undesired, often dose-limiting effect elsewhere in the CNS. However, these substances could have significant therapeutic benefit if their delivery in the brain could be localized. One way to provide selective targeting would be to utilize the BBB itself to prevent the penetration of the agent into undesired locations, while opening the barrier locally at the desired target site.

Focused ultrasound has been proposed for BBB disruption for chemotherapy by Patrick *et al.* (Patrick *et al.*, 1990), based on the observation that ultrasound induced thermal lesions are surrounded by a rim of brain tissue with a compromised BBB. However, in all cases within this study, the BBB opening was associated with tissue destruction. Several investigators have explored the potential of ultrasound to open the BBB; firstly, by using cavitation effects (Vykhodtseva *et al.*, 1995; Mourad, 2001), and secondly, by inducing thermal exposures around focal lesions (Patrick *et al.*, 1990; Hynynen *et al.*, 1997) or near the threshold for damage in the brain under MRI thermometry guidance (Hynynen *et al.*, 1997, Vykhodtseva *et al.*, Vykhodtseva *et al.*, 2001). None of these methods, however, has allowed us to disrupt the BBB predictably without irreversible damage. The main challenge in using ultrasound exposures to open the BBB is in ensuring that the targeted energy delivery is localized only at the blood vessel walls *without* damaging the adjacent neural elements. We have developed a hypothesis that the BBB can be opened reproducibly by localizing the cavitation-generated mechanical stresses to the blood vessel walls, by injecting gas bubbles into the blood stream just prior to sonication. The use of gas bubbles assures a reproducible bubble size population in the sonicated tissue volume. Since the bubbles are intravascular, any adverse effects to the adjoining brain tissue should be minimal.

Our recent studies (Hynynen *et al.*, 2001a; Sheikov *et al.*, 2004) demonstrated this approach *in vivo* by injecting a gas bubble-based ultrasound contrast agent (Optison®, GE Healthcare) into the blood stream followed by low power ultrasound pulses. Focal BBB opening was detected by using MRI contrast agents (Figs. 21 and 22). The corresponding histology study showed that at the lowest power levels used, the sonications did not cause neuronal damage to the brain. In addition, the opening was reversible and was completely healed at the 6 hr following the sonications, with no observable, long-term effects (Hynynen *et al.*, 2005). Furthermore, the power levels used were orders of magnitude lower than that required for generating tissue ablation or the cavitation threshold. The threshold for the opening was found to be frequency-dependent (Fig. 23). Transmission electron microscopy investigation has shown the passage of large molecular tracers (horseradish peroxidase, molecular weight: 40,000, and immunoglobulin) and the apparent activation of transcellular passage, as well as tight junction opening (Fig. 24). Initial experiments have demonstrated that this method can be used to selectively enhance the delivery of doxyrubicin in the targeted brain tissue (Treat *et al.*, 2004).

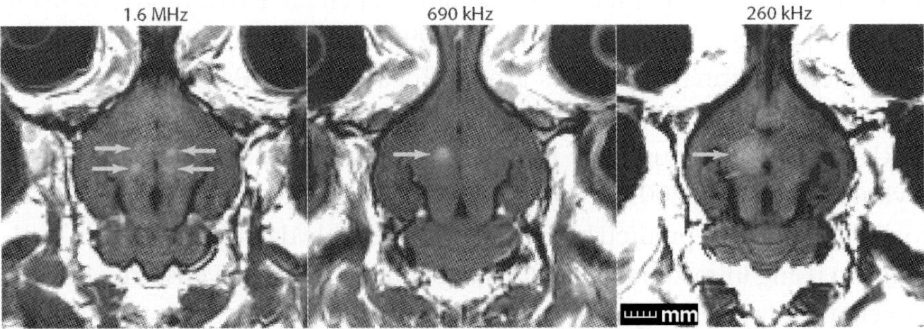

Fig. 21. Focal opening of the blood-brain barrier in the rabbit after sonication as demonstrated by T1-weighted contrast enhanced MR images. The scans were performed across the focal plane of the ultrasound beam, and the BBB disruption is demonstrated as a localized increase in the MR signal after the contrast injection. Examples of the BBB disruption with three different frequencies are shown. The 1.63 MHz sonications were performed in four spots of the brain. The lower frequency sonications were performed only in one location due to the increased exposure volume. As the frequency decreases, the focal size increases and the ability to focus through the skull bone is facilitated.

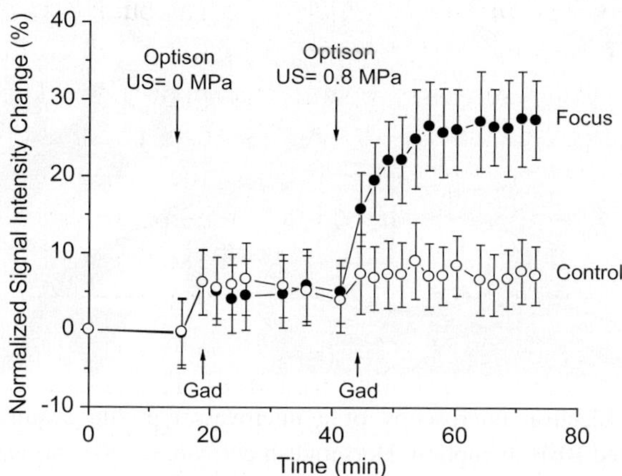

Fig. 22. The signal intensity measured inT1-weighted images due to contrast enhancement in the focal location together with the signal intensity of the same non-sonicated anatomical location in the contralateral hemisphere of a rabbit brain as a function of time (frequency 0.69 MHz) (Hynynen *et al.*, 2005). The time points of ultrasound and MRI contrast injections and the sonication are given.

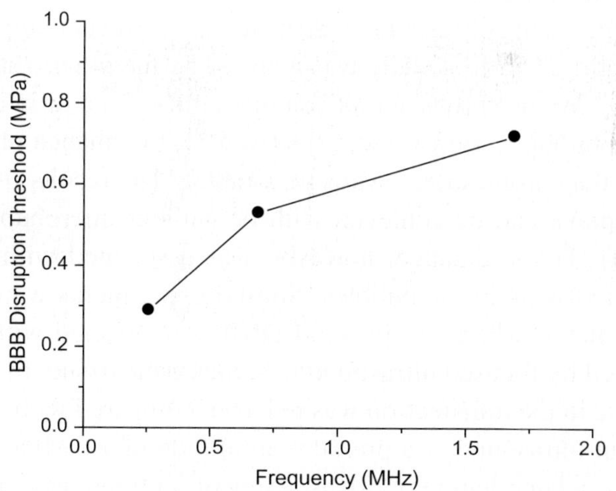

Fig. 23. The estimation of the threshold for BBB disruption vs. the ultrasound frequency in rabbit brain *in vivo*.

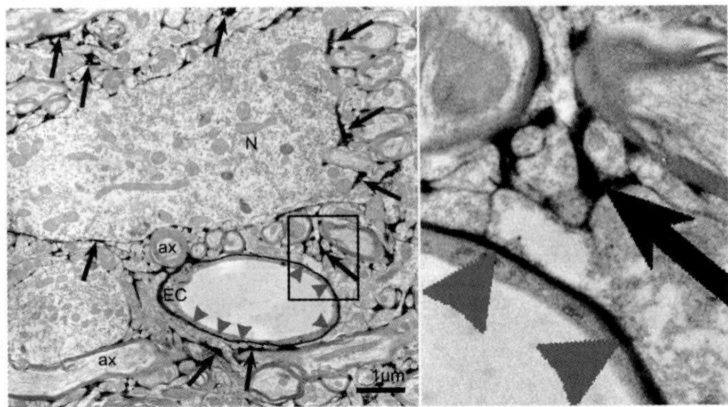

Fig. 24. Left: Electron microscopy of a microvessel profile acquired 60 min after ultrasound-induced BBB disruption. Horseradish peroxidase (40 kDa) has penetrated outside the endothelium, in the basement membrane, which appears heavily infiltrated (arrowheads), and is evident everywhere in the interstitial spaces of neuropil (the dark zones, some of which are pointed with arrows). N — cytoplasm of an adjacent neuron; ax - cross and longitudinal sections of myelinated axons.

4.4. *Gene therapy*

Ultrasound has been explored extensively for enhancing gene therapy, as reported in the other chapters of this book. We will only summarize our *in vivo* experience using ultrasound, with a view toward eventually using MRI-guided targeting. Our first study was inspired by the *in vitro* study by Kim *et al.*, (1996). We used focused ultrasound, either alone or in combination with a microbubble contrast agent (Optison®), to enhance plasmid DNA uptake into the carotid artery walls of a rabbit. The results indicated that enhanced uptake can be achieved with or without microbubbles (Huber *et al.*, 2003). Tissue damage, however, was associated with the sonications delivered without the bubbles. Similar experiments were performed in the pig's heart, where the plasmid DNA was injected with microbubbles, followed by focused ultrasound to sonicate the tissue. In this case, an 88% increase in the transfection was reached, compared with control locations without ultrasound at a pressure amplitude of 1.6 MPa, a frequency of 0.89 MHz, a burst length of 50 ms, a repetition frequency of 1 Hz, and a sonication duration of 60 s (Silcox, 2004). This work supports by the earlier and parallel studies (Bednarski *et al.*, 1997; Bednarski *et al.*, 1998) that have shown the potential of MRI guided targeting for gene therapy.

We have also investigated the feasibility of utilizing a heat shock protein promoter to induce heat-activated gene therapy in a canine model (Silcox *et al.*, 2005). In these experiments, the prostate in three dogs was injected with recombinant adenoviral vector, with a human hsp70B promoter and firefly luciferase. Two days after the injection, MRI monitored temperature exposures were produced using an unfocused, transrectal ultrasound applicator (Smith *et al.*, 1998). The results suggest that the thermal exposure was able to activate the gene therapy and that the exposures can be monitored and targeted using MR imaging and thermometry. Although these experiments are very preliminary, they demonstrate that MRI-guided ultrasound heating can be used to target gene therapy. Earlier and more extensive MRI-guided ultrasound temperature activated gene therapy work has been conducted by Moonen *et al.* (Guilhon *et al.*, 2003; Moonen *et al.*, 1997).

5. Conclusions

MRI guidance and monitoring allows accurate targeting of the FUS beam deep into the tissue. The ability to monitor the thermal exposure provides online information to control the exposure. This method is already FDA-approved for the thermal coagulation of the uterine fibroids, and offers promise for the treatment of other solid tumors. It may also provide a non-invasive method for deep brain tumor surgery, functional disorders, and vascular malformations. Ultrasound exposures can be controled to achieve a wide variety of potentially therapeutic effects beyond thermal coagulation. These include targeted blood-brain barrier disruption, thrombolysis, vascular occlusions, etc. All of these interventions will benefit from MRI targeting, at least initially, when the methods are clinically tested. If methods are ultimately developed that will reliably quantify temperature elevations using ultrasound imaging, most of the work done using MRI can then be directly transferred.

References

Abbott NJ, Romero IA. Transporting therapeutics across the blood-brain barrier. *Mol Med Today* (1996) **2**: 106–113.

Alexandrov AV, Molina CA, Grotta JC, Garami Z, Ford SR, J. Alvarez-Sabin, Montaner J, Saqqur M, Demchuk AM, Moye LA, Hill MD, Wojner AW.

Ultrasound-enhanced systemic thrombolysis for acute ischemic stroke. *N Engl J Med* (2004) **351**: 2170–2178.

Apfel RE. Possibility of microcavitation from diagnostic ultrasound. *IEEE Trans Ultrason Ferroelectr Freq Contr UFFC* (1986) **33**: 139–142.

Apfel RE. Acoustic cavitation: A possible consequence of biomedical use of ultrasound. *Br J Cancer* (Suppl)**V**: 140–146 (1995).

Atar S, Luo H, Birnbaum Y, Hansmann D, Siegel RJ. The use of transducer-tipped ultrasound catheter for recanalization of thrombotic arterial occlusions. *Echocardiography* (2001) **18**: 233–237.

Aubry JF, Tanter M, Gerber J, Thomas JL, Fink M. Optimal focusing by spatio-temporal inverse filter. II. Experiments. Application to focusing through absorbing and reverberating media. *J Acoust Soc Am* (2001) **110**: 48–58.

Aubry JF, Tanter M, Pernot M, Thomas JL, Fink M. Experimental demonstration of noninvasive transskull adaptive focusing based on prior computed tomography scans. *J Acoust Soc Am* (2003) **113**: 84–93.

Bednarski MD, Lee JW, Callstrom MR, King CP. *In vivo* target-spesific delivery of macromolecular agents with MR-guided focused ultrasound. *Radiology* (1997) **204**: 263–268.

Bednarski MD, Lee JW, Yuh EL, Li KCP. *In vivo* target-spesific delivery of genetic materials with MR-guided focused ultrasound. *Ultrasonics* (1998) **30**: 325–330.

Behnia B, Suthar M, Webb AG. Closed-loop feedback control of phsed-array microwave heating using thermal measurements from magnetic resonance imaging. *Con Magnetic Reson* (2002) **15**: 101–110.

Billard BE, Hynynen K, Roemer RB. Effects of physical parameters on high temperature ultrasound hyperthermia. *Ultrasound Med Biol* (1990) **16**: 409–420.

Buchanan MT, Hynynen K. Design and experimental evaluation of an intracavitary ultrasound phased array system for hyperthermia. *IEEE Trans Biomed Eng* (1994) **41**: 1178–1187.

Burov AK. High intensity ultrasonic oscillations for the treatment of malignant tumors in animal and man. *Dokl Akad Nauk SSSR* (1956) **106**: 239–241.

Burov AK, Adreevskaya G. The effect of ultra-acoustic oscillation of high intensity on malignant tumors in animals and man. *Dokl Akad Nauk SSSR* (1956) **106**: 445–448.

Cain CA. Umemura SA. Concentric-ring and sector vortex phased array applicators for ultrasound hyperthermia therapy. *IEEE Trans Microwave Theory Tech MTT* (1986) **34**: 542–551.

Carr MM, Mahoney JL, Bowen CVA. Extremity arteriovenous malformations: Review of a series. *CJS* (1994) **37**: 293–299.

Chapelon JY, Ribault M, Vernier F, Souchon R, Gelet A. Treatment of localised prostate cancer with transrectal high intensity focused ultrasound. *Eur J Ultrasound* (1999) **9**: 31–38.

Chaussy C, Thuroff S. The status of high-intensity focused ultrasound in the treatment of localized prostate cancer and the impact of a combined resection. *Curr Urol Rep* (2003) **4**: 248–252.

Chavrier F, Chapelon JY, Gelet A, Cathignol D. Modeling of high-intensity focused ultrasound-induced lesions in the presence of cavitation bubbles. *J Acoust Soc Am* (2000) **108**: 432–440.

Chen L, Bouley D, Yuh E, D'Arceuil H and Butts K. Study of focused ultrasound tissue damage using MRI and histology. *J Magn Reson Imaging* (1999) **10**: 146–153.

Chung A, Hynynen K, Cline HE, Jolesz FA. Quantification of thermal exposure using proton resonance frequency shift. *Proc SMR 4th Meeting* (1996a) 1751.

Chung A, Hynynen K, Cline HE, Colucci V, Oshio K, Jolesz F. Optimization of spoiled gradient-echo phase imaging for *in vivo* localization of focused ultrasound beam. *Magn Reson Med* (1996b) **36**: 745–752.

Chung A, Jolesz FA, Hynynen K. Thermal dosimetry of a focused ultrasound beam *in vivo* by MRI. *Med Phys* (1999) **26**: 2017–2026.

Clement GT, Sun J, Giesecke T, Hynynen K. A hemisphere array for non-invasive ultrasound brain therapy and surgery. *Phys Med Biol* (2000) **45**: 3707–3719.

Clement GT, White J, Hynynen K. Investigation of a large-area phased array for focused ultrasound surgery through the skull. *Phys Med Biol* (2000) Apr; **45**(4): 1071–1083.

Clement GT, Hynynen K. A non-invasive method for focusing ultrasound through the human skull. *Phys Med Biol* (2002a) **47**: 1219–1236.

Clement GT, Hynynen K. Correlation of ultrasound phase with physical skull properties. *Ultrasound Med Biol* (2002b) **28**: 617–624.

Clement GT, Hynynen K. Micro-receiver guided transcranial beam steering. *IEEE Trans Ultrason Ferroelectr Freq Control* (2002c) **49**: 447–453.

Cline HE, Hynynen K, Schneider E, Hardy CJ, Maier SE, Watkins RD, Jolesz FA. (1995) Simultaneous magnetic resonance phase and magnitude temperature maps in muscle. *Proc SMR* 3rd Meeting, 1174.

Cline HE, Hynynen K, Schneider E, Hardy CJ, Maier SE, Watkins RD, Jolesz FA. Simultaneous magnetic resonance phase and magnitude temperature maps in muscle. *Magn Reson Med* (1996) **35**: 309–315.

Cline HE, K. Hynynen, Watkins RD, Adams WJ, Schenck JF, Ettinger RH, Freund WR, Vetro JP, Jolesz FA. A focused ultrasound system for MRI guided ablation. *Radiology* (1995) **194**: 731–737.

Cline HE, Schenck JF, Watkins RD, Hynynen K, Jolesz FA. Magnetic resonance guided thermal surgery. *Magn Reson Med* (1993) **31**: 628–636.

Coakley A. Acoustical detection of single cavitation events in a focussed field in water at 1 MHz. *J Acoust Soc Am* (1971) **49**: 792–801.

Coleman DJ, Lizzi FL, Driller J, Rosado AL, Chang S, Iwamoto T, Rosenthal D. Therapeutic ultrasound in the treatment of glaucoma. *Ophthalmology* (1985) **92**: 339–346.

Connor CW, Clement GT, Hynynen K. A unified model for the speed of sound in cranial bone based on genetic algorithm optimization. *Phys Med Biol* (2002) **47**: 3925–3944.

Crotty KL, Orihuela E, Warren MM. Recent advances in the diagnosis and treatment of renal arteriovenous malformations and fistulas. *J Urology* (1993) **150**: 1355–1359.

Crum LA, Fowlkes JB. Acoustic cavitation generated by microsecond pulses of ultrasound. *Nature* (1986) **319**: 52–54.

Damianou C, Hynynen K. Focal spacing and near-field heating during pulsed high temperature ultrasound hyperthermia treatment. *Ultrasound Med Biol* (1993) **19**: 777–787.

Damianou C, Hynynen K, Fan X. Evaluation of accuracy of a theoretical model for predicting the necrosed tissue volume during focused ultrasound surgery. *IEEE Trans Ultrason Ferroelectr Freq Contr* (1995) **42**: 182–187.

Darkazanli A, Hynynen K, Unger E, Schenck JF. On-line monitoring of ultrasound surgery with MRI. *J Mag Res Image* (1993) **3**: 509–514.

Daum DR, Hynynen K. Thermal dose optimization via temporal switching in ultrasound surgery. *IEEE Trans Ultrason Ferroelectr Freq Contr* (1998) **45**: 208–215.

Daum DR, Hynynen K. A 256 Element Ultrasonic Phased Array System for Treatment of Large Volumes of Deep Seated Tissue. *IEEE Trans Ultrason Ferroelect Freq Contr* (1999) **46**: 1254–1268.

Daum D, Buchanan MT, Fjield T, Hynynen K. Design and evaluation of a feedback based phased array system for ultrasound surgery. *IEEE Trans Ultrason Ferroelectr Freq Contr* (1998) **45**: 431–438.

Daum DR, Hynynen K. Sherical phased array design optimized for ultrasound surgery. *Proc IEEE Ultrasonics Symp* (1997) **2**: 1315–1318.

Daum DR, Hynynen K. Theoretical design of a spherically sectioned phased array for ultrasound surgery of the liver. *Eur J Ultrasound* (1999) **9**: 61–69.

Daum DR, Smith NB, King R, Hynynen K. *In vivo* demonstration of noninvasive, thermal surgery of the liver and kidney using an ultrasonic phased array. *Ultrasound Med Biol* (1999) **25**: 1087–1098.

Delon-Martin C, Vogt C, Chigner E, Guers C, Chapelon JY, Cathignol D. Venous thrombosis generation by means of high-intensity focused ultrasound. *Ultrasound Med Biol* (1995) **21**: 113–119.

Deng CX, Lizzi FL, Kalisz A, Rosado A, Silverman RH, Coleman JD. Study of ultrasonic contrast agents using a dual-frequency band technique. *Ultrasound Med Biol* (2000) **26**: 819–831.

Diederich C, Hynynen K. Induction of hyperthermia using an intracavitary multi-element ultrasonic applicator. *IEEE Trans Biomed Eng* (1989) **36**: 432–438.

Diederich C, Hynynen K. The development of intracavitary ultrasonic applicators for hyperthermia: A theoretical and experimental study. *Med Phys* (1990) **17**: 626–634.

Diederich C, Hynynen K. The feasibility of using electrically focussed ultrasound arrays to induce deep hyperthermia via body cavities. *IEEE Trans Ultrason Ferroelectr Freq Contr* (1991) **38**: 207–219.

Doolittle ND, Miner ME, Hall WA, Siegal T, Jerome E, Osztie E, McAllister LD, Bubalo JS, Kraemer DF, Fortin D, Nixon R, Muldoon LL, Neuwelt EA. Safety and efficacy of a multicenter study using intraarterial chemotherapy in conjunction with osmotic opening of the blood-brain barrier for the treatment of patients with malignant brain tumors. *Cancer* (2000) Feb; **88**(3): 637–647.

Dorr LN, Hynynen K. The effect of tissue heterogeneities and large blood vessels on the thermal exposure induced by short high power ultrasound pulses. *Int J Hyperthermia* (1992) **8**: 45–59.

Ebbini ES, Cain CA. Multiple-focus ultrasound phased-array pattern synthesis: Optimal driving-signal distributions for hyperthermia. *IEEE Trans Ultrason Ferroelectr Freq Contr* (1989) **36**: 540–548.

Fan X, Hynynen K. Control of the necrosed tissue volume during noninvasive ultrasound surgery using a 16 element phased array. *Med Phys* (1995) **22**: 297–308.

Fan X, Hynynen K. A study of various parameters of spherically curved phased arrays for noninvasive ultrasound surgery. *Phys Med Biol* (1996a) **41**: 591–608.

Fan X, Hynynen K. Ultrasound surgery using multiple sonications — treatment time considerations. *Ultrasound Med Biol* (1996b) **22**: 471–482.

Fjield T, Fan X, Hynynen K. A parametric study of the concentric-ring transducer design for MRI guided ultrasound surgery. *J Acoust Soc Am* (1996a) **100**: 1220–1230.

Fjield T, Fan X, Hynynen K. The combined concentric-ring and sector-vortex phased-array for MRI guided ultrasound surgery. *J Ultrasound Med* (1996b) **15**: s35.

Fjield T, Hynynen K. The combined concentric-ring and sector-vortex phased array for MRI guided ultrasound surgery. *IEEE Trans Ultrason Ferroelectr Freq Contr* (1997) **44**: 1157–1167.

Fosmire H, Hynynen K, Drach GW, Stea B, Swift P, Cassady JR. Feasibility and toxicity of transrectal ultrasound hyperthermia in the treatment of locally-advanced adenocarcinoma of the prostate. *Int J Radiat Oncol Biol Phys* (1993) **26**: 253–259.

Foster RS, Bihrle R, Sanghvi NT, Fry FJ, Donohue JP. High-intensity focused ultrasound in the treatment of prostatic disease. *Eur Urol* (1993) **23**: 29–33.

Frizzell LA, Linke CA, Carstensen EL, Fridd CW. Thresholds for focal ultrasonic lesions in rabbit kidney, liver and testicle. *IEEE Trans Biomed Eng* (1977) BME-**24**: 393–396.

Fry FJ. Transkull transmission of an intense focused ultrasonic beam. *Ultrasound Med Biol* (1977) **3**: 179–184.

Fry FJ, Barger JE. Acoustic properties of the human skull. *J Acoust Soc Am* (1978) **63**: 1576–1590.

Fry FJ, Goss SA. Further studies of the transkull transmission of an intense focused ultrasound beam: Lesion produced at 500 kHz. *Ultrasound Med Biol* (1980) **6**: 33–38.

Fry WJ, Barnard JW, Fry FJ. Ultrasonically produced localized selective lesions in the central nervous system. *Am J Phys Med* (1955) **34**: 413–423.

Fry WJ, Barnard JW, Fry FJ, Krumins RF, Brennan JF. Ultrasonic lesions in the mammalian central nervous system. *Science* (1955) **122**: 517–518.

Fry WJ, Fry FJ. Fundamental neurological research and human neurosurgery using i.ntense ultrasound. *IRE Trans Med Electron* (1960) ME-**7**: 166–181.

Gelet A, Chapelon JY, Margonari J, Theillere Y, Gorry F, Souchon R, Bouvier R. High-intensity focused ultrasound on human benign prostatic hypertrophy. *Eur Urol* (1993) **23**: 44–47.

Gelet A, Chapelon JY, Bouvier R, Souchon R, Pangaud C, Abdelrahim AF, Cathignol D, Dubernard JM. Treatment of prostate cancer with transrectal focused ultrasound: early clinical experience. *Eur Urol* (1996) **29**: 174–183.

Gianfelice D, Khiat A, Amara M, Belblidia A, Boulanger Y. MR imaging-guided focused US ablation of breast cancer: Histopathologic assessment of effectiveness — initial experience. *Radiology* (2003) **227**: 849–855.

Gianfelice D, Khiat A, Amara M, Belblidia A, Boulanger Y. MR imaging-guided focused ultrasound surgery of breast cancer: Correlation of dynamic contrast-enhanced MRI with histopathologic findings. *Breast Cancer Res Treat* (2003) **82**: 92–101.

Gianfelice D, Khiat A, Boulanger Y, Amara M, Belblidia A. Feasibility of magnetic resonance imaging-guided focused ultrasound surgery as an adjunct to tamoxifen therapy in high-risk surgical patients with breast carcinoma. *J Vasc Interv Radiol* (2003) **14**: 1275–1282.

Gianfelice DC, Mallouche H, Lepanto L, Poisson R, Nassif E, Breton G. MR-guided focused ultrasound ablation of primary breast neoplasms: Works in progress. *Radiology* **213(P)**: 106–107 (1999).

Graham SJ, Chen L, Leitch M, Peters RD, Bronskill MJ, Foster FS, Henkelman RM, Plewes DB. Quantifying tissue damage due to focused ultrasound heating observed by MRI. *Magn Reson Med* (1999) **41**: 321–328.

Guilhon E, Voisin P, De Zwart JA, Quesson B, Salomir R, Maurange C, Bouchaud V, Smirnov P, de H, Verneuil, Vekris A, Canioni P, Moonen CT. Spatial and temporal control of transgene expression *in vivo* using a heat-sensitive promoter and MRI-guided focused ultrasound. *J Gene Med* (2003) **5**: 333–342.

Guthkelch AN, Carter LP, Cassady JR, Hynynen K, Iacono RP, Johnson PC, Obbens EAMT, Roemer RB, Seeger JF, Shimm DS, Stea B. Treatment of malignant braintumors with focussed ultrasound hyperthermia and radiation: Results of a phase I trial. *J Neuro-Oncology* (1991) **10**: 271–284.

Hazle JD, Stafford RJ, Price RE. Magnetic resonance imaging-guided focused ultrasound thermal therapy in experimental animal models: Correlation of ablation volumes with pathology in rabbit muscle and VX2 tumors. *J Magn Reson Imaging* (2002) **15**: 185–194.

Heimburger RF. Ultrasound augmentation of central nervous system tumor therapy. *Indiana Med* (1985) **78**: 469–476.

Helft G, Bara L, Bloch MF, Samama MM. Comparative time course of thrombolysis induced by intravenous boluses and infusion of staphylokinase and tissue plasminogen activator in a rabbit arterial thrombosis model. *Blood Coagul Fibrinolysis* (1998) **9**: 411–417.

Hindley J, Gedroyc WM, Regan L, Stewart E, Tempany C, Hynnen K, Macdanold N, Inbar Y, Itzchak Y, Rabinovici J, Kim K, Geschwind JF, Hesley G, Gostout B, Ehrenstein T, Hengst S, Sklair-Levy M, Shushan A, Jolesz F. MRI guidance of focused ultrasound therapy of uterine fibroids: Early results. *AJR Am J Roentgenol* (2004) **183**: 1713–1719.

Hindman JC. Proton resonance shift of water in the gas and liquid states. *J Chem Phys* (1966) **44**: 4582–4592.

Holland CK, Apfel RE. Thresholds for transient cavitation produced by pulsed ultrasound in a controlled nuclei environment. *J Acoust Soc Am* (1990) **88**: 2059–2069.

Holt RG, Roy RA. Measurements of bubble-enhanced heating from focused, MHz-frequency ultrasound in a tissue-mimicking material. *Ultrasound Med Biol* (2001) **27**: 1399–1412.

Huber PE, Jenne JW, Rastert R, Simiantonakis I, Sinn HP, Strittmatter HJ, von D, Fournier, Wannenmacher MF, Debus J. A new noninvasive approach in breast cancer therapy using magnetic resonance imaging-guided focused ultrasound surgery. *Cancer Res* (2001) **61**: 8441–8447.

Huber PE, Mann MJ, Melo LG, Ehsan A, Kong D, Zhang L, Rezvani M, Peschke P, Jolesz F, Dzau VJ, Hynynen K. Focused ultrasound (HIFU) induces localized enhancement of reporter gene expression in rabbit carotid artery. *Gene Ther* (2003) **10**: 1600–1607.

Hurwitz MD, Kaplan ID, Svensson GK, Hynynen K, Hansen MS. Feasibility and patient tolerance of a novel transrectal ultrasound hyperthermia system for treatment of prostate cancer. *Int J Hyperthermia* (2001) **17**(1): 31–37.

Hutchinson E, Dahleh M, Hynynen K. The feasibility of MRI feedback control for intracavitary phased array hyperthermia treatments. *Int J Hyperthermia* (1998) **14**: 39–56.

Hutchinson EB, Buchanan MT, Hynynen K. Evaluation of an aperiodic phased array for prostate thermal therapies. *IEEE Ultrasonics Symp* (1995) **2**: 1601–1604.

Hutchinson EB, Buchanan MT, Hynynen K. Design and optimization of an aperiodic ultrasound phased array for intracavitary prostate thermal therapies. *Med Phys* (1996) **23**: 767–776.

Hutchinson EB, Hynynen K. Intracavitary phased arrays for non-invasive prostate surgery. *IEEE Trans Ultrason Ferroelectr Freq Contr* (1996) **43**: 1032–1042.

Hutchinson EB, Hynynen K. Intracavitary ultrasound phased arrays for prostate thermal therapies: MRI compatibility and *in vivo* testing. *Med Phys* (1998) **25**: 2392–2399.

Hynynen K. Demonstration of enhanced temperature elevation due to nonlinear propagation of focussed ultrasound in dog's thigh *in vivo*. *Ultrasound Med Biol* (1987) **13**: 85–91.

Hynynen K. Hot spots created at skin-air interfaces during ultrasound hyperthermia. *Int J Hyperthermia* (1990) **6**: 1005–1012.

Hynynen K. The threshold for thermally significant cavitation in dog's thigh muscle *in vivo*. *Ultrasound Med Biol* (1991) **17**: 157–169.

Hynynen K. *Proc 6th Int Congress Hyperthermic Oncology* (1992).

Hynynen K, Chung A, Colucci V, Jolesz FA. *In vivo* vascular effects of MRI guided focused ultrasound exposures. *Proc SMR 3rd Meeting* (1995).

Hynynen K, Chung A, Culucci V, Jolesz FA. Potential adverse effects of high intensity focused ultrasound exposure on blood vessel *in vivo*. *Ultrasound Med Biol* (1996a) **22**: 193–201.

Hynynen K, Chung A, Fjield T, Buchanan MT, Daum D, Colucci V, Lopath P, Jolesz F. Feasibility of using ultrasound phased arrays for MRI monitored noninvasive surgery. *IEEE Trans Ultrason Ferroelectr Freq Contr* (1996b) **43**: 1043–1053.

Hynynen K, Clement GT, McDannold N, Vykhodtseva N, King R, White PJ, Vitek S, Jolesz FA. 500-element ultrasound phased array system for noninvasive focal surgery of the brain: A preliminary rabbit study with *ex vivo* human skulls. *Magn Reson Med* (2004) **52**: 100–107.

Hynynen K, Colucci V, Chung A, Jolesz FA. Noninvasive artery occlusion using MRI guided focused ultrasound. *Ultrasound Med Biol* (1996c) **22**: 1071–1077.

Hynynen K, Damianou C, Darkazanli A, Unger E, Levy M, Schenck JF. On-line MRI monitored noninvasive ultrasound surgery. *Proc 14th annual EMB Soc Mtg* (1992) 350–351.

Hynynen K, Damianou CA, Culucci V, Unger E, Cline HE, Jolesz AF. MR monitoring of focused ultrasonic surgery of renal cortex: Experimental and simulation studies. *J Mag Res Image* (1995) **5**: 259–266.

Hynynen K, Darkanzanli A, Damianou C, Unger E, Schenck JF. Tissue thermometry during ultrasound exposure. *Eur Urol* (1993) **23**: 12–16.

Hynynen K, Darkazanli A, Damianou C, Unger E, Schenck JF. The usefulness of contrast agent and GRASS imaging sequence for MRI guided noninvasive ultrasound surgery. *Invest Radiol* (1994) **29**: 897–903.

Hynynen K, Darkazanli A, Unger E, Schenck JF. MRI-guided noninvasive ultrasound surgery. *Med Phys* (1993) **20**: 107–115.

Hynynen K, DeYoung D. Temperature elevation at muscle-bone interface during scanned, focussed ultrasound hyperthermia. *Int J Hyperthermia* (1988) **4**: 267–279.

Hynynen K, Freund W, Cline HE, Chung A, Watkins R, Vetro J, Jolesz FA. A clinical noninvasive MRI monitored ultrasound surgery method. *RadioGraphics* (1996d) **16**: 185–195.

Hynynen K, Jolesz FA. Demonstration of potential noninvasive ultrasound brain therapy through intact skull. *Ultrasound Med Biol* (1998) **24**: 275–283.

Hynynen K, McDannold N. MRI guided and monitored focused ultrasound thermal ablation methods: A review of progress. *Int J Hyperthermia* (2004) **20**: 725–737.

Hynynen K, McDannold N, Sheikov NA, Jolesz FA, Vykhodtseva N. Local and reversible blood-brain barrier disruption by noninvasive focused ultrasound at frequencies suitable for trans-skull sonications. *NeuroImage* (2005) **24**: 12–20.

Hynynen K, McDannold N, Clement GT, Jolesz FA, Zadicario E, Killiany R, Moore T, Rosene DL. Pre-clinical testing of a phased array ultrasound system for MRI-guided noninvasive surgery of the brain — A primate study. *Eur J Radiol* (2006), in press.

Hynynen K, McDannold N, Vykhodtseva N, Jolesz FA. Noninvasive MR imaging-guided focal opening of the blood-brain barrier in rabbits. *Radiology* (2001) **220**: 640–646.

Hynynen K, Pomeroy O, Smith DN, Huber PE, McDannold NJ, Kettenbach J, Baum J. Singer S, Jolesz FA. MR imaging-guided focused ultrasound surgery of fibroadenomas in the breast: A feasibility study. *Radiology* (2001) **219**: 176–185.

Hynynen K, Roemer R, Anhalt D, Johnson C, Xu ZX, Swindell W, Cetas TC. A scanned focussed multiple transducer ultrasonic system for localized hyperthermia treatments. *Int J Hyperthermia* (1987) **3**: 21–35.

Hynynen K, Shimm D, Anhalt D, Stea B, Sykes H, Cassady JR, Roemer RB. Temperature distributions during clinical scanned, focussed ultrasound hyperthermia treatments. *Int J Hyperthermia* (1990) **6**: 891–908.

Hynynen K, Sun J. Trans-skull ultrasound therapy: The feasibility of using image derived skull thickness information to correct the phase distortion. *IEEE Trans Ultrason Ferroelectr Freq Contr* (1998) **46**: 752–755.

Hynynen K, Vykhodtseva NI, Chung A, Sorrentino V, Colucci V, Jolesz FA. Thermal effects of focused ultrasound on the brain: Determination with MR Imaging. *Radiology* (1997) **204**: 247–253.

Ishihara Y, Calderon A, Watanabe H, Okamoto K, Suzuki Y, Kuroda K. A precise and fast temperature mapping using water proton chemical shift. *Magn Reson Med* (1995) **34**: 814–823.

Kim HJ, Greenleaf JF, Kinnick RR, Bronk JT, Bolander ME. Ultrasound-mediated transfection of mammalian cells. *Hum Gene Ther* (1996) **7**: 1339–1346.

Kowalski ME, Behnia B, Webb AG, Jin JM. Optimization of electromagnetic phased-arrays for hyperthermia via magnetic resonance temperature estimation. *IEEE Trans Biomed Eng* (2002) **49**: 1229–1241.

Kremkau FW. Cancer therapy with ultrasound: A historical review. *J Clin Ultrasound* (1979) **7**: 287–300.

Kroll RA, Neuwelt EA. Outwitting the blood-brain barrier for therapeutic purposes: osmotic opening and other means. *Neurosurgery* (1998) **42**: 1083–1099.

Kuroda K, Abe K, Tsutsumi S, Ishihara Y, Suzuki Y, Sato K. Water proton magnetic resonance spectroscopic imaging. *Biomed Thermol* (1995) **13**: 43–62.

Kuroda K, Chung A, Hynynen K, Jolesz FA. Calibration of water proton chemical shift with temperature for noninvasive temperature imaging during focused ultrasound surgery. *J Mag Res Image* (1998) **8**: 175–181.

Kuroda K, Suzuki Y, Ishihara Y, Okamoto K. Temperature mapping using water proton chemical shift obtained with 3D-MRSI: Feasibility *in vivo*. *Magn Reson Med* (1996) **35**: 20–29.

Lardo AC, McVeigh ER, Jumrussirikul P, Berger RD, Calkins H, Lima J, Halperin HR. Visualization and temporal/spatial characterization of cardiac radiofrequency ablation lesions using magnetic resonance imaging. *Circulation* (2000) **102**: 698–705.

Lele PP. A simple method for production of trackless focal lesions with focused ultrasound: Physical factors. *J Physiol* (1962) **160**: 494–512.

Lele PP. Cavitation and its effects on organized mammalian tissues, in *Ultrasound: Its applications in medicine and biology*. Part II. pp. 737–741, Elsevier, Amsterdam 1978.

Lin WL, Roemer RB, Hynynen K. Theoretical and experimental evaluation of a temperature controller for scanned focused ultrasound hyperthermia. *Med Phys* (1990) **17**: 615–625.

Liu H-L, McDannold N, Hynynen K. Focal Beam Distortion and Treatment Planning in Abdominal Focused Ultrasound Surgery. *Med Phys* (2005).

Lynn JG, Putnam TJ. Histology of cerebral lesions produced by focused ultrasound. *Am J Path* (1944) **20**: 637–652.

Lynn JG, Zwemer RL, Chick AJ, Miller AE. A new method for the generation and use of focused ultrasound in experimental biology. *J Gen Physiol* (1942) **26**: 179–193.

Mahoney K, Fjield T, McDannold N, Clement G, Hynynen K. Comparison of modelled and observed *in vivo* temperature elevations induced by focused ultrasound: Implications for treatment planning. *Phys Med Biol* (2001) **46**(7): 1785–1798.

McDannold N. Quantitative MRI-based temperature mapping based on the proton resonant frequency shift: review of validation studies. *Int J Hyperthermia* (2005).

McDannold N, Hynynen K, Wulf D, Wulf G, Jolesz F. MRI evaluation of thermal ablation of tumors with focused ultrasound. *J Mag Res Imag* (1998) **8**: 91–100.

McDannold N, Jolesz FA, Hynynen K. The use of MRI *in vivo* to monitor thermal build-up during focused ultrasound surgery. *Radiology* (1999) **211**: 419–426.

McDannold N, King RL, Hynynen K. MRI monitoring of heating produced by ultrasound absorption in the skull: *In vivo* study in pigs. *Magn Reson Med* (2004) **51**: 1061–1065.

McDannold N, Moss M, Killiany R, Rosene DL, King RL, Jolesz FA, Hynynen K. MRI-guided focused ultrasound surgery in the brain: Tests in a primate model. *Magn Reson Med* (2003) **49**: 1188–1191.

McDannold N, Vykhodtseva N, Hynynen K. The use of Optison® in conjunction with focused ultrasound to create lesions in the brain at low power levels: An MRI/histology study in rabbits. *Radiology* (2006), in press.

McDannold NJ, Hynynen K, Jolesz FA. MRI monitoring of the thermal ablation of tissue: Effects of long exposure times. *J Magn Reson Imaging* (2001) **13**: 421–427.

McDannold NJ, King RL, Jolesz FA, Hynynen KH. Usefulness of MR imaging-derived thermometry and dosimetry in determining the threshold for tissue damage induced by thermal surgery in rabbits. *Radiology* (2000) **216**: 517–523.

McGough RJ, Ebbini ES, Cain CA. Direct computation of ultrasound phased-array driving signals from a specified temperature distribution. *IEEE Trans Ultrason Ferroelectr Freq Contr* (1992) **39**: 825–835.

McNichols RJ, Gowda A, Kangasniemi M, Bankson JA, Price RE, Hazle JD. MR thermometry-based feedback control of laser interstitial thermal therapy at 980 nm. *Lasers Surg Med* (2004b) **34**: 48–55.

McNichols RJ, Gowda A, Kangasniemi M, Bankson JA, Price RE, Hazle JD. MR thermometry-based feedback control of laser interstitial thermal therapy at 980 nm. *Lasers Surg Med* (2004a) **34**: 48–55.

Melodelima D, Lafon C, Prat F, Theillere Y, Arefiev A, Cathignol D. Transoe-sophageal ultrasound applicator for sector-based thermal ablation: first *in vivo* experiments. *Ultrasound Med Biol* (2003) **29**: 285–291.

Melodelima D, Salomir R, Mougenot C, Prat F, Theillere Y, Moonen C, Cathignol D. Intraluminal ultrasound applicator compatible with magnetic resonance imaging "real-time" temperature mapping for the treatment of oesophageal tumours: An *ex vivo* study. *Med Phys* (2004) **31**: 236–244.

Moonen C, Madio D, de J, Zwart, Olson A, DesPres D, van P, Gelderen, Mandel M, Voisin P, Canioni P, Vekris A, Arveiller B, de H, Verneuil. MRI-guided focused ultrasound as a potential tool for control of gene therapy. *Eur Radiol* (1997) **7**: 1165.

Mougenot C, Salomir R, Palussiere J, Grenier N, Moonen CT. Automatic spatial and temporal temperature control for MR-guided focused ultrasound using fast 3D MR thermometry and multispiral trajectory of the focal point. *Magn Reson Med* (2004) **52**: 1005–1015.

Mourad PD. Ultrasound induced Blood brain barrier opening. *J Acoust Soc Am* (2001).

Muldoon LL, Pagel MA, Kroll RA, Roman-Goldstein S, Jones RS, Neuwelt EA. A physiological barrier distal to the anatomic blood-brain barrier in a model of transvascular delivery [see comments]. *AJNR Am J Neuroradiol* (1999) **20**: 217–222.

Nag S. Morphology and molecular properties of cellular components of normal cerebral vessels. *Meth Mol Med* (2003) **89**: 3–36.

Oka M. Surgical application of high-intensity focused ultrasound. *Clin All Round(Jpn)* (1960) **13**: 1514.

Palussiere J, Salomir R, Le B, Bail, Fawaz R, Quesson B, Grenier N, Moonen CT. Feasibility of MR-guided focused ultrasound with real-time temperature mapping and continuous sonication for ablation of VX2 carcinoma in rabbit thigh. *Magn Reson Med* (2003a) **49**: 89–98.

Palussiere J, Salomir R, Le B, Bail, Fawaz R, Quesson B, Grenier N, Moonen CT. Feasibility of MR-guided focused ultrasound with real-time temperature mapping and continuous sonication for ablation of VX2 carcinoma in rabbit thigh. *Magn Reson Med* (2003b) **49**: 89–98.

Pardridge WM. Drug and gene delivery to the brain: The vascular route. *Neuron* (2002) **36**: 555–558.

Parker DL. Applications on NMR imaging in hyperthermia: An evaluation of the potential for localized tissue heating and noninvasive temperature monitoring. *IEEE Trans Biomed Eng* (1984) **31**: 161–167.

Patrick JT, Nolting MN, Goss SA, Dines KA, Clendenon JL, Rea MA, Heimburger RF. Ultrasound and the blood-brain barrier. *Adv Exp Med Biol* (1990) **267**: 369–381.

Peters RD, Hinks RS, Henkelman RM. *Ex vivo* tissue-type independence in proton-resonance frequency schift MR thermometry. *Magn Reson Med* (1998) **40**: 454–459.

Quesson B, De Zwart JA and Moonen CT. Magnetic resonance temperature imaging for guidance of thermotherapy. *J Magn Reson Imaging* (2000) **12**: 525–533.

Richards ED, Tyner CF, Shealy CN. Focused ultrasonic spinal commissurotomy: Experimental evaluation. *J Neurosurg* (1966) **24**: 701–707.

Rivens IH, Rowland IJ, Denbow M, Fisk NM, ter Haar GR and Leach MO. Vascular occlusion using focused ultrasound surgery for use in fetal medicine. *Eur J Ultrasound* (1999) **9**: 89–97.

Rosenschein U, Frimerman A, Laniado S, Miller HI. Study of the mechanism of ultrasound angioplasty from human thrombi and bovine aorta. *Am J Cardiol* (1994) **74**: 1263–1266.

Salomir R, Palussiere J, Vimeux FC, De Zwart JA, Quesson B, Gauchet M, Lelong P, Pergrale J, Grenier N, Moonen CT. Local hyperthermia with MR-guided focused ultrasound: Spiral trajectory of the focal point optimized for temperature uniformity in the target region. *J Magn Reson Imaging* (2000) **12**: 571–583.

Sanghvi NT, Fry FJ, Bihrle R, Foster RS, Phillips MH, Syrus J, Zaitsev A, Hennige C. *Proc Ultrasonics Symp* (1995).

Sanghvi NT, Fry FJ, Bihrle R, Foster RS, Phillips MH, Syrus J, Zaitsev AV, Hennige CW. Noninvasive surgery of prostate tissue by high-intensity focused ultrasound. *IEEE Trans Ultrason Ferroelectr Freq Contr* (1996) **43**: 1099–1110.

Sapareto SA, Dewey WC. Thermal dose determination in cancer therapy. *Int J Radiat Oncol Biol Phys* (1984) **10**: 787–800.

Schenck JF, Jolesz FA, Roemer PB, Cline HE, Lorensen WE, Kikinis R, Silverman SG, Hardy CJ, Barber WD, Laskaris ET. Superconducting open-configuration MR imaging system for image-guided therapy. *Radiology* (1995) **195**: 805–814.

Seip R, Chen W, Carlson R, Frizzell LA, Warren G, Smith NB, Saleh K, Gerber G, Shung KK, Guo H, Sanghvi NT, ter Haar GR, Rivens IH. (2005) AIP. *Proc 4th Int Symp Therapeutic Ultrasound*, Sept 18–20, 2004, Kyoto, Japan.

Sheikov N, McDannold N, Vykhodtseva N, Jolesz F, Hynynen K. Cellular mechanisms of the blood-brain barrier opening induced by ultrasound in presence of microbubbles. *Ultrasound Med Biol* (2004) **30**: 979–989.

Silcox C, The use of ultrasound to facilitate the delivery of genetic-based therapeutic strategies. MS Thesis, MIT, 2004.

Silcox CE, Smith RC, King R, McDannold N, Bromley P, Walsh K, Hynynen K. MRI-guided ultrasonic heating allows spatial control of exogenous luciferase in canine prostate. *Ultrasound Med Biol* (2005) **31**: 965–970.

Simon RH, Ho SY, Lange SC, Uphoff DF, D'Arrigo JS. Applications of lipid-coated microbubble ultrasonic contrast to tumor therapy. *Ultrasound Med Biol* (1993) **19**: 123–125.

Smith NB, Buchanan MT, Hynynen K. Transrectal ultrasound applicator for prostate heating monitored using MRI thermometry. *Int J Radiat Oncol Biol Phys* (1998) **43**: 217–225.

Smith NB, Hynynen K. The feasibility of using focused ultrasound for transmyocardial revascularization. *Ultrasound Med Biol* (1998) **24**: 1045–1054.

Smith NB, Merilees NK, Hynynen K, Dahleh M. Control system for an MRI compatible intracavitary ultrasound array for thermal treatment of prostate disease. *Int J Hyperthermia* (2001) **17**: 271–282.

Smith NB, Webb AG, Ellis DS, Wilmes LJ, O'Brien WD. Experimental verification of theoretical *in vivo* ultrasound heating using cobalt detected magnetic resonance. *IEEE Trans Ultrason Ferroelectr Freq Contr* (1995) **42**: 489–491.

Smith SW, Phillips DJ, von Ramm OT and Thurstone FL. Some advances in acoustic imaging through skull, in *Symposium on Biological Effects and Characterizations of Ultrasound Sources*. vol. FDA 78–8048. (Eds. Hazzard DG and Litz ML,) pp. 37–52, HEW, FDA, Rockville, MA 1977.

Sokka SD, Gauthier TP, Hynynen K. Theoretical and experimental validation of a dual-frequency excitation method for spatial control of cavitation. *Phys Med Biol* (2005) **50**: 2167–2179.

Sokka SD, Hynynen K. The feasibility of MRI-guided whole prostate ablation with a linear aperiodic intracavitary ultrasound phased array. *Phys Med Biol* (2000) **45**: 3373–3383.

Sokka SD, King R, Hynynen K. MRI-guided gas bubble enhanced ultrasound heating in *in vivo* rabbit thigh. *Phys Med Biol* (2003) **48**: 223–241.

Sommer FG, Sumanaweera TS, Glover G. Tissue ablation using an acoustic waveguide for high-intensity focused ultrasound. *Med Phys* (1997) **24**: 537–538.

Stafford RJ, Hazle JD, Glover GH. Monitoring of high-intensity focused ultrasound-induced temperature changes *in vitro* using an interleaved spiral acquisition. *Magn Reson Med* (2000) **43**: 909–912.

Stepanow B, Huber P, Brix G, Debus J, Bader R, van G, Kaick and Lorenz WJ. Fast MRI temperature monitoring: Application in focused ultrasound therapy of malignant tissue *in vivo*. (1995) *Proc SMR 3rd Meeting*, 1172.

Stewart EA, Gedroyc WM, Tempany CM, Quade BJ, Inbar Y, Ehrenstein T, Shushan A, Hindley JT, Goldin RD, David M, Sklair M, Rabinovici J. Focused ultrasound treatment of uterine fibroid tumors: Safety and feasibility of a noninvasive thermoablative technique. *Am J Obstet Gynecol* (2003) **189**: 48–54.

Strickberger SA, Tokano T, Kluiwstra JU, Morady F, Cain C. Extracardiac ablation of the canine atrioventricular junction by use of high-intensity focused ultrasound. *Circulation* (1999) **100**: 203–208.

Sun J, Hynynen K. Focusing of ultrasound through a human skull: A numerical study. *J Acoust Soc Am* (1998a) **104**: 1705–1715.

Sun J, Hynynen K. The potential of transskull ultrasound therapy and surgery using the maximum available skull surface area. *J Acoust Soc Am* **104**: 2519–2527 (1998b).

Suzuki T, Fujimoto K, Aida S, Isihara Y, Watanabe H, Okamoto K, Iorita N, Shirai S, Orikasa S. MRI monitoring during high-intensity focused ultrasound treatment. *Proc SMR 3rd Meeting* (1995).

Tachibana K, Tachibana S. Prototype therapeutic ultrasound emitting catheter for accelerating thrombolysis. *J Ultrasound Med* (1997) **16**: 529–535.

Tempany CM, Stewart EA, McDannold N, Quade BJ, Jolesz FA, Hynynen K. MR imaging-guided focused ultrasound surgery of uterine leiomyomas: A feasibility study. *Radiology* (2003) **226**: 897–905.

J.-L. Thomas and Fink MA. Ultrasonic beam focusing through tissue inhomogeneities with a time reversal mirror: application to transskull therapy. *IEEE Trans Ultrason Ferroelectr Freq Contr* (1996) **43**: 1122–1129.

Tran BC, Seo J, Hall TL, Fowlkes JB, Cain CA. Microbubble-enhanced cavitation for noninvasive ultrasound surgery. *IEEE Trans Ultrason Ferroelectr Freq Control* (2003) **50**: 1296–1304.

Treat LH, McDannold N, Vykhodtseva N, Hynynen K. Transcranial MRI-guided focused ultrasound-induced blood-brain barrier opening in rats, in *Proc IEEE Int Conf Ultrasonics, Ferroelectrics, Frequency Control* (2004) pp. 998–1000.

Uchida T, Sanghvi NT, Gardner TA, Koch MO, Ishii D, Minei S, Satoh T, Hyodo T, Irie A, Baba S. Transrectal high-intensity focused ultrasound for treatment of patients with stage T1b-2n0m0 localized prostate cancer: A preliminary report. *Urology* (2002) **59**: 394–398.

S.-I. Umemura, K.-I. Kawabata, Sasaki K. *In vitro* and *in vivo* enhancement of sonodynamically active cavitation by second-harmonic superimposition. *J Acoust Soc Am* (1997) **101**: 569–577.

Umemura S, Kawabata K, Sasaki K. Enhancement of sonodynamic tissue damage production by second-harmonic superimposition: Theoretical analysis of its mechanism. *IEEE Trans Ultrason Ferroelectr Freq Contr* (1996) **43**: 1054.

Vaezy S, Marti R, Mourad P, Crum L. Hemostasis using high intensity focused ultrasound. *Eur J Ultrasound* (1999) **9**: 79–87.

Vaezy S, Martin R, Keilman G, Kaczkowski P, Chi E, Yazaji E, Caps M, Poliachik S, Carter S, Sharar S, Cornejo C, Crum L. Control of splenic bleeding by using high intensity ultrasound. *J Trauma* (1999) **47**: 521–525.

Vaezy S, Martin R, Schniedl U, Caps M, Taylor S, Beach K, Carter S, Kaczkowski P, Kielman G, Helton S, Chandler W, Mourad P, Rice M, Roy R, Crum L. Liver hemostasis using high-intensity focused ultrasound. *Ultrasound Med Biol* (1997) **23**: 1413–1420.

Vaezy S, Martin R, Yaziji H, Kaczkowski P, Keilman G, Carter S, Caps M, Chi EY, Bailey M, Crum L. Hemostasis of punctured blood vessels using high-intensity focused ultrasound. *Ultrasound Med Biol* (1998) **24**: 903–910.

Vallancien G, Harouni M, Veillon B, Mombet A, Prapotnich D, Bisset MJ, Bougaran J. Focused extracorporeal pyrotherapy: Feasibility study in man. *J Endourol* (1992) **6**: 173–180.

Vanne A, Hynynen K. MRI feedback temperature control for focused ultrasound surgery. *Phys Med Biol* (2003) **48**: 31–43.

Vimeux FC, De Zwart JA, Palussiere J, Fawaz R, Delalande C, Canioni P, Grenier N, Moonen CT. Real-time control of focused ultrasound heating based on rapid MR thermometry. *Invest Radiol* (1999) **34**: 190–193.

Vykhodtseva N, McDannold N, Martin H, Bronson RT, Hynynen K. Apoptosis in ultrasound-produced threshold lesions in the rabbit brain. *Ultrasound Med Biol* (2001) **27**: 111–117.

Vykhodtseva N, Sorrentino V, Jolesz FA, Bronson RT, Hynynen K. MRI detection of the thermal effects of focused ultrasound on the brain. *Ultrasound Med Biol* (2000) Jun 1; **26**(5): 871–880.

Vykhodtseva NI, Hynynen K, Damianou C. The effect of pulse duration and peak intensity during focused ultrasound surgery: A theoretical and experimental study in rabbit brain *in vivo*. *Ultrasound Med Biol* (1994) **20**: 987–1000.

Vykhodtseva NI, Hynynen K, Damianou C. Histologic effects of high intensity pulsed ultrasound exposure with subharmonic emission in rabbit brain *in vivo*. *Ultrasound Med Biol* (1995) **21**: 969–979.

Wallance S, Chuang VP, Swanson D, Bracken B, Hersh E, Ayala A, Johnson D. Embolization of renal carcinoma. *Radiology* (1981) **138**: 563.

Wallance S, Gianturco C,erson JH, Goldstein HM, Davis LJ, Bree RL. Therapeutic vascular oclusion using stell coil technique: Clinical application. *AJR* (1976) **127**: 381.

Wan H, VanBaren P, Ebbini ES, Cain CA. Ultrasound Surgery: Comparison of strategies using phased array systems. *IEEE Trans Ultrason Ferroelectr Freq Contr* (1996) **43**: 1085–1098.

Watmough DJ, Lakshmi R, Ghezzi F, Quan KM, Watmough JA, Khizhnyak E, Pashovkin TN, Sarvazyan AP. The effect of gas bubbles on the production of ultrasound hyperthermia at 0.75 MHz: A phantom study. *Ultrasound Med Biol* (1993) **19**(3): 231–241.

Watson BD, Dietrich WD, Prado R, Ginsberg MD. Argon Laser-induced arteral photothrombosis: Characterization and possible application to therapy of arteriovenous malformations. *J Neurosurg* (1987) **66**: 748–754.

Wu F, Chen WZ, Bai J, Zou JZ, Wang ZL, Zhu H, Wang ZB. Pathological changes in human malignant carcinoma treated with high- intensity focused ultrasound. *Ultrasound Med Biol* **27**: 1099–1106 (2001a).

Wu F, Chen WZ, Bai J, Zou JZ, Wang ZL, Zhu H, Wang ZB. Pathological changes in human malignant carcinoma treated with high-intensity focused ultrasound. *Ultrasound Med Biol* **27**: 1099–1106 (2001b).

Xu Z, Fowlkes JB, Rothman ED, Levin AM, Cain CA. Controlled ultrasound tissue erosion: the role of dynamic interaction between insonation and microbubble activity. *J Acoust Soc Am* (2005) **117**: 424–435.

Xu Z, Ludomirsky A, Eun LY, Hall TL, Tran BC, Fowlkes JB, Cain CA. Controlled ultrasound tissue erosion. *IEEE Trans Ultrason Ferroelectr Freq Control* (2004) **51**: 726–736.

Yin X, Epstein LM, Hynynen K. Feasibility of noninvasive transesophageal cardiac thermal ablation using an ultrasound phased array, in *Proc IEEE Int Conference Ultrasonics, Ferroelectrics Frequency Control* (2004) pp. 126–129.

Young FR. *Cavitation* (1989) McGraw-Hill Book Company: New York.

Young IR, Hand JW, Oatridge A, Prior MV, Forse GR. Further observations on the measurement of tissue T1 to monitor temperature *in vivo* by MRI. *Magn Reson Med* (1994) **31**: 342–345.

VI

SONOPORATION, GENE TRANSFECTION, ANTICANCER DRUG AND ANTIBODY DELIVERY USING ULTRASOUND

Junru Wu

In this chapter, a brief review of the current techniques of *in vitro* and *in vivo* targeting delivery is presented. The technique of sonoporation is demonstrated. Possible physical mechanisms and *in vitro* applications of sonoporation in DNA, anticancer drug and antibody deliveries are discussed. The delivery efficiency using sonoporation is compared with that using electroporation, a currently widely used targeting delivery method *in vitro*.

1. Introduction

Gene therapy as well as drug and antibody targeting delivery are two emerging technologies in medicine. They are changing and will continue to change how medicine is delivered. An ideal *in vivo* technique should be able to deliver macromolecules, including pharmaceutical drugs, antibodies or DNA to their specific site of action. For pharmaceutical drug and antibodies, the dosage delivered should be at therapeutically relevant levels. Targeting delivery (TD) offers enormous advantages compared with conventional deliveries. For example, since conventional methods lack target specificity, some highly toxic anticancer drugs delivered conventionally may severely damage healthy tissues and organs undesirably. Targeting delivery not only increases drug efficacy but also minimizes any possible side effect of the conventional delivery method. Although it has great potential, TD also faces serious technical challenge. Major difficulties to TD include barriers from cell membranes, as well as from nuclear membranes for DNA, and also for antibodies and drugs if their targets are located in the cell nuclei. Barriers for cell membranes are difficult to overcome for most cases and barriers from membranes of cell nuclei are sometimes formidable.

Gene transfection is the process of introducing recombinant DNA into eukaryotic cells and subsequently integrating it into the recipient cell's chromosomal DNA. Current gene transfection techniques may be divided into two categories: viral and non-viral. The former achieves transfection by using a virus and the latter does not. Several viral systems (adenovirus and retrovirus) have been used to deliver genes into primary cells from specific tissues *in vitro*, but their use for *in vivo* gene delivery has faced several problems such as an immune response against the virus and the poor specificity of cell target. Here, primary cells are those isolated from a specific tissue, *e.g.*, spleen and lymph nodes. They can be maintained transiently in culture *in vitro* in the presence of specific growth factors, but eventually they will die. Non-primary cells are those isolated from tissues and transformed with given oncogenic proteins that allow the cells to grow indefinitely in culture *in vitro* in the absence of specific growth factors. Most cell lines available commercially, such as Jurkat cells, are non-primary cells; they are inexpensive and easily obtainable.

Existing non-viral transfection approaches include calcium phosphate infusion, electroporation, particle bombardment and lipofection. Lack of target specificity is a major problem to the most existing delivery techniques. Recently, applications of nanoparticles as targeting drug delivery carriers have been investigated (Vasir *et al.*, 2005). Nanoparticles including the nano-sized (<1000 nm) polymeric particles, liposomes and micelles. The application of liposome has shown great potential in gene transfection (Lasic, 1993) because of its properties, and biocompatibility with cell membranes and the possible addition of special ligands on their surface.

A new non-viral and controllable transfection tool to deliver macromolecules, including lipsomes and other nanoparticles, safely and efficiently into targets desired *in vivo* as well *in vitro* is urgently needed.

It has been demonstrated that ultrasound assisted by encapsulated microbubbles (EMB) can make cell membranes temporarily "open", deliver DNA and other macromolecules into cell nuclei and make affected cells transfected (Bao *et al.*, 1997; Greenleaf *et al.*, 1998; Lawrie *et al.*, 2000;

Lu *et al.*, 2003; Miller *et al.*, 1999, 2003; Ward *et al.*, 1999, 2000; Wu *et al.*, 2002; Wu 2002). Most EMB used in applications belong to ultrasound (US) imaging contrast agents used clinically. The ultrasound technique associated with this process is often called "sonoporation."

In this chapter, we demonstrate the effects of sonoporation, discuss its possible physics mechanisms and *in vitro* applications of sonoporation in DNA, anticancer drug and antibody deliveries, and also compare the delivery efficiency using sonoporation with that using electroporation — a currently widely used method *in vitro*.

2. Demonstration of Sonoporation

Optison® (GE Healthcare, Chicago, IL, USA), one type of EMB, is an US imaging contrast agent that has been used in the USA and other countries to enhance tissue echogenicity for US imaging. It consists of micrometer-size (mean diameter $\approx$2–5 μm) denatured hollow albumin microspheres of shell thickness approximately 15 nm. The microbubbles are filled with octafluoropropane gas and the microbubble stock concentration is approximately 6.5×10^8/mL. Demonstrations (Ward *et al.*, 1999) of the feasibility of sonoporation were successfully achieved by using 2 mL cervical cancer cell (HeLa S3) suspensions of cell concentration 2×10^5/mL mixed with 140 μL Optison® EMB, and exposing them to ultrasound tonebursts of moderate pressure amplitude (spatial peak-pressure amplitude $= 0.2$ MPa, central frequency $= 2$ MHz, pulse repetition frequency $= 10$ kHz, on cycles/off cycles $= 20/180$). It should be noted that the cell concentration used here was lower (2×10^5/mL) than those of other studies reported in the literature. The bubble to cell ratio was approximately 230. The sample was supplemented with 10% fluorescein isothiocyanate — dextran (FITC-dextran) before US exposure. These fluorescent-labeled dextran molecules (FITC-dextran) played a role of a marker and have an average molecular weight of 500,000 Da. Normally they are unable to enter the cells. It was found that they were entrapped, once they overcome the cell membrane barriers and entered the cells. The fluorescent light of wavelength 530 nm transmitted by FITC and excited by 440 nm light, made these cells visible under the epifluorescent mode of a microscope. The sample described earlier was centrifuged after it was exposed to the US for a period of time.

The cells were then washed with RPMI (serum-free) to remove any Optison® and FITC-dextran from the solution. The cells were resuspended in the 0.4 mL RPMI and 0.1 mL Trypan Blue dye, gently mixed and counted using a hemacytometer. A stained cell observed under a microscope indicated that the plasma membrane was damaged (lethal sonoporation) and the cell was unable to exclude the Tryban Blue dye. A fluorescent cell, however, indicated that the plasma membrane, previously compromised by US, allowed the FITC-dextran to enter the cell, but had since been repaired (reparable sonoporation) and prevented the FITC-dextran from leaving the cell and the Trypan Blue from entering the cell. It was observed that about 15% of the cells showed fluorescent (reparably sonoporated) and 12% of the cells were stained (lethally sonoporated) after 5 minutes of US exposure.

3. The Effects of Optison® Concentration

In order to explore the possible physical mechanisms of sonoporation, Ward *et al.* (2000) further studied the effects of EMB concentration on sonoporation using Jurkat lymphocytes (subclone of T cells). For this study, it was hypothesized that EMB and cells were evenly distributed in the suspension. Under this assumption, the nearest bubble-bubble spacing is equal to the nearest bubble-cell spacing. When the bubble-to-cell ratio was changed from 0–230 by changing EMB or cell numbers, the nearest bubble-to-cell spacing, r, changes. The mathematical relationship between the percentage of cells exhibiting reparable or lethal sonoporation, as indicated by fluorescence or Trypan Blue staining respectively, versus r was found to be $1/r^3$ (Ward *et al.*, 2000) as shown in Fig. 1. This result suggests that the bubble-cell interaction is relatively short-ranged, decaying as $1/r^3$. Only the cells that move very close to pulsating bubbles experience this significant interaction with the bubbles. The probability of this short-range interaction decays quickly as the spacing, r, increases. It should be noted that this result was derived from relatively low cell concentration cases.

4. Microstreaming Generated by EMBs Near Cells

A steady and direct current (DC) flow can be generated in a liquid by an acoustic field and is known as acoustic streaming (Nyborg, 1978;

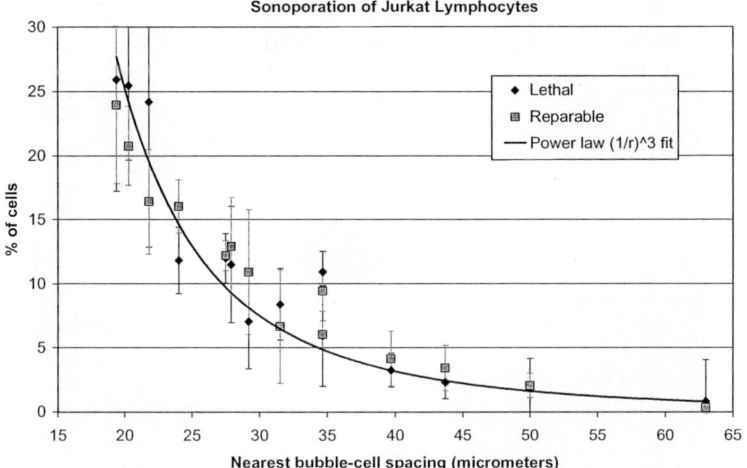

Fig. 1. Percentage of cells exhibiting reparable or lethal sonoporation as indicated by fluorescence and Trypan Blue staining respectively. Each data point represents the average and standard deviation of four independent trials. A $1/r^3$ (1/spacing^3) function is fit to all the data with an R-value of 0.9448 (Ward *et al.*, 2000).

Wu and Du, 1993). A small-scale and boundary-associated acoustic streaming is also named microstreaming (Elder, 1959). Vigorous microstreaming was observed near EMBs of ultrasound contrast agents near a solid boundary (Gormley and Wu, 1998) as shown in Fig. 2. Shear stress resulting from microstreaming near pulsating bubbles (Nyborg, 1978; Lewin and Bjørnø, 1982; Wu, 2002) may generate bioeffects if cells are present in a microstreaming field (refer to Chap. II for detailed description). Based on a linear theory, microstreaming established in the vicinity of a pulsating bubble (Nyborg, 1958) near a solid boundary has a sharp velocity (time-independent) drop across a thin boundary layer whose thickness, δ, is described by

$$\delta = \sqrt{\eta/(\pi f \rho)}, \tag{1}$$

where η and ρ are the viscosity and density of a liquid respectively, and f is the frequency. The velocity gradient, G, associated with the drop is approximately given by

$$G = 2\pi f \varepsilon_0^2/(R_0 \delta), \tag{2}$$

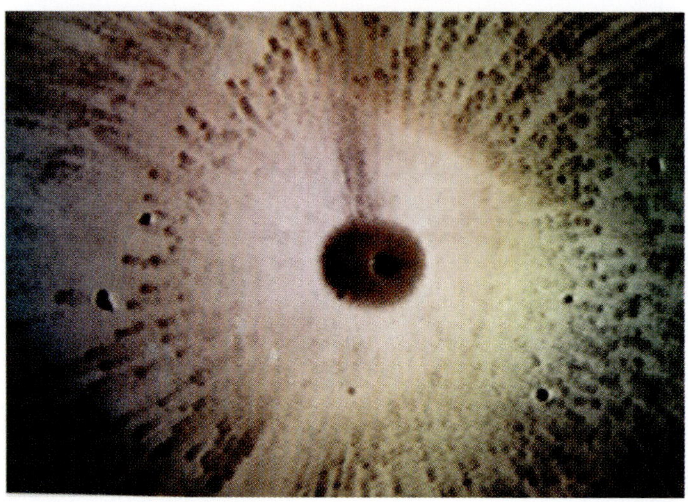

Fig. 2. Acoustic streaming pattern near a pulsating encapsulated microbubble (in the central position) of radius $10\,\mu$m that was in a 160-kHz standing wave field. The 1-μm latex particles were used as tracers (Reprinted with permission from Gomley, G. and Wu, J., Observation of acoustic streaming near Albunex sphere, *J Acoust Soc Am* **104:** 3115–3118, 1998. Copyright 2006, Acoustical Society of America).

where ε_0 equals to $R(t) - R_0$, with $R(t)$ being the amplitude of the time-dependent instantaneous radius of a pulsating bubble, is the radial displacement amplitude of a vibrating bubble of the equilibrium radius, R_0. Thus, the shear stress, S, incurred from the velocity gradient is given by

$$S = \eta G = 2\pi^{3/2}\varepsilon_0^2(\rho f^3 \eta)^{1/2}/R_0. \tag{3}$$

A nonlinear differential equation (RPNNP equation) for $R(t)$ was solved (Wu, 2002). It was developed and modified by Rayleigh, Plesset, Noltingk, Neppiras and Portisky to describe the nonlinear oscillations of a bubble driven by ultrasonic waves. Applying the above described model for microstreaming, the shear stress generated by the microstreaming of an EMB near a cell was calculated. The calculated results suggest that oscillating EMB of few-micron radii driven by 1–2 MHz ultrasound of the acoustic pressure amplitude as low as 0.1 MPa, may generate shear stress surpassing the threshold to cause reparable sonoporation after 5 minutes exposure. On the other hand, some EMB that have mechanically weak shells may break into free bubbles under 0.1 MPa after US exposure of a short time. When that happens, the oscillating free bubbles of the same order of size would generate shear stress that is a few hundred-fold higher than that generated by EMB. For the mathematical detail, please refer to the Appendix. It is thus possible that the free bubbles were the primary sources of the stress which caused some cells to suffer lethal sonoporation. It should be pointed out that if we shorten the exposure time, a much higher acoustic pressure amplitude would be needed to achieve similar effects. Under such conditions, more violent inertial cavitation may dominate (NCRP, 2002).

5. Delivery of DNA Using Sonoporation and Electroporation

Currently, electroporation may be the most widely used gene transfection tool for *in vitro* research; commercial electroporation devices are available. Electroporation uses high-voltage electrical pulses to make cell membranes transiently permeable, permitting cellular uptake of foreign macromolecules (Neumann *et al.*, 1989). Like viral and the other nonviral transfection techniques, it also suffers from the lack of site specificity, difficulties in control and optimization in applications *in vivo*. Although for electroporation, transfection efficiency, which may be defined as the number of cells transfected divided by the number of cells surviving the electroporation or sonoporation, is reasonable for non-primary cells, its transfection efficiency on primary cells was unsatisfactorily low.

Due to its lack of target specificity and safety concerns, electroporation has limited applications *in vivo*. An experimental study for cell suspensions using non-primary cells (Jurkat lymphocytes) and primary cells (human peripheral blood mononuclear cells) has been performed recently (Pepe *et al.*, 2004), to compare cell viability and transfection efficiency between sonoporation and electroporation. The experimental methods used are briefly described as follows.

5.1. *Plasmid DNA preparation*

The plasmid DNA was prepared with a Concert™ Nucleic Acid Purification System (Gibco BRL® Life Technologies®, Paisley, UK) following the Company's protocol. In summary, *E. coli* bacteria were made to express CMV-GFP plasmid. The *E. coli* were then cultured to produce a large quantity of usable DNA, and then lysed. The lysate was passed through a plastic column, which separated the plasmid DNA from genomic DNA. Plasmid DNA concentration was verified with a BioPhotometer (Eppendorf, Hamburg, Germany).

5.2. *Cell preparation*

Blood was drawn from a healthy donor following a protocol approved by the Institutional Review Board, and human peripheral blood mononuclear cells (PBMC), a type of primary cells, were extracted in the following manner. The whole blood was mixed with PBS equally. A volume of 9 mL of this mixture was added to 3 mL of Histopaque®-1077 in 15 mL tubes, without mixing the two. These samples were centrifuged at 1900 RPM for 20 minutes. The PBMC layer was removed from the tube samples and placed in a 50mL tube. A buffer (PBS/BSA/EDTA) was added (1:1 ratio) to the PBMC, and the tube was centrifuged for 5 minutes at 1000 RPM, 4°C. The supernatant was aspirated, and the remaining cells were resuspended with RPMI (rich medium for mammalian cell culture) and put on ice.

Jurkat lymphocytes were incubated in a humidified 37°C, 5% CO_2 atmosphere in 25 cm^2 tissue culture flasks (Becton-Dickson, Oxnard, CA, USA) in a solution of RPMI (liquid tissue culture medium containing a nutrient blend of amino acids, vitamins, carbohydrates, organic and inorganic supplements and salts) and Medium 1640 (GIBCOBRL, Grand Island, NY, USA), supplemented with 10% fetal bovine serum (FBS).

5.3. *Ultrasound exposure and calibration*

For ultrasound exposures, both primary and non-primary cells were prepared in the same manner. The cells were counted with a hemacytometer (Hausser Scientific Co., Horsham, PA) and diluted to a concentration of 10^6/mL in RPMI, supplemented with 25 μg CMV-GFP (Green Fluorescent Protein prepared as described above), used as a marker to detect fluorescent cells. One mL of this solution was placed in a 12×75 mm culture tube (VWR Scientific, West Chester, PA, USA) with 100 μL Optison®; its initial bubble concentration obtained from the commercial vial is 5.0–8.0×10^8/mL. The final bubble concentration is 4.5–7.3×10^7/mL.

The transducer used was a 2.5 cm diameter Panametrics A 304 S planar non-focusing transducer (Panametrics, MA, USA), driven by a Hewlett Packard 3314A function generator (Hewlett Packard, CA), and an ENI A-300 RF power amplifier (ENI, Rochester, NY, USA). The center frequency was 2 MHz. For a pulsed mode (PULSE US), the transducer was driven intermittently, the duty cycle was 10% (on cycles/off cycles = 20/180, pulse repetition frequency = 10 kHz). The test tube was situated at the near-field, 1 cm distance from the source transducer; the beam-width is about 2.5 cm, much greater than the test tube diameter.

Each sample tube was rotated at 200 rpm by a DC motor throughout the exposure period, and the rotation helps to mix cells with Optison® bubbles better. The test tube sample was lowered into a glass tank filled with distilled water kept at human body temperature (37°C) and aligned axially with the ultrasound transducer. Samples were exposed to pulsed US. The control samples were either exposed to pulsed US with Optison® in the same fashion but without GFP added (PULSE US, NO GFP), or sham-exposed(No US, GFP). Ultrasound exposure was performed quickly after a sample was prepared and the bubbles and cell suspension were mixed.

The *in situ* spatial peak-pressure amplitude after attenuation correction was 1.5 MPa for PULSE US. The acoustic pressure was measured by a needle pvdf (0.2 mm diameter) hydrophone (NTR Systems, Seattle, Washington, USA) that was calibrated by measuring the acoustic radiation force generated by the transducer using an electronic balance and scanning a two-dimensional sound field *in situ* (Beissner, 1992). The attenuation of the test tube was found by measuring the amplitude of short ultrasound pulse with/without placing the test tube before the hydrophone (note that the ultrasound was attenuated twice using this method and the standing wave effect is small, as the reflection coefficient of acoustic pressure of the test tube was measured to be less than 0.1). Since the sample tube was placed in near field, the nonlinear distortion of the waveform was not serious, and the peak positive and peak negative pressures are found to be equal.

Each sample was exposed to ultrasound in the following way. A sample with 100 μL fresh Optison® added was first exposed to the ultrasound for 10 seconds. Fresh Optison® (100 μL) was added again immediately before a second 10-second exposure. This was repeated one more time so that each sample was exposed to ultrasound for a total of 30 seconds with fresh ($100\,\mu l$) Optison® added for each of the three 10-second exposures.

5.4. *Electroporation procedure*

Primary or nonprimary cells with $25\,\mu g$ CMV-GFP added were placed in $800\,\mu L$ Gene Pulser® Cuvettes for electroporation exposure with Gene Pulser® II Apparatus (BIO-RAD, Herinles, CA, USA), a commercial product designed for cell electroporation. Following suggestions from the manufacturer and based on the parameter optimization results for this commercial system to achieve the optimum transfection and viability performance as reported previously (Chow *et al.*, 1999), electroporation parameters were set as $950\,\mu F$, $250\,V$. The spacing between the two electrodes was $0.4\,cm$. The peak electric field was calculated as $E = V/d = 250\,V/0.4\,cm = 625\,V/cm$. Time constants obtained for exposures were consistently in the range of $11\,ms$–$14\,ms$.

5.5. *Flow cytometer*

A flow cytometer (Coulter EPICS ELITE ESP, Beckman Couiter International, Inc., Miami, FL.) housed in the University Medical College was used for counting the percentages of viable cells and cells with fluorescence. The percentage of cells with fluorescence is defined as the delivery efficiency. Immediately after applications of US, the cells were washed twice and re-suspended in PBS for flow analysis.

5.6. *Experimental results*

Experimental results are presented by tables. Each column represents the mean $\pm$ one standard deviation (SD) of the three samples ($n = 3$) prepared in the same manner described above and treated identically. To measure cell loss and viability immediately after sonoporation and electroporation treatments and the effects of incubation after their treatments, Jurkat cell samples initially prepared with a cell concentration of 10^6/mL were sham-exposed (no US) + incubated for 20 hours (second column in Table 1), or sonoporated using PULSE US, GFP (third column), or sonoporated using PULSE

Table 1. Cell (Jurkat) loss and viability after electroporation and sonoporartion.

	No US, GFP + Incu	PULSE US, GFP	PULSE US, GFP + Incu	GFP, Electro	GFP, Electro + Incu
Concentration ($\times 10^6$/mL)	2.0 ± 0.40	0.46 ± 0.09	0.72 ± 0.08	0.49 ± 0.04	0.8 ± 0.36

US, GFP + incubated for 20 hours (4th column), or electroporated (5th column), or electroporated + incubated for 20 hours (6th column) respectively. Viable cells for each case were counted using a hemacytometer (i.e., if cells looked round and healthy and their diameters were greater than 10 μm, they were counted as viable cells), and typical results are shown in Table 1. The mean of viable cell concentration of samples which were sham-exposed was doubled, reaching 2×10^6/mL $\pm 4 \times 10^5$/mL. The mean of viable cell concentrations of those samples which were sonoporated (third column) or electroporated (5th column) were 4.60×10^5/mL $\pm 0.90 \times 10^5$/mL and 4.9×10^5/mL $\pm 0.4 \times 10^5$/mL respectively. The mean of viable cell concentrations of those samples which were sonoporated + incubated (4th column) or electroporated + incubated (6th column), were 7.2×10^5/mL $\pm 0.8 \times 10^5$/mL and 8.0×10^5/mL $\pm 3.6 \times 10^5$/mL respectively.

Examining column 3 and column 5, cell concentrations were reduced to about 46% and 49% of the initial value (10^6/mL) respectively for sonoporation and electroporation. However, the reductions were statistically indistinguishable between sonoporation and electroporation treatments ($P < 0.23$). Comparing column 3 and column 4, for sonoporation, the number of viable cells increased approximately 56% after 20 hours incubation and the growth is significant ($P < 0.04$). Comparing column 5 and column 6, for electroporation, the viable cells grew ~63% after incubation and the growth is significant ($P < 0.036$). The number of viable cells after sonoporation + incubation (column 4), and that after electroporation + incubation (column 6), are statistically indistinguishable ($P < 0.30$). Similar results were obtained for PBMC cells. The results shown in Table 1 indicate that cells surviving electroporation and sonoporation still grew, and their growth rates were statistically indistinguishable.

A flow cytometer can give us the percentages of viable cells and cells showing fluorescence in a sample. Tables 2 and 3 present the mean

Table 2. Comparison of transfection and viability of Jurkat cells between electroporation and sonoporartion.

	PULSE US, No GFP	PULSE US, GFP	Electrical, GFP
Fluorescent (%)	1.10 ± 0.20	7.53 ± 0.40	15.83 ± 3.50
Cell Viability (%)	43.9 ± 0.35	50.8 ± 4.15	65.8 ± 2.30

Table 3. Comparison of transfection and viability of PBMC between electroporation and sonoporartion.

	PULSE US, No GFP	PULSE US, GFP	Electrical, GFP
Fluorescent (%)	0.13 ± 0.06	2.73 ± 0.21	0.43 ± 0.06
Cell Viability (%)	63.0 ± 0.84	64.8 ± 1.51	53.7 ± 1.53

percentage of viable cells and the mean percentage of fluorescent cells of Jurkat cells and PBMC, respectively, after PULSE US, No GFP, PULSE US, GFP + incubation and Electrical, GFP + incubation, as given by a flow cytometer. The fluorescent signal is an indication of cell transfection.

Table 2 shows that significantly higher percentage of Jurkat cells survived electroporation ($65.8\% \pm 2.3\%$) than sonoporation ($50.8 \pm 4.15\%$) for "PULSE US, GFP" and "PULSE US, No GFP" ($43.9 \pm 0.35\%$). A Two-Sample Assuming Unequal Variances t-Test between "PULSE US, GFP" and "Electrical, GFP" resulted in $P < 0.006$. Table 2 also indicated that significantly ($P < 0.03$) more Jurkat cells showed fluorescence after electroporation ($15.83 \pm 3.50\%$) than sonoporation ($7.53 \pm 0.40\%$). They are both significantly higher than "PULSE US, No GFP" case ($1.10 \pm 0.20\%$); for both cases, $P < 0.01$.

Table 3 shows that significantly more PBMC survived after sonoporation ($64.8 \pm 1.51\%$) for "PULSE US, GFP" than electroporation ($53.7 \pm 1.53\%$); a Two-Sample Assuming Unequal Variances t-Test between "PULSE US, GFP" and "Electrical, GFP" resulted in $P < 0.0004$. Table 3 also indicates that significantly ($P < 0.015$) more PBMC showed fluorescence after sonoporation ($2.73 \pm 0.21\%$) than electroporation ($0.43 \pm 0.06\%$). They are both significantly higher than the "PULSE US, No GFP" case ($0.13 \pm 0.06\%$).

It was shown that right after the treatment, the viable cell concentration was reduced to $46\% \pm 9\%$ and $49\% \pm 4\%$, and subsequently increased to $72\% \pm 8\%$ and $80\% \pm 36\%$ of their initial value (1×10^6/mL), after 20 hours of incubation for sonoporation and electroporation respectively (Pepe, 2004). These numbers were statistically indistinguishable ($p < 0.05$) between sonoporation and electroporation. It was also demonstrated that compared with sonoporation, electroporation had superior cell viability ($65.8 \pm 2.3\%$ *vs* $50.8 \pm 4.15\%$) and transfection efficiency ($15.83 \pm 3.5\%$ *vs* $7.53 \pm 0.4\%$) for Jurkat lymphocytes (nonprimary cells), and sonoporation was better in terms of viability ($64.8 \pm 1.51\%$ *vs* $53.7 \pm 1.53\%$) and transfection efficiency ($2.73 \pm 0.21\%$ *vs* $0.43 \pm 0.06\%$) for human peripheral blood mononuclear cells (PBMC) (primary cells). In *in vitro* applications of DNA delivery, it has been shown that sonoporation is a promising alternative to electroporation.

Our experimental results suggest that sonoporation is more effective than electroporation in transfection for one type of primary cells. This finding makes sonoporation an attractive alternative tool. Further studies are needed to verify this result for other primary cells.

In our experiments, 25 μg CMV-GFP per mL cell sample was used. In our preliminary tests, we varied the concentration of CMV-GFP to maximize the transfection efficiency. We found that 25 μg CMV-GFP per mL was the optimum concentration; this finding was in agreement with the conclusion reached by Greenleaf *et al.* (1998). We also tried different *in situ* spatial peak-pressure amplitude for our experiments and found that 1.5 MPa for PULSE US modes provided the best combination of transfection efficiency and cell viability (*i.e.*, high transfection efficiency and minimal cell death). It is known (Wu & Tong, 1998) that Optison® is not stable under ultrasonic excitations, with a relatively high acoustic pressure. The majority of EMB are destroyed after a short time of exposure of moderate ultrasound intensity. The life-time of most Optison® is probably quite short for the exposure level used. It is more effective using the multiple-exposure procedure by adding fresh Optison® between two exposures.

Electroporation is a relatively mature technique compared with sonoporation (Neumann, 1989). The choice for electroporation parameters used in this study was based on several publications (Chow *et al.*, 1999; Eksioglu-Demiralp *et al.*, 2003). In general, high voltage would generate high transfection efficiency and also low cell viability. Particularly, Eksioglu-Demiralp *et al.* (2003) did an extensive study, and they found that for the same commercial system, the same parameters as used in this study gave the optimum transfection and viability for Jurkat and PBMC.

6. Delivery of Antibodies and Anticancer Drug Using Sonoporation and Electroporation

Instead of the delivery of plasmid DNA into cell nuclei, antibodies such as anti-rabbit IgG conjugated with fluorophore (Alexafluor 647, Molecular Probes, Eugene, Oregon), anti-mouse IgD conjugated with fluorescein isothyocyanate-dextran (FITC, Pharmingen, San Diego, CA) and the anticancer drug Adriamycin hydrochloride (ADR), also known as doxorubicin hydrochloride (Sigma-Aldrich, St. Louis, MO 63103), were delivered into the cytoplasm of PBMC and Jurkat lymphocytes.

It was reported that the commercial ADR drug has been used successfully to produce regression in disseminated neoplastic conditions such as acute lymphoblastic leukemia, acute myeloblastic leukemia, soft tissue and bone sarcomas, breast carcinoma, ovarian carcinoma, transitional cell bladder carcinoma, thyroid carcinoma, gastric carcinoma, Hodgkin's disease, malignant lymphoma and bronchogenic carcinoma, *etc.* ADR provided by Sigma-Aldrich has a molecular weight of 580 Da. It shows fluorescence at 585 nm, excited by photons of 470 nm wavelength. Fluorophore (Alexafluor 647) and FITC were used as markers for detection of the successful delivery of the antibody.

Antibodies play an essential role in immunity. Antibodies are often used as clinical therapy to block the interaction of soluble molecules with their receptors, and to prevent the initiation of the signaling pathways triggered by the receptor. Antibodies can also be used to block intracellular pathways when they recognize proteins involved in signaling pathways, transcription factors, and cytoskeleton *etc.* Antibodies are usually hydrophobic and large in size; it has been a challenge to send them into the cytoplasm of a cell because of the protection of the cell membrane. Direct microinjection of antibodies has been frequently done in adherent cells of large size, but microinjection is almost impossible in small suspension cells such as lymphocytes. The molecular weight of antibodies varies. For example, IgG, the major immunoglobulin in human serum, has a molecular weight of 150,000 Da and another immunoglobulin in the blood serum, IgD, has a molecular weight of 180,000 Da.

6.1. *Cell preparation*

Refer to Sec. 5.2.

6.2. *Ultrasound exposure and calibration*

For US exposures, both Jurkat cells and PBMC were prepared in the same manner. The cells were counted with a hemacytometer (Hausser Scientific Co., Horsham, PA) and diluted to a concentration of 10^6/mL in RPMI supplemented with 15 μL anti rabbit IgG, conjugated with Alexafluor 647 of 2 mg/mL concentration, or 20 μL anti mouse IgD conjugated with FITC of 0.5 mg/mL. For the ADR case, we added 0.1 μL of 10 mg/mL concentration to each 1 mL sample. This brought the sample concentration to 1 in 10,000 by volume. The ADR is added right before the application of US. In all cases, one mL of the solution was placed in a 12×75 mm culture tube (VWR Scientific, West Chester, PA, USA) with 100 μL Optison®; its initial bubble concentration obtained from the commercial vial is $5.0 - 8.0 \times 10^8$/mL. The final bubble concentration is 4.5–7.3×10^7/mL.

The US exposure system, exposure time and parameters are described in Sec. 5.3.

6.3. *Flow Cytometer*

Refer to Sec. 5.5.

6.4. *Experimental results and discussion*

Figures 3 and 4 contain typical pictures showing that anti mouse IgD conjugated with fluorescein isothyocyanate-dextran (FITC) was delivered into Jurkat lymphocytes and PBMC respectively; they were observed and captured using a confocal microscope (objective $\times$ 60) (Bio Rad, MRC 1024 ES CLSM, Hercules, CA). For both cases, pictures on the left panel are for a

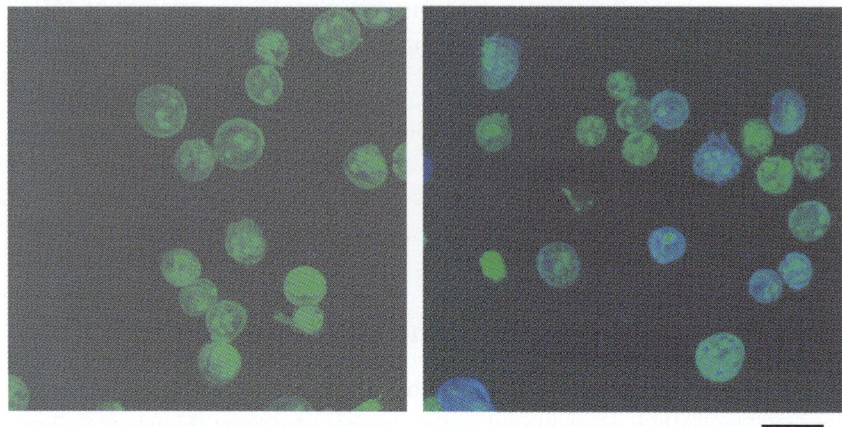

30 µm

Fig. 3. Pictures taken from a confocal microscope (objective × 60) (Bio Rad, MRC 1024 ES CLSM, Hercules, CA) show that anti mouse IgD conjugated with fluorescein isothyocyanate-dextran (FITC) was delivered into Jurkat lymphocytes. A picture on the left is for a control case (sham-exposed) and that on the right is for a case after sonoporation. The scale bar is 30 μm long.

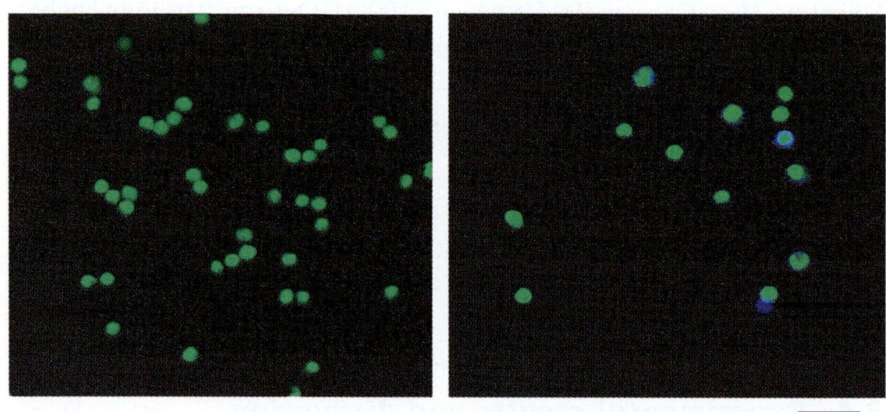

30 µm

Fig. 4. Pictures taken from a confocal microscope (objective × 60) (Bio Rad, MRC 1024 ES CLSM, Hercules, CA) show that anti mouse IgD conjugated with fluorescein isothyocyanate-dextran (FITC) was delivered into PBMC. A picture on the left is for a control case (sham-exposed) and that on the right is for a case after sonoporation. The scale bar is 30 μm long.

control case (sham-exposed) and those on the right panel are for a case after sonoporation. The initial color of cells was green as shown in the pictures for the control case, and became blue or partially blue after anti mouse IgD, conjugated with fluorescein isothyocyanate-dextran (FITC), was delivered into them as shown in the picture on the right.

Experimental results obtained using a flow cytometer are presented by tables. Data in each column represents the mean $\pm$ one standard deviation (SD) of three samples ($n = 3$) prepared in the same manner described above and treated identically. Table 4 summarized the results of the delivery of goat anti rabbit IgG and anti mouse IgD into Jurkat lymphocytes using sonoporation. The second and 4th columns listed the results of the control (sham-exposed); the delivery efficiency baseline was $1.6 \pm 0.0\%$ and cell viability was $87.2\pm0.62\%$ for IgG, and the delivery efficiency baseline was $1.33\pm0.31\%$ and cell viability was $92.0\pm0.42\%$ for IgD. The third and 5th columns are for the results for IgG and IgD deliveries respectively using US. The delivery efficiency and viability are now $78.60\pm3.6\%$ and $81.1\pm0.44\%$ for IgG, and $34.9 \pm 1.80\%$ and $65.7 \pm 2.21\%$ for IgD. If we subtract the delivery efficiency baseline (control) from the data, we obtain the net delivery efficiency 77.0% for IgG and 33.57% for IgD. Table 5 shows the results of delivery of goat anti rabbit IgG and anti mouse IgD into PBMC *via* sonoporation. Again, the second and 4th columns are for the controls of IgG and IgD respectively; the delivery efficiencies were $11.3\pm0.81\%$ (baseline) and cell viability was $81.1 \pm 2.32\%$ for IgG, and the delivery efficiencies were $1.66 \pm 0.06\%$ (baseline) and cell viability was $67.9 \pm 4.30\%$ for IgD. The third and 5th columns were for IgG and IgD delivery using US. The delivery efficiency and viability now are $57.50 \pm 4.32\%$ and $61.1 \pm 4.32\%$ for IgG, and $32.5 \pm 4.36\%$ and $61.8 \pm 3.89\%$ for IgD. The net delivery

Table 4. Antibody delivery efficiency and cell viability for Jurkat lymphocytes.

	NO US, Goat Anti-Rabbit IgG	US, Goat Anti-Rabbit IgG	NO US, Anti-Mouse IgD	US, Anti-Mouse IgD
Efficiency (%)	1.60 ± 0.00	78.60 ± 3.60	1.33 ± 0.31	34.9 ± 1.80
Cell Viability (%)	87.2 ± 0.62	81.1 ± 0.44	92.0 ± 0.42	65.7 ± 2.21

Table 5. Antibody delivery efficiency and cell viability for PBMC.

	NO US, Goat Anti-Rabbit IgG	US, Goat Anti-Rabbit IgG	NO US, Anti-Mouse IgD	US, Anti-Mouse IgD
Efficiency (%)	11.3 ± 0.81	57.5 ± 4.23	1.66 ± 0.06	32.5 ± 4.36
Cell Viability (%)	81.1 ± 2.32	61.1 ± 4.23	67.9 ± 4.30	61.8 ± 3.89

efficiencies are 46.2% (57.50% − 11.3%) and 30.84% (32.5%–1.66%) for IgG and IgD respectively.

The delivery efficiencies measured by the flow cytometer are correlated with the ratio of the number of cells shown in blue and the total number of cells on the right panel accurately shown in Figs. 3 and 4. From the data, we also conclude that the delivery efficincy was higher for Jurkat cells than that for PBMC.

Table 6 summarizes the results of anti cancer drug (ADR) delivery into Jurkat cells. Drug delivery efficiency is defined as the number of cells that showed fluorescence divided by the total number of cells. Columns 2–4 are three different control cases involving no US, no ADR; US, no ADR and no US, ADR. Delivery efficiencies for all three are 0.17 ± 0.14, 0.29 ± 0.08, and 0.42 ± 0.36 respectively. Column 5 shows that with US and ADR, the delivery efficiency reached 4.80 ± 2.04%, much higher than that of any control case. A t-test assuming unequal variance was applied between US + ADR case, and in any of the control case, we obtained $p = 0.03$ (one-tail).

Obviously, for the US, No ADR case, the percentage of dead cells is relatively high, *i.e.*, sonoporation without ADR also killed about 24.1% cells, yet the delivery efficiency for this case is small (0.29 ± 0.08%).

Table 6. Anticancer drug (ADR) delivery efficiency for Jurkat lymphocytes.

	No US, No ADR	US, No ADR	No US, ADR	US, ADR
Live Cell (%)	93.2 ± 1.56	72.1 ± 4.03	91.5 ± 0.79	62.3 ± 8.99
Dead Cells (%)	5.49 ± 1.50	24.1 ± 3.97	5.99 ± 0.45	33.87 ± 9.39
Drug Delivery Efficiency (%)	0.17 ± 0.14	0.29 ± 0.08	0.42 ± 0.04	4.80 ± 2.04

One may also note that a sum of the number of live cells and that of dead cells is slightly less than 100%. This is because there were some cells scattered outside of the gates chosen during analysis of the flow cytometer data; errors incurred due to those cells are negligibly small.

6.5. *Discussion and summary*

Our experimental results suggest that sonoporation may be a promising technique in delivering DNA, antibodies and anticancer drugs into the cells. Optimization of the acoustic parameters to maximize the delivery efficacy and more experiments to test other cells, antibodies and anti cancer drugs are certainly needed. Our results also indicate that sonoporation is less effective in delivering DNA and antibodies into primary (PBMC), than nonprimary cells (Jurkat cells). In general, it seems to be true that it is much more difficult to deliver foreign microscopic objects into primary cells than non-primary cells; electroporation technique also demonstrated this same pattern (Pepe *et al.*, 2004). This phenomenon may be related to the fast replication and multiplication nature of nonprimary cells.

Our results also suggest that the threshold US amplitude to generate reparable sonoporation is US exposure time dependent. The longer the exposure time, the smaller the US amplitude needed. The possible physical mechanisms causing the sonoporation described in this chapter are believed to be bubble activity related. Particularly, when a moderate US amplitude (0.1–0.2 MPa at 1 or 2 MHz) is used, EMB may oscillate steadily as shown in Fig. 2. If cells are very close to the oscillating EMB, the shear stress introduced by the EMB at the cell membrane may be large enough to cause the reparable sonoporation (refer to Appendix). In this case, the exposure time may be in the order of minutes or tens minutes. Its advantage is the ease in controling but the delivery efficiency may be low. On the other hand, if larger US amplitude is used, more EMB would vibrate vigorously and break into free bubbles, and it would require shorter US exposure time to cause the reparable sonoporation, introducing more lethal sonoporation.

To verify that shear stress generated by the microstreaming near an oscillating EMB, that may be the source of reparable sonoporation, we designed an experiment using a vibrating Mason horn to generate shear stress (Wu *et al.*, 2002). A Mason horn was made in our laboratory consisting of a stainless steel stepped (exponentially tapered) bar glued to a cylindrical PZT tube transducer (3 mm thickness, 10.5 cm long and 2.5 cm diameter). This vibrator was tuned to 21.4 kHz. The total length of the cylindrical metallic probe was 17 cm and the tip diameter of the smallest section of the probe was 400 μm. The Mason horn was driven by a Hewlett Packard 3314A function generator (Agilent Technologies, Palo Alto, CA) and an ENI 2100L RF power amplifier (ENI, Rochester, NY). The oscillation of the tip was along the transverse direction and the transverse displacement was measured using a calibrated microscope. Near the tip of the Mason horn, a symmetrical microstreaming pattern was generated as shown in Fig. 5. The shear stress produced near the tip of the Mason horn due to the microstreaming was then calculated using Eq. (3), after the displacement amplitude of the Mason horn, ε_0, was measured. Here, Ro in the equation is the radius of the tip of the Mason horn.

Reparable sonoporation was observed in Jurkat lymphocytes in suspension exposed to the vibrating Mason horn tuned to 21.4 KHz. Its transverse displacement amplitude was 7.8 μm. It was found that the shear stress associated with microstrearning surrounding the Masonhorn tip was the primary reason for the cell reparable sonoporation. The threshold shear stress was determined to be 12 ± 4 Pa, for exposure time up to 7 min. It was also found that the shorter the exposure time, the greater the threshold.

The measured acoustic pressure amplitude generated by the vibrating Mason horn was 4,100 Pa, too low to produce inertial cavitation.

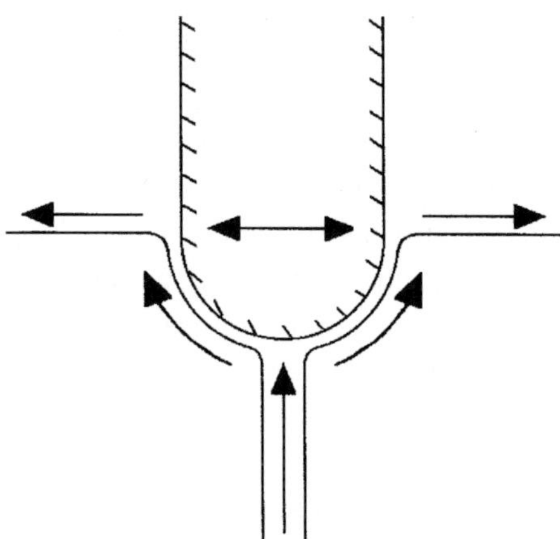

Fig. 5. Microstreaming pattern observed around the Mason horn tip (Wu *et al.*, 2002).

Furthermore, no bubble or bubble activity was observed during insonification *via* usual observation, or by the hydrophone as a passive cavitation detector (Roy *et al.*, 1990). These facts suggest that the microstreaming was the primary source of the reparable sonoporation observed.

Appendix

A theoretical model has been developed to describe the acoustic response of an EMB (de Jong *et al.*, 1994) that has a surrounding layer of human serum albumin. The human serum albumin layer of the encapsulated gas bubbles introduces two parameters relevant to the bubble behaviors in a sound field: S_p, a shell elastic parameter and S_f, a shell friction factor. The values of S_p and S_f are estimated to be 8 N/m and 4×10^{-6} Ns/m respectively (de Jong *et al.*, 1994). The nonlinear differential equation (RPNNP equation) to describe nonlinear bubble oscillations was developed and modified by Rayleigh, Plesset, Noltingk, Neppiras and Poritsky. By introducing S_p and S_f, the following equation was used by de Jong:

$$\ddot{R} R \rho + \frac{3}{2} \rho \dot{R}^2 = (p_0 + 2\sigma/R_0)(R_0/R)^{3\kappa} - p_0 - 2\sigma/R$$
$$- 2S_p(1/R_0 - 1/R)$$
$$- [4\eta/R^2 + S_f/(4\pi R^3)]\dot{R} R + P_{ac}, \qquad (A.1)$$

where σ is surface tension of a liquid, p_0 is the atmospheric pressure, κ is polytropic exponent, and P_{ac} is time varying applied acoustic pressure. For megahertz frequencies the viscous damping dominates (Coakley and Nyborg, 1978) and therefore only this mechanism has been considered here.

Under the linear approximation, the resonance frequency of an encapsulated gas bubble can be calculated as

$$f_r = \frac{1}{2\pi} \sqrt{\frac{3\kappa}{\rho R_0^2} \left(p_0 + \frac{2\sigma}{R_0} \right) - \frac{2\sigma}{\rho R_0^3} + \frac{2S_p}{\rho R_0^3}}. \qquad (A.2)$$

Table A.1 lists the numerical values of f_r versus R_0 when S_p changes. The albumin shell of Optison® bubbles increases the resonance frequency of the bubbles significantly. For example, for $R_0 = 2\,\mu$m, f_r increases from 2.04 MHz to 7.40 MHz when S_p increases from 0 (free bubbles) to 8 N/m (Optison). If the mean radius of the microbubbles of Optison® is between 1 to 2.5 μm, the corresponding resonance frequency should be in the range

Table A.1. Resonance frequency *vs* radius for various S_p.

$R_0(\mu m)$	$S_p = 8\,\text{N/m}$	$S_p = 4.2\,\text{N/m}$	$S_p = 0$
	F_0 (MHz)	F_0 (MHz)	F_0 (MHz)
0.50	58.20	42.90	11.7
1.00	20.70	15.40	4.74
1.50	11.30	8.50	2.87
2.00	7.40	5.60	2.04
2.50	5.30	4.00	1.57
3.00	4.10	3.10	1.28
3.50	3.30	2.50	1.07
4.00	2.70	2.00	0.93
4.50	2.30	1.70	0.81
5.00	1.90	1.50	0.72
5.50	1.70	1.30	0.65
6.00	1.50	1.20	0.59
6.50	1.30	1.00	0.55
7.00	1.20	0.90	0.50
7.50	1.10	0.85	0.47
8.00	0.99	0.78	0.44
8.50	0.91	0.72	0.41
9.00	0.84	0.66	0.39
9.50	0.78	0.62	0.36
10.00	0.72	0.58	0.35

of 5.3 to 20.7 MHz, which usually lies at the high end of, or beyond the range of diagnostic ultrasound frequencies.

If we let $P_{ac} = p \sin 2\pi f_0 t$, $\rho = 998\,\text{kg/m}^3$, $\eta = 0.00128\,\text{Pa s}$ (measured value for the suspension, see Wu *et al.*, 2001), $\sigma = 0.072\,\text{N/m}$, $\kappa = 1.4$ (it was suggested to the author to use 1.09 instead of 1.4 because Optison$^{®}$ bubbles contain C_3F_8. It turned out that the results were insensitive to κ values in this case), $S_p = 8\,\text{N/m}$, $S_f = 4 \times 10^{-6}\,\text{Ns/m}$, $R(0) = R_0$ (R_0 is the equilibrium radius of the bubble), and $\dot{R}(0) = 0$, Eq. (A.1) can be solved numerically using Mathematica$^{®}$ (Wolfram Research, Inc., Champaign, Illinois). Figure A.1 is a plot of $(R - R_0)/R_0$ versus normalized time (in the unit of $1/f_0$) for $p = 0.1$ MPa and 0.4 MPa and $R_0 = 2\,\mu m$. The results show that since the frequency of acoustic field ($f_0 = 1$ or 2 MHz) is far from resonance frequency ($f_r = 7.8$ MHz), the change

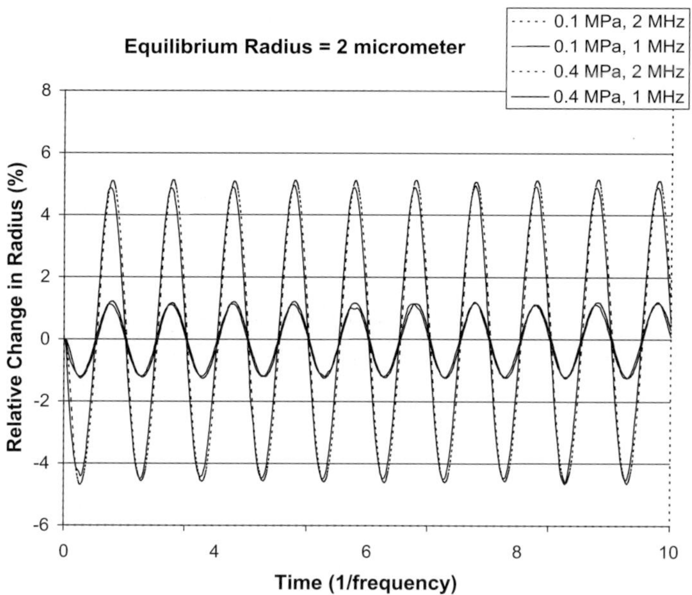

Fig. A.1. Percentage change in radius versus time of encapsulated bubbles (2.0 micron radius) driven by various combinations of external acoustic pressure amplitudes.

of radius is relatively small for both 1 MHz and 2 MHz. For most cases (not shown), the response of Optison$^{®}$ bubbles to the acoustic fields is not symmetric; the positive amplitude $(+)$ of $(R - R_0)/R_0$ is not necessarily equal to the negative amplitude $(-)$ of $(R - R_0)/R_0$. Using the results of numerical calculations, response curves of Optison$^{®}$ (radial displacement versus equilibrium radius for various p and f_0) can be plotted. Figure A.2 contains results of the response curves for $+$ amplitude and $-$ amplitude of $(R - R_0)/R_0$ versus R_0. The response curves show that when $p = 0.4$ MPa, the peak radii, 5.1 and 8.0 μm, corresponding to 1 MHz and 2 MHz, respectively are very close to resonance radii predicted by the linear approximation (see Table A.1). After the Optison bubble response to the ultrasonic field is calculated, the time average shear stress associated with the microstreaming near the bubble with a cell attached can be calculated using Eq. (3). The result is plotted in Fig. A.2. Figure A.3 shows shear stress as a function of R_0 when the amplitude of acoustic field is 0.4 MPa. The shear stress, for example, associated with 1 and 2 MHz is 170 Pa and 530 Pa respectively for R_0 equal to 2.5 μm.

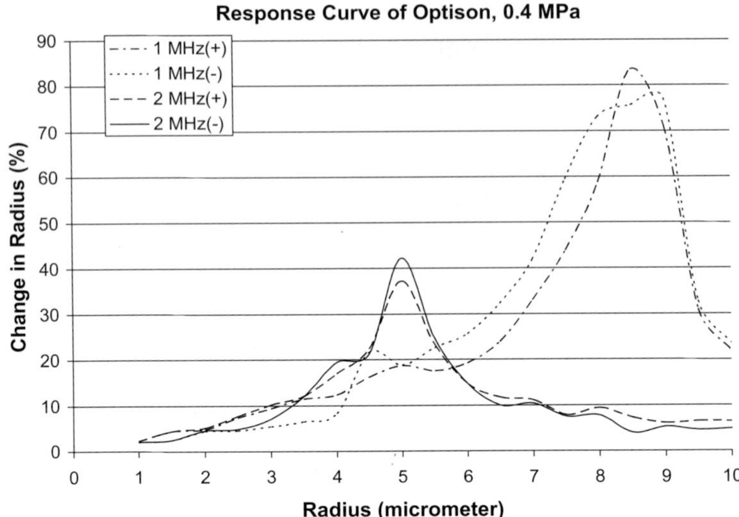

Fig. A.2. Percentage change in radius versus radius of encapsulated bubbles driven by 0.4 MPa ultrasound at 1 and 2 MHz.

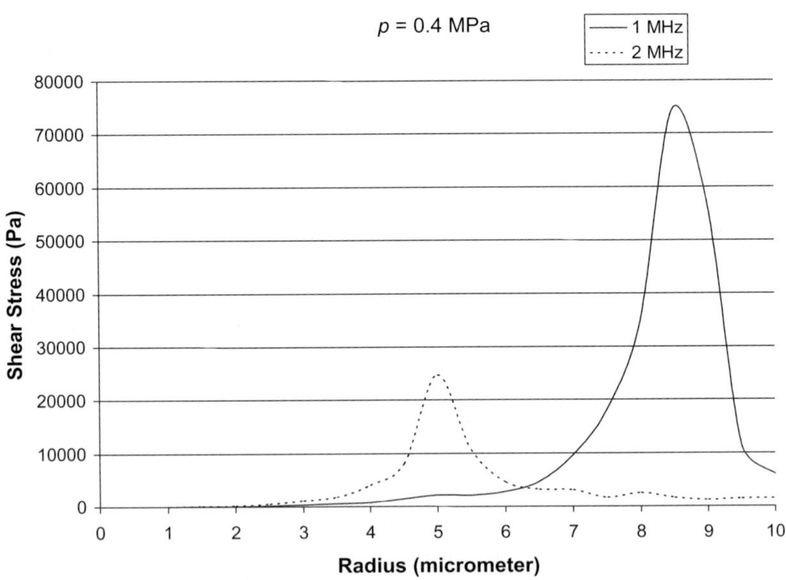

Fig. A.3. Shear stress versus radius of encapsulated bubbles driven by 0.4 MPa ultrasound at 1 and 2 MHz.

When the encapsulated bubbles break into free bubbles ($S_p = 0$), the free bubbles respond to the ultrasound field more vigorously than their parent encapsulated microbubbles since they are closer to resonance size bubble (see $S_p = 0$ cases as shown in Table A.1). Figure A.4 contains numerical solutions of Eq. (A.1) for free bubbles of $R_0 = 2\,\mu$m responding to 1 MHz and 2 MHz ultrasound fields of 0.1 MPa acoustic pressure amplitude. The relative change of radius $(R - R_0)/R_0$ reached 300% and 50% respectively for 1 MHz and 2 MHz ultrasound. It was only about 3% for encapsulated bubbles under the same conditions as shown in Fig. A.1. The shear stress associated with microstreaming is proportional to the square of the radial displacement as indicated by Eq. (3). In contrast to encapsulated bubbles cases discussed above, Fig. A.4 also suggests that for free bubbles of $R_0 = 2\,\mu$m, 1 MHz ultrasound generates higher shear stress than 2 MHz. Furthermore, other phenomena such as high local temperature and internal gas pressure, shock wave formation etc. related to vigorous bubble oscillations may also occur (Apfel, 1997). Therefore, it is conceivable that during the early stage of ultrasound exposure (the first few seconds), the inertial cavitation of free bubbles may play an important role in lethal

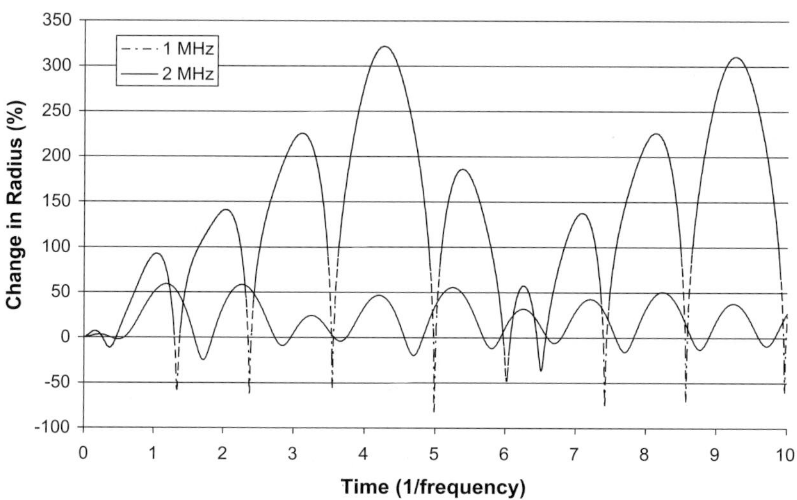

Fig. A.4. Percentage change in radius versus time of free bubbles (2.0 micron radius) driven by 1 and 2 MHz ultrasound of 0.1 MPa.

sonoporation and fragmentation of cells. According to our experience, a portion of Optison® bubbles actually broke up at the acoustic pressure level of 0.1 MPa. This process usually takes place swiftly; the time scale is about a second. For effects of longer time exposure, up to 10 min, microstreaming surrounding encapsulated bubbles may play an important role in reparable sonoporation.

References

Apfel RE. Sonic effervescence: A tutorial on acoustic cavitation, *J Acoust Soc Am* (1997) **101**: 1227–1237.

Bao S, Thrall BD, Miller DL. Transfection of a reporter plasmid into cultured cells by sonoporation *in vitro*. *Ultrasound Med Biol* (1997) **23**: 953–959.

Beissner K. Radiation force and force balance, in *Ultrasonic Exposimetry*, Ziskin M, Lewin P (eds.) (1992) CRC Press: Roca Raton, FL.

Coakley WT, Nyborg WL. Cavitation: Dynamics of gas bubbles, in *Ultrasound: Its Applications in Medicine and Biology, Part I*, Fry FJ (ed.) (1978) Elsevier Scientific Publishing Co., Amsterdam.

Chow CW, Rincon M, Davis RJ. Requirement for transcription factor NFAT in interleukin-2 expression. *Mol Cell Biol* (1999) **19**: 2300–2307.

Eksioglu-Demiralp E, Kitada S, Carson D, Garland J, Andreef M, Reed JC. A method for functional evaluation of caspase activation pathways in intact lymphoid cells using electroporation-mediated protein delivery and flow cytometric analysis, *J Immunol Meth* (2003) **275**: 41–56.

De Jong N, Cornet R, Lancee CT. Higher harmonics of vibrating gas-filled microspheres. Part one: Simulations. *Ultrasonics* (1994) **32**: 447–453.

Elder AE. Cavitation microstreaming. *J Acoust Soc Am* (1959) **31**: 54–64.

Greenleaf WJ, Bolander ME, Sarkar G, Goldring MB, Greenleaf JF. Artificial cavitation nuclei significantly enhance acoustically induced cell transfection. *Ultrasound Med Biol* (1998) **24**: 587–595.

Lasic DD. *Liposomes: From Physics to Applications* (1993) Elsevier Scientific Publishing Co., Amsterdam.

Lawrie A, Brisken AF, Francis SE. Microbubble-enhanced ultrasound for vascular gene delivery. *Gene Ther* (2000) **7**: 2023–2027.

Lewin PA, Bjørnø L. Acoustically induced shear stress in the vicinity of microbubbles in tissue. *J Acoust Soc Am* (1982) **71**: 728–734.

Lu QL, Liang HD, Partridge T, Blomley MJ. Microbubble ultrasound improves the efficiency of gene transduction in skeletal muscle *in vivo* with reduced tissue damage. *Gene Ther* (2003) **10**: 396–405.

Miller DL, Bao S, Morris JE. Sonoporation of cultured cells in the rotating tube exposure system. *Ultrasound Med Biol* (1999) **25**: 143–149.

Miller DL, Dou C, Song J. DNA transfer and cell killing in epidermoid cells by diagnostic ultrasound activation of contrast agent gas bodies *in vitro*. *Ultrasound Med Biol* (2003) **29**: 601–607.

NCRP. Exposure criteria for medical diagnostic ultrasound: II. Criteria based on all known mechanisms, *National Council on Radiation Protection and Measurements* (2002) NCRP Publications, Bethesda, MD.

Neumann E, Sowers AE, Jordan CA. *Electroporation and Electrofusion in Cell Biology* (1989) Plenum Press: New York.

Nyborg WL. Acoustic streaming near a boundary. *J Acoust Soc Am* (1958) **30**: 329–339.

Pepe J, Rincon M, Wu J. Experimental comparison of sonoporation and electroporation in cell transfection applications. *Acoust Res Lett* (2004) **5**: 62–67.

Roy AR, Madanshetty SI, Apfel RE. An acoustic backscattering technique for the detection of transient cavitation produced by microsecond pulses of ultrasound. *J Acoust Soc Am* (1990) **87**: 2451–2458.

Vasir JK, Reddy MK, Labhasetwar VD. Nanosystems in drug targeting: Opportunities and challenges. *Curr Nanosci* (2005) **1**: 47–64.

Ward M, Wu J, Chiu JF. Ultrasound-induced cell lysis and sonoporation by enhanced by contrast agents. *J Acoust Soc Am* (1999) **105**: 2951–2957.

Ward M, Wu J, Chiu JF. Experimental study on effects of Optison concentration on sonoporation *in vitro*. *Ultrasound Med Biol* (2000) **26**: 1169–1175.

Wu J, Du G. Acoustic streaming generated by a focused Gaussian beam and finite amplitude of tonebursts. *Ultrasound Med Biol* (1993) **19**: 167–176.

Wu J, Ross JR, Chiu JF. Reparable sonoporation generated by microstreaming. *J Acoust Soc Am* (2002) **111**: 1460–1464.

Wu J, Tong J. Experimental study of stability of contrast agents. *Ultrasound Med Biol* (1998) **24**: 257–265.

Wu J. Theoretical study on shear stress generated by microstreaming surrounding contrast agents attached to living cells. *Ultrasound Med Biol* (2002) **28**: 125–129.

Endnote

Permission is given by Elsevier to reproduce the following figures:
Figure 1 is reprinted from Fig. 7 from *Ultrasound Med Biol* **V26**: 1169–1175, Ward *et al.* "Experimental study on effects of Optison...," ©2000 World Federation of Ultrasound in Medicine and Biology. Figs. A.1, A.2, A.3 and A.4 are reprinted from Figs. 1, 3, 5(a) and 6 from *Ultrasound Med Biol* **V28**: 125–129, Wu: "Theoretical study on shear stress...," ©2002 World Federation of Ultrasound in Medicine and Biology.

VII

LOW-FREQUENCY SONOPHORESIS: ULTRASOUND-MEDIATED TRANSDERMAL DRUG DELIVERY

Samir Mitragotri

Transdermal drug delivery offers an attractive mode of drug administration. However, applications of transdermal drug delivery are limited due to low skin permeability. Application of ultrasound enhances skin permeability to a variety of molecules (sonophoresis). The enhancement induced by ultrasound is particularly significant at low frequencies ($f < 100\,\text{kHz}$, low-frequency sonophoresis). This chapter summarizes mechanisms and applications of low-frequency sonophoresis. *In vitro*, *in vivo*, as well as clinical studies demonstrating the effect of low-frequency ultrasound on transdermal drug delivery and glucose extraction are summarized. Mechanistic insights gained through a number of investigations are also reviewed. Reports on the synergistic effect of low-frequency ultrasound with other enhancers including chemicals and iontophoresis are also summarized. Finally, safety considerations of low-frequency sonophoresis are reviewed.

1. Introduction

Transdermal drug delivery offers several advantages over traditional drug delivery systems such as oral delivery and injections, especially in regard to protein delivery (Prausnitz *et al.*, 2004). These advantages include:

1.1. *Avoiding drug degradation in the gastrointestinal tract*

Orally administered drugs are highly susceptible to gastro-enteric and first pass metabolism. On the other hand, in the case of transdermal drug delivery, the drug diffuses through the skin and is absorbed by the capillary network under the skin. Accordingly, the gastro-intestinal metabolism of the drug is avoided.

1.2. *Better patient compliance*

Transdermal drug devices are easier to handle and use than injections. In addition, the pain associated with injections can also be avoided. These characteristics of transdermal drug delivery offer a significant advantage in cases where frequent drug doses are required, for example, in the case of insulin delivery.

1.3. *Sustained release of the drug can be obtained*

Transdermal drug delivery can provide sustained release of drugs over a sufficiently long time of approximately one week. Hence, it is possible to maintain a steady drug concentration in the blood. This is especially important for drugs with a narrow therapeutic window.

Transdermal drug delivery, however, suffers from the severe limitation that the permeability of the skin is very low. Therefore, it is difficult to deliver drugs across the skin at a therapeutically relevant rate. This, in fact, is the main reason why only a handful of low-molecular weight drugs are clinically administered by this route today. Development of transdermal products for macromolecules is primarily hindered by low skin permeability. Evolved to impede the flux of toxins into the body, skin naturally offers a very low permeability to the movement of foreign molecules across it. A unique hierarchical structure of lipid-rich matrix with embedded corneocytes in the upper strata ($15 \, \mu m$) of skin, stratum corneum (SC), is responsible for this barrier (Fig. 1). Overcoming this barrier safely and

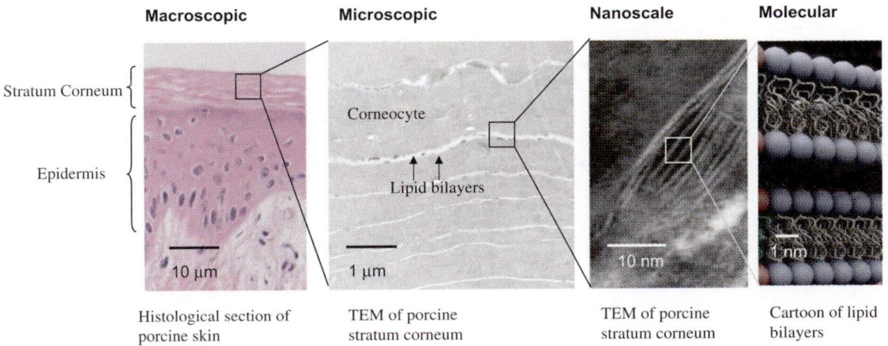

Fig. 1. Hierarchical organization of skin structure. (a) shows presence of stratum corneum and epidermis in a histological section of the skin. (b) shows a transmission electron micrograph (TEM) of corneocytes. (c) show the regions of intercellular lipid bilayers in TEM. (d) shows a schematic of intercellular lipid bilayers.

reversibly is a fundamental problem that persists in the field of transdermal delivery.

2. Ultrasound in Medical Application

Ultrasound is used in various medical therapies (Fig. 2) (Mitragotri, 2005) including lithotripsy (Coleman & Saunders, 1993), hyperthermia (Diederich & Hynnen, 1999), thrombolysis (Alexandrov, 2002), lipoplasty (Goes & Landecker, 2002), wound healing (Speed, 2001), fracture healing (Hadjiargyrou *et al.*, 1998), drug delivery (sonophoresis (Tezel *et al.*, 2001; Mitragotri & Langer, 1995a; Tang & Langer, 2002a), sonoporation (Guzman *et al.*, 2001; Sundaram & Mitragotri, 2002; Miller & Quddus, 2000; Wu *et al.*, 2002), triggered drug release (Nelson *et al.*, 2002; Price & Kaul, 2002; Kwok *et al.*, 2001; Kost & Leong, 1989), and targeted drug delivery (Linder, 2002; Unger *et al.*, 2001). A majority of these applications have emerged in the last decade. Ultrasound also has been used to enhance transdermal transport of various drugs including macromolecules (Tezel *et al.*, 2001; Mitragotri & Langer, 1995b; Tang *et al.*, 2002; Benson *et al.*, 1988; Benson *et al.*, 1989; Benson, 1991; Bommannan *et al.*, 1992a, b; Byl *et al.*, 1993; Cameroy, 1966; Ciccone *et al.*, 1991; Griffin & Touchstoe; Griffin *et al.*, 1967; Griffin & Touchstone, 1968;

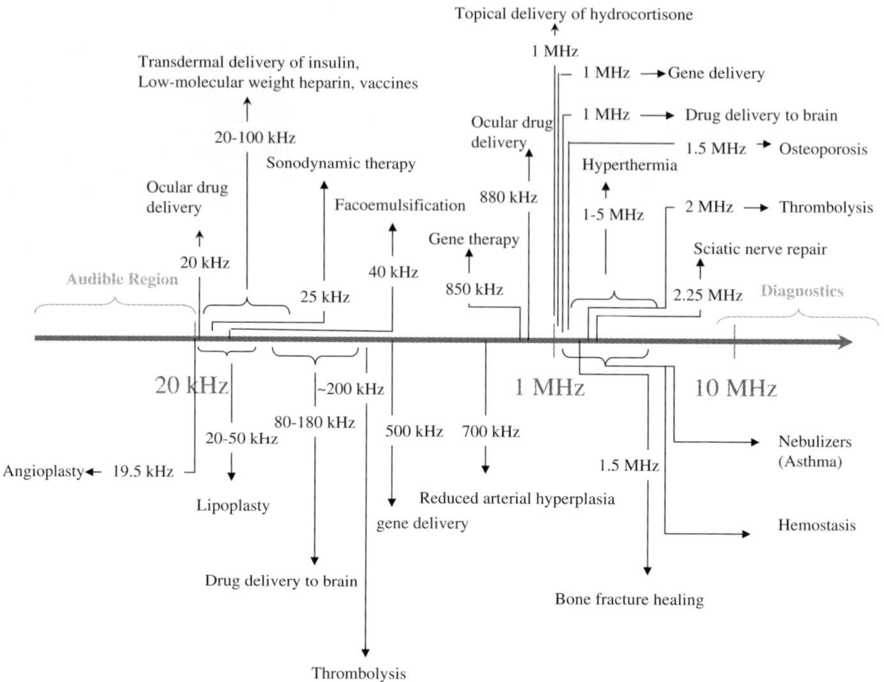

Fig. 2. Adopted from Mitragotri (2005). A partial summary of ultrasound frequencies used for medical applications. Each item in the figure corresponds to one or more literature reports. The figure provides an overview of the conditions used for medical ultrasound applications and does not necessarily depict optimal or recommended conditions. For many applications, more than one condition has been used. Only selected conditions are represented in figure for clarity. Ultrasound parameters other than frequency that are also critical to medical applications including the intensity (or pressure amplitude) and duty cycle (pulse width and repetition frequency) are not listed in the figure for clarity. A significant clustering of applications is found around a frequency of 1 MHz.

Griffin & Touchstone, 1972; Johnson *et al.*, 1996; Kleinkort & Wood, 1975; Kost & Langer, 1993; Kost *et al.*, 1996; Kost *et al.*, 1999; Kost *et al.*, 2000; Le *et al.*, 2000; Machluf & Kost, 1993; Menon *et al.*, 1994; Mitragotri, 1995; Mitragotri & Langer 1995b; Mitragotri *et al.* 1996a, b; Mitragotri, *et al.*, 1997; Mitragotri *et al.*, 2000, b; Mitragotri & Kost, 2000a, b; Mitragotri, 2000; Quillen, 1980; Roitt *et al.*, 1998; Tezel *et al.*, 2001; Terahara *et al.*, 2002; Tang *et al.*, 2002; Tang *et al.*, 2001; Tezel *et al.*, 2002a, b; Tezel *et al.*, 2003; Tachibana, 1992; Tachibana & Tachibana, 1993;

Tachibana & Tachibana 1991; Williams, 1990; Alvarez-Roman *et al.*, 2003; Merrino *et al.*, 2003; Merriono *et al.*, 2003; Weimann *et al.*, 2002; Joshi & Raje, 2002; Machet & Boucaud, 2002). This type of enhancement is termed sonophoresis, indicating the enhanced transport of molecules under the influence of ultrasound. Ultrasound at various frequencies in the range of 20 kHz–16 MHz has been used to enhance skin permeability. However, transdermal transport enhancement induced by low-frequency ultrasound ($f < 100$ kHz) has been found to be more significant than that induced by high frequency ultrasound (Tezel *et al.*, 2001; Mitragotri & Langer, 1995a; Boucaud *et al.*, 2002).

3. Historical Overview of Sonophoresis

The first published report on sonophoresis dates back to 1950's. Fellinger and Schmidt (1954) reported successful treatment of polyarthritis of the hand's digital joints, using hydrocortisone ointment with sonophoresis. It was subsequently shown that hydrocortisone injection combined with ultrasound "massage" yielded better outcome, compared with simple hydrocortisone injections for bursitis treatment (Coodley, 1960). Cameroy (1966) reported success using carbocaine sonophoresis for closed Colle's fractures. In a series of publications, Griffin *et al.* showed improved treatment of elbow epicondylitis, bicipital tendonitis, shoulder osteoarthritis, shoulder bursitis and knee osteoarthritis by combined application of hydrocortisone and ultrasound (Griffin *et al.*, 1967; Griffin & Touchstone, 1968; Griffin & Touchstone, 1972; Griffin, 1966). Improved dermal penetration using ultrasound was also reported for local anesthetics (Benson *et al.*, 1988; McElnay *et al.*, 1985; Moll *et al.*, 1979).

Studies demonstrated that ultrasound enhanced the percutaneous absorption of methyl and ethyl nicotinate by disordering the structured lipids in the stratum corneum. Similar conclusions were reached by Hofman and Moll (1993) who studied the percutaneous absorption of benzyl nicotinate. While several investigators reported positive effect of ultrasound on drug permeation, lack of an effect of ultrasound on skin permeation was also reported in certain cases. For example, Williams reported no detectable effect of 1.1 MHz ultrasound on the rate of penetration of three anesthetic preparations through human skin (Williams, 1990).

Levy *et al.* (1989) showed that 3–5 minutes of ultrasound exposure (1 MHz, 1.5 W/cm^2) increased transdermal permeation of mannitol and physostigmine across hairless rat skin *in vivo* by up to 15-fold. They also reported that the lag time typically associated with transdermal drug delivery was nearly-completely eliminated after exposure to ultrasound. Mitragotri *et al.* reported *in vitro* permeation enhancement of several low-molecular weight drugs under the same ultrasound conditions (Mitragotri & Langer, 1995a).

Bommanan *et al.* (1992) hypothesized that since the absorption coefficient of the skin varies directly with the ultrasound frequency, high frequency ultrasound energy would concentrate more in the epidermis, thus leading to higher enhancements. In order to assess this hypothesis, they studied the effect of high-frequency ultrasound (2 MHz–16 MHz) on the permeability of salicylic acid (dissolved in a gel) through hairless guinea pig skin *in vivo*. They found that a 20 minute application of ultrasound (0.2 W/cm^2) at a frequency of 2 MHz did not significantly enhance the amount of salicylic acid penetrating the skin. However, 10 MHz ultrasound under the otherwise same conditions resulted in a 4-fold increase and 16 MHz ultrasound resulted in ~2.5-fold increase in transdermal salicylic acid transport (Bommannan *et al.*, 1992a, b).

4. Low-Frequency Sonophoresis

Low-frequency sonophoresis has been a topic of extensive research only in the last 10 years or so. Tachibana *et al.* (1991, 1992, 1993) reported that application of low-frequency ultrasound (48 kHz) enhanced transdermal transport of lidocaine and insulin across hairless rat skin *in vivo*. They found that the blood glucose level of a hairless rat immersed in a beaker filled with insulin solution (20 U/ml) (1 U ~ 40 μg) and placed in an ultrasound bath (48 kHz, 5000 Pa), decreased by 50% in 240 minutes (Tachibana & Tachibana, 1991). They also showed that the application of ultrasound under similar conditions prolonged the anesthetic effect of transdermally administrated lidocaine in hairless rats (Tachibana & Tachibana, 1993) and enhanced transdermal insulin transport in rabbits. Mitragotri *et al.* (1995a, 1996b) showed that the application of ultrasound at even lower frequencies (20 kHz) enhances transdermal transport of various low-molecular weight drugs including corticosterone and high-molecular weight proteins such as insulin, γ-interferon, and erythropoietin across the human skin *in vitro*. Quantitatively, Mitragotri *et al.* compared the enhancement ratios (ratio of sonophoretic and passive permeabilities measured *in vitro* across human cadaver skin) induced by therapeutic ultrasound (1 MHz) and low-frequency ultrasound (20 kHz) for four permeants, butanol, corticosterone, salicylic acid, and sucrose. They found that the enhancement induced by low-frequency ultrasound is up to 1000-fold higher than that induced by therapeutic ultrasound (Mitragotri *et al.*, 1996b).

Low-frequency sonophoresis can be classified into two categories: simultaneous sonophoresis and pretreatment sonophoresis. Simultaneous sonophoresis corresponds to a simultaneous application of drug and ultrasound to the skin. This was the first mode in which low-frequency sonophoresis was shown to be effective. This method enhances transdermal transport in two ways: (i) enhanced diffusion through structural alterations of the skin and (ii) convection induced by ultrasound. Transdermal transport enhancement induced by this type of sonophoresis decreases after ultrasound is turned off (Mitragotri & Kost, 2000). Although this method can be used to achieve a temporal control over skin permeability, it requires that patients use a wearable ultrasound device for drug delivery. In pretreatment sonophoresis, a short application of ultrasound is used to permeabilize skin prior to drug delivery. The skin remains in a state of high permeability for several hours. Drugs can be delivered through permeabilized skin during this period. In this approach, the patient does not need to wear the ultrasound device.

5. Sonophoresis: Choice of Parameters

The enhancement induced by low-frequency sonophoresis is determined by four main ultrasound parameters, frequency, intensity, duty cycle, and application time. A detailed investigation of the dependence of permeability enhancement on frequency and intensity in the low-frequency regime (20 kHz < f < 100 kHz) has been reported by Tezel *et al.* (2001). At each

254 *S. Mitragotri*

frequency, there exists an intensity below which no detectable enhancement is observed. This intensity is referred to as the threshold intensity. Once the intensity exceeds this threshold, the enhancement increases strongly with the intensity until another threshold intensity, referred to as the decoupling intensity is reached. Beyond this intensity, the enhancement does not increase with further increase in intensity due to acoustic decoupling. The threshold intensity for porcine skin increased from $\sim 0.11\,\mathrm{W/cm^2}$ at 19.6 kHz to more than $2\,\mathrm{W/cm^2}$ at 93.4 kHz. At a given intensity, the enhancement decreased with increasing ultrasound frequency.

The dependence of enhancement on intensity, duty cycle, and application time can be combined into a single parameter, total acoustic energy, fluence delivered from the transducer, $E = It$, where I is the ultrasound intensity ($\mathrm{W/cm^2}$) during each pulse and t is the total "on time" (seconds). As a general trend, no significant enhancement is observed until a threshold energy fluence dose is reached (Fig. 3). The threshold energy fluence doses for various frequencies were found to be $10\,\mathrm{J/cm^2}$ for 19.6 kHz, $63\,\mathrm{J/cm^2}$ at 36.9 kHz, $103\,\mathrm{J/cm^2}$ at 58.9 kHz, $304\,\mathrm{J/cm^2}$ for 76.6 kHz, and $1{,}305\,\mathrm{J/cm^2}$ at 93.4 kHz. Thus, the threshold energy fluence dose increased by about

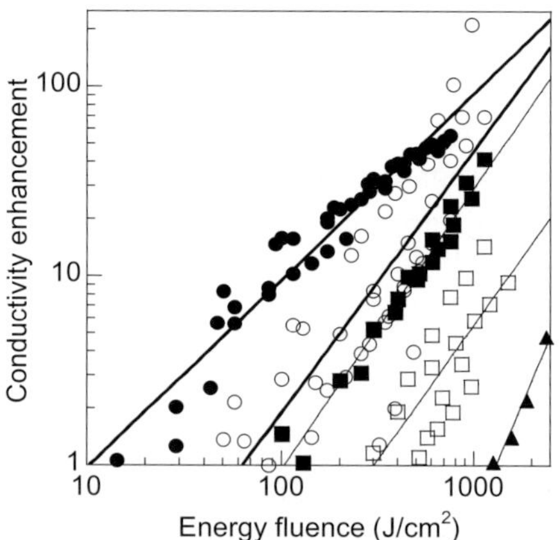

Fig. 3. Adopted from Tezel *et al.* (2001). Dependence of skin conductivity (indicator of skin permeability) on ultrasound energy density at five frequencies (filled circles — 19.6 kHz, open circles — 36.9 kHz, closed squares — 58.9 kHz, open squares — 76.6 kHz and closed triangles — 93.4 kHz).

130-fold, as the frequency increased from 19.6 kHz to 93.4 kHz. The dependence of enhancement on energy fluence after the threshold is different for different frequencies. For extremely high-energy doses (*e.g.*, 10^4 J/cm^2), the enhancement induced by all the frequencies is comparable. However, for lower energy fluence doses, the differences between various different frequencies are significant and the choice of frequency may affect the effectiveness of sonophoresis.

In addition to frequency and energy fluence, sonophoretic enhancement also depends on additional parameters including the distance between the transducer and the skin, gas concentration in the coupling medium, and the transducer geometry. Detailed dependence of enhancement on these parameters has not yet been studied.

6. Macromolecular Delivery

6.1. *Peptides and proteins*

Low-frequency sonophoresis has been shown to deliver several macromolecular drugs. Tachibana and Tachibana demonstrated that a 5 minute exposure to ultrasound (40 kHz, 3000–5000 Pa) induced a significant reduction of blood glucose levels in rats exposed to insulin (Tachibana & Tachibana, 1991). Specifically, the glucose level decreased to 34% of the initial value at lower pressures and to 22% of the initial value at higher acoustic pressures. Comparable results were obtained in rabbits at somewhat higher frequencies (*e.g.*, 150 kHz). Mitragotri *et al.* performed *in vitro* and *in vivo* evaluation of the effect of low-frequency ultrasound on transdermal delivery of proteins (Mitragotri & Langer, 1995a). Application of low-frequency ultrasound (20 kHz, 125 mW/cm^2, 100 msec pulses applied every second) enhanced transdermal transport of proteins including insulin, γ-interferon, and erythropoietin across human cadaver skin *in vitro* (Mitragotri & Langer, 1995a). Ultrasound under the same conditions delivered therapeutic doses of insulin across hairless rat skin *in vivo* from a chamber glued on the rat's back and filled with an insulin solution (100 U/ml) (Mitragotri & Langer, 1995a). A simultaneous application of insulin and ultrasound from outside (20 kHz, 225 mW/cm^2, 100 msec pulses applied every second) reduced the blood glucose level of diabetic hairless rats from approximately 400 mg/dL to 200 mg/dL in 30 minutes.

A corresponding increase in plasma insulin levels was observed during sonophoresis. Boucaud *et al.* (2002) also demonstrated a dose-dependent hypoglycemia in hairless rats exposed to ultrasound and insulin. At an energy dose of 900 J/cm^2, ~75% reduction in glucose levels was reported. Pretreatment of skin by low-frequency ultrasound (20 kHz, ~7 W/cm^2) has also been shown to enhance skin permeability to insulin (Mitragotri & Kost, 2004). More recently, Smith *et al.* (2003) have demonstrated ultrasonic transdermal insulin delivery in rabbits and rats with a low-profile two-by-two ultrasound array based on the cymbal transducer. In rats, the blood glucose decreased by 233 ± 22 mg/dL in 90 minutes after 5 minutes of pulsed ultrasound exposure. In rabbits, the glucose level was found to decrease to 133 ± 36 mg/dL from the initial baseline in 60 minutes.

6.2. *Low-molecular weight heparin*

Low-frequency ultrasound has also been shown to deliver low molecular weight heparin (LMWH) across the skin (Mitragotri & Kost, 2000b). Transdermal LMWH delivery was measured by monitoring aXa activity in the blood. No significant aXa activity was observed when LMWH was placed on non-treated skin. However, significant amount of LMWH was transported transdermally after ultrasound pretreatment. Anti-Factor X activity (aXa) in the blood increased slowly for ~2 hours, after which it increased rapidly before achieving a steady state after 4 hours at a value of about 2 U/ml (Mitragotri & Kost, 2000b). Effect of transdermally delivered LMWH was observed well beyond 6 hours in contrast to intravenous or subcutaneous injections, which resulted only in transient biological activity.

6.3. *Oligonucleotides*

Low-frequency ultrasound (LFS) has also been shown to enhance dermal penetration of oligonucleotides (ODN) (Tezel *et al.*, 2004). A 10-minute application of ultrasound (20 kHz and 2.4 W/cm^2) increased skin ODN permeability to 4.5×10^{-5} cm/hour, compared with nearly undetectable values across non-treated skin. A significant amount of ODN was also localized in the skin. Greater enhancements of ODN delivery were obtained by simultaneous application of ultrasound and ODN. Experiments performed with FITC-labeled ODN revealed that ODN is largely localized in the superficial layers of the skin. An estimate of local concentration of ODN in the skin was performed. Assuming a depth of penetration of 100–1000 μm, the estimated concentration of ODN in the skin at the end of ultrasound application was 0.53–5.3% of the donor concentration. ODN penetration into the skin due to LFS was heterogeneous. Heterogeneity of dermal penetration was visualized by monitoring penetration of a dye, sulforhodamine B (SRB) that was incorporated in the coupling medium. SRB penetration clearly indicated 4–5 intensely stained spots ($\sim$1 mm in diameter), which were termed as Localized Transport Pathways, LTPs. To further ensure that ODN penetrated into skin without losing integrity, skin exposed to ISIS 13920 in the presence of ultrasound was assessed using immunohistochemistry (Fig. 4). No visible staining was observed in the case of passive delivery, however, the skin treated with LFS was heavily stained, suggesting penetration of oligonucleotide delivery. ODN was localized in the epidermis as well as the dermis. Furthermore, microscopy studies suggested that ODN penetrated into epidermal cells. This is a particularly appealing feature since viable epidermal cells are an attractive target for ODN delivery.

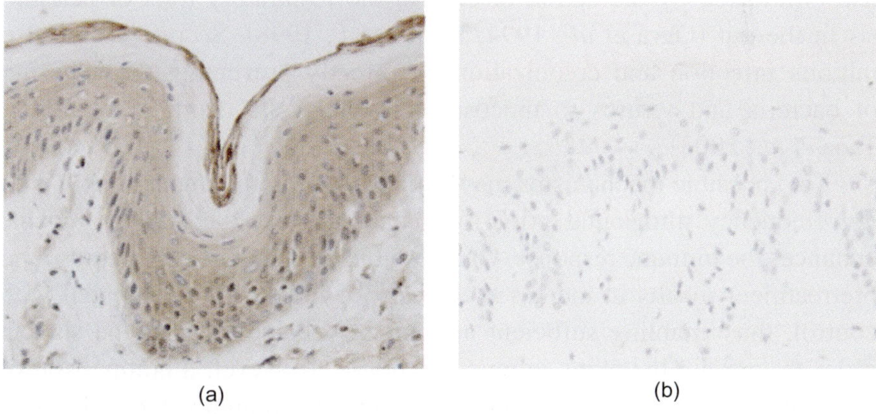

(a)   (b)

Fig. 4. Adopted from Tezel *et al.* (2004). (a) Penetration of oligonucleotides into porcine skin (Immunohistochemical staining) after ultrasound treatment. (b) Oligonucleotides penetration into control samples (no ultrasound).

6.4. *Vaccines*

Recently, low-frequency sonophoresis has also been used to deliver vaccines across the skin (Tezel *et al.*, 2005). Transcutaneous immunization (TCI) promises to be a potent novel vaccination technique since topical immunization elicits both systemic and mucosal immunity (Gockel *et al.*, 2000). The latter is of great importance, since a significant number of pathogens invade the host via mucosal surfaces (Ogra *et al.*, 1994). TCI is based on the premise that systemic and mucosal immune responses can be initiated by the stimulation of the Langerhans cells (LCs) in the skin.

Ultrasonic delivery of TTx generated strong IgG titers in animals. Delivery of 1.3 μg of TTx generated an immune response comparable to that induced by 10 μg subcutaneous injection. Studies have shown that IgG antibody titers generated by only 5 μg subcutaneous injection are sufficient for protection against a lethal dose of tetanus toxin (Scharton-Kersten *et al.*, 2000). Ultrasonic delivery of TTx also generated a strong mucosal immune response. A large number of TTx specific plasma cells were found in the intestine (unpublished data). Secretory IgA produced by local antibody secreting cells (ASC), *i.e.*, B-lymphocytes, is an important line of defense for mucosal surfaces such as the respiratory or intestinal track. The polymeric structure of the secretory IgA results in effective cross-linking of large antigens, which are then easily trapped in mucus and eliminated by the action of cilia in the respiratory tract or peristalsis in the gut (Ogra *et al.*, 1994; Roitt *et al.*, 1998). Secretory IgA also inhibits infection and colonization by directly preventing the adhesion of bacteria and viruses to mucosal epithelial cells (Roitt *et al.*, 1998; Tana *et al.*, 2003).

Two possible mechanisms may explain why pretreatment of skin with low-frequency ultrasound prior to contacting with the antigen vaccine enhances the immune response. One possible mechanism is that ultrasound pretreatment results in increased delivery of the vaccine compared with control, thus enabling sufficient amount of vaccine to enter the skin in order to activate the skins immune response. However, a comparison of the response obtained by TCI and subcutaneous immunization shows that IgG titers elicited by TCI are almost 10-fold more effective per dose compared with subcutaneous injections. The second mechanism involves the involvement of the Langerhans cells (LC) and the immune cells of the

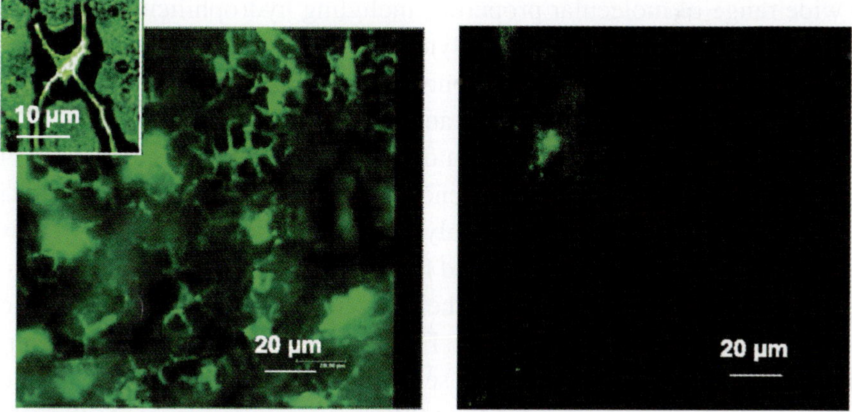

Fig. 5. Adopted from Tezel *et al.* (2005). Assessment of activation of skin's Langerhans cells with ultrasound treatment. (a) Mice skin stained with FITC-conjugated 2G9 antibody that reacts with the I-A^d and I-E^d MHC class II alloantigens 24 hours post ultrasound treatment. (a) Ultrasound + tetanus toxoid. (b) Control samples (no ultrasound).

skin that effectively capture the antigen and present it to the immune system. Clear activation of LCs was observed after ultrasonic TTx delivery (Fig. 5). LC activation is partly induced by the entry of the antigen and partly by the direct effect of ultrasound on skin. Mechanisms responsible for ultrasound-induced activation of LCs are not clear, although barrier disruption or release of pro-inflammatory signals by the keratinocytes are possible candidates.

7. Transdermal Extraction of Analytes Using Sonophoresis

Low-frequency ultrasound skin pretreatment has also been used to extract glucose and other analytes from the skin (*i.e.,* transport in the opposite direction; from the interstitial compartment through the skin into a reservoir filled with water placed on the top of the pretreated skin). Several analytes including glucose, calcium, albumin, urea, lactate, triglycerides, and dextran (the last analyte was injected intravenously) were extracted after the application of partial vacuum (10 inch Hg) across ultrasound-exposed rat skin for 15 minutes (Mitragotri *et al.*, 2000a, b). These analytes cover a wide range of molecular properties including hydrophilicity and molecular weight. For example, the analytes cover a molecular weight range of 62 (urea) to 70,000 (dextran). Concentrations of various analytes in the chamber at the end of extraction ranged from 0.2% to 3% of their serum values. Note that the volume of fluid Phosphate Buffered Saline (PBS) in the receiving chamber was 1 ml. Hence, the extracted analytes got diluted in this volume. Concentrations of analytes in the receiving chamber (relative to their serum concentration) varied from analyte to analyte. This variation originates from the differences in their interstitial fluid (ISF) concentration relative to the serum concentration. For example, while glucose concentration in the ISF is comparable to its serum value, average ISF concentration of triglycerides in rats is only about 30% of its serum value. On the other hand, the ISF concentration of lactate is about two times higher than its serum concentration. It was shown that ultrasound-followed-by-vacuum application extracts $\sim$10 μl of ISF in 15 minutes. This corresponds to a convective volumetric flow of 25.7 μl/cm^2/hour.

Correlation between analyte concentrations in sonophoretically extracted fluid and blood were analyzed in detail using glucose. In these experiments, rat skin was exposed to ultrasound. Multiple extractions were performed using partial vacuum (10 in Hg for 5 minutes applied every 20 minutes) over a period of 2 hours. The first transdermal flux was used to calculate the calibration factor. Blood glucose levels of rats were varied by infusing insulin intravenously at a rate of 10 mU/min for 2 hours. Transdermally extracted glucose flux correlated well with the changes in the blood glucose level in the hypo- and hyperglycemic range. The relationship between the predicted and measured glucose values was linear ($r = 0.97$). Similar results were reported by Kost *et al.* (2000) in the tests performed in human volunteers. Specifically, ultrasound was used to permeabilize skin of human volunteers. A short application of ultrasound permeabilized the skin for about 15 hours. During this period, interstitial fluid was extracted every 30 minutes. Concentration of glucose in the extracted fluid was measured and compared with blood glucose values. The results showed a good correlation between glucose in the interstitial fluid and in the blood. Furthermore, patients reported no pain upon ultrasound application. More recently, Kost *et al.* reported clinical studies performed on diabetic volunteers where ultrasound was used to permeabilize the skin and glucose was collected by diffusion instead of vacuum through the permeabilized skin. Glucose flux through sonicated site averaged 11 nmol/cm^2/hours.

8. Mechanism of Low-Frequency Sonophoresis

A general discussion of mechanisms for biological effects of ultrasound is presented in Chap. II. The present section is devoted specifically to mechanisms of low-frequency ultrasound.

Significant attention has been devoted to understanding the mechanisms of low-frequency sonophoresis (Tezel & Mitragotri, 2003; Mitragotri *et al.* 1995; Tang *et al.*, 2002; Merino *et al.*, 2003). A consensus has been reached that acoustic cavitation, the formation and collapse of gaseous cavities, is responsible for low-frequency sonophoresis (Tezel & Mitragotri, 2003; Tang *et al.*, 2002). Below, we summarize the current conclusions of the mechanistic investigations of sonophoresis.

During low-frequency sonophoresis, cavitation is predominantly induced in the coupling medium (*i.e.*, the liquid present between the ultrasound transducer and the skin (Tezel *et al.*, 2002a)). The maximum radius reached by the free cavitating bubbles is related to the frequency and acoustic pressure amplitude. Under the conditions used for low-frequency sonophoresis ($f \sim 20$–100 kHz and pressure amplitudes ~ 1–2.4 bar), the maximum bubble radius is estimated to be between 10–100 μm. Hence, cavitation is unlikely to occur within the 15 μm thick SC during low-frequency sonophoresis. Accordingly, cavitation in the coupling medium is of primary interest during low-frequency sonophoresis.

Two types of cavitation, stable or inertial, have been evaluated for their role in sonophoresis (Fig. 6). Stable cavitation corresponds to periodic growth and oscillations of bubbles, while inertial cavitation corresponds to violent growth and collapse of cavitation bubbles (Suslick, 1989). Using acoustic spectroscopy, stable as well as inertial cavitation has been quantified. (Tang & Langer, 2002a; Tezel *et al.*, 2002b). The overall dependence of inertial cavitation on ultrasound intensity was found to be similar to that of conductivity enhancement (Tang & Langer, 2002a; Tezel *et al.*, 2002b). Specifically, ultrasound intensity above the threshold value is required before inception of inertial cavitation is observed. This threshold

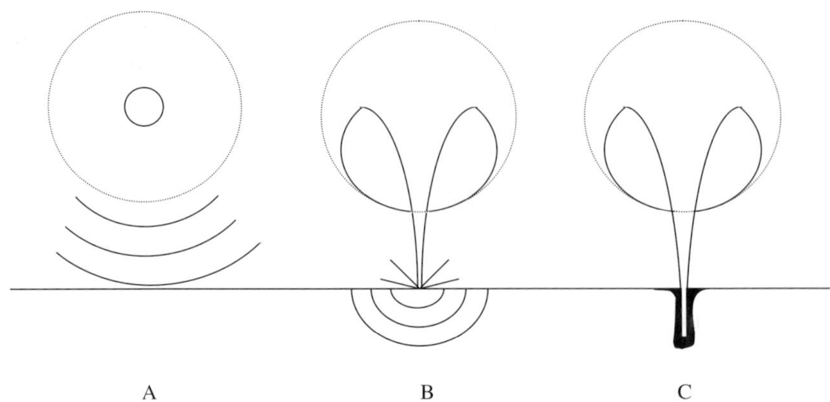

Fig. 6. Adopted from Tezel and Mitragoni (1995). Three possible modes through which inertial cavitation may enhance SC permeability. (A) Spherical collapse near the SC surface emits shock waves, which can potentially disrupt the SC lipid bilayers. (B) Impact of an acoustic microjet on the SC surface. The microjet possessing a radius about one tenth of the maximum bubble diameter impacts the SC surface without penetrating into it. The impact pressure of the microjet may enhance SC permeability by disrupting SC lipid bilayers. (C) Microjets may physically penetrate into the SC and enhance the SC permeability.

corresponds to minimum pressure amplitude required to induce the rapid growth and collapse of cavitation nuclei. Beyond this threshold, white noise (indicator of inertial cavitation) increased linearly with ultrasound intensity, although at any given intensity, inertial cavitation activity decreased rapidly with ultrasound frequency (Tezel *et al.*, 2002b). The threshold intensity for the occurrence of inertial cavitation increased with increasing ultrasound frequency. This dependence reflects the fact that the growth of cavitation bubbles becomes increasingly difficult with increasing ultrasound frequency. Tezel *et al.* (2002) showed that regardless of the intensity and frequency, skin conductivity enhancement correlated universally with a measure proportional to the total acoustic energy fluence. These data suggested a strong role played by inertial cavitation in low-frequency sonophoresis.

Inertial cavitation occurs in the bulk coupling medium as well as near the skin surface. Inertial cavitation at both locations may potentially be responsible of conductivity enhancement. Three mechanisms by which inertial cavitation events might enhance SC permeability were proposed

(Tezel & Mitragotri, 2003). These include bubbles that collapse symmetrically and emit a shock wave, which can disrupt the SC lipid bilayers and acoustic microjets that might impact the SC without penetration. Impact of microjets may also be responsible for SC lipid bilayer disruption. Microjets resulting from collapsing bubbles near the SC surface may also potentially penetrate into the SC and disrupt the structure.

Inertial cavitation in the vicinity of a surface is fundamentally different from that away from the surface. Specifically, collapse of spherical cavitation bubbles in the bulk solution is symmetric and results in the formation of a shock wave. This shock wave can potentially disrupt the structure of the lipid bilayers. However, the amplitude of the shock wave decreases rapidly with the distance. Collapse of cavitation bubbles near boundaries (especially rigid ones) has been extensively studied in the literature (Blake & Gibson, 1985). Specifically, Naude and Ellis showed that cavitation bubbles travel under the influence of ultrasound field towards the boundary and collapse near the boundary depending on its proximity to the surface (Naude & Ellis, 1961). The collapse of cavitation bubbles near the boundary is asymmetric due to the difference in the surrounding condition on either side of the bubble. Specifically, the asymmetry in the surroundings leads to the generation of asymmetry in the pressure, which ultimately leads to the formation of a liquid microjet directed towards the surface. The diameter of the microjet is much smaller than that of the maximum bubble radius. There have been several estimates of the speed of the liquid microjet when it strikes the surface [between 50 and 180 m/s (Benjamin & Ellis, 1966; Lauterborn & Bolle, 1975; Plesset & Chapman, 1971)].

In a recent study, Tezel *et al.* (2003) evaluated the effect of spherical collapses, as well as microjets, on skin permeability enhancement. They concluded that both types of cavitation events may be responsible for sonophoresis. Regardless of the precise mode of collapse, about 10 collapses/second/cm^2 in the form of spherical collapses or microjets near the surface of the stratum corneum were suggested to explain experimentally observed conductivity enhancements. They also reported that bubble collapses close to the stratum corneum surface ($\sim$50 μm) contribute to sonophoresis.

Disruption of SC lipid bilayers due to bubble-induced shock waves or microjet impact may enhance skin permeability by at least two mechanisms.

Firstly, a moderate level of disruption decreases the structural order of lipid bilayers and increases solute diffusion coefficient (Mitragotri, 2001). At a higher level of disruption, lipid bilayers may loose structural integrity and facilitate penetration of the coupling medium into the SC. Since many sonophoresis experiments reported in the literature are performed using coupling media comprising aqueous solutions of surfactants, disruption of SC lipid bilayers enhances incorporation of surfactants into lipid bilayers. Incorporation of excessive water and surfactants further promotes bilayer disruption, thereby opening pathways for solute permeation (Black, 1993; Walters, 1990). Recently, Alvarez-Roman reported that lipid extraction also plays a role in low-frequency sonophoresis (Alvarez-Roman *et al.*, 2003). They reported that about 30% of the stratum corneum lipids were removed during low-frequency sonophoresis.

Ultrasound has also been shown to induce convective flow across the skin. Morimoto *et al.* (2005) reported that 41 kHz ultrasound has the potential to induce convective solvent flow to increase the skin permeation of hydrophilic calcein in excised hairless rat skin. Similar conclusions have also been reached by Tang *et al.* (2001). The precise origin of convective flow is not clear, although cavitation is indicated to play a significant role.

9. Synergistic Effect of Ultrasound and Other Mechanism

While ultrasound has been shown to enhance transdermal drug transport, its combinations with other penetration enhancers has been shown to be more effective. Over the last 10 years, several papers have been published to support this hypothesis. In addition to increasing transdermal transport, a combination of enhancers should also reduce the severity of the enhancers required to achieve the desirable drug flux. Specifically, the enhancement induced by these enhancers depends on their strength. However, the highest strength of the enhancer that can be applied on the skin is typically limited by safety. By combining two or more enhancers, one can reduce the strength of individual enhancers required to achieve the desired enhancement. Hence, a combination of two or more enhancers may not only increase the total enhancement, but can also increase the safety of enhancers by reducing the strength of individual enhancers.

9.1. *Ultrasound and chemical enhancers*

Literature reports have confirmed the synergistic effect between ultrasound and chemical enhancers. Johnson *et al.* (1996) performed a study of the synergistic effect of therapeutic ultrasound (1 MHz, 2 W/cm^2) with a series of chemical enhancer formulations, including (i) polyethylene glycol 200 dilaurate (PEG), (ii) isopropyl myristate (IM), (iii) glycerol trioleate (GT), (iv) ethanol/pH 7.4 phosphate buffered saline in a one-to-one ratio (50% EtOH), (v) 50% EtOH saturated with linoleic acid (LA/EtOH), and (vi) phosphate buffered saline (PBS), using corticosterone as a model drug. A combination of LA/EtOH and ultrasound was most effective in enhancing transdermal drug transport. The combination of LA/EtOH with ultrasound increased corticosterone flux by up to 13,000-fold (LA/EtOH), relative to the passive flux from PBS. This enhancement was substantially higher than that induced by LA/EtOH alone (900-fold) or ultrasound alone (5-fold). Johnson *et al.* (1996) suggested that the primary mechanism of the synergistic effect of ultrasound and chemicals was due to the mixing of the chemical enhancer with SC lipids upon ultrasound application.

Recently, synergistic effect of low-frequency ultrasound (20 kHz) and surfactants has also been reported (Mitragotri *et al.*, 2000c; Tezel *et al.*, 2001). Surfactants also reduced the threshold ultrasound energy fluence required to induce a detectable change in skin permeability. Specifically, in the absence of surfactants, the threshold ultrasound energy fluence for producing a detectable change in skin impedance is about 141 J/cm^2. Addition of 1% SLS to the solution decreased the threshold to about 18 J/cm^2 (Mitragotri *et al.*, 2000c). Various possible mechanisms of this synergistic effect were investigated. These include (i) surfactants enhance ultrasound-induced cavitation, (ii) ultrasound drives more surfactants into the skin, and (iii) ultrasound may enhance dispersion of surfactants within the SC lipids. The latter two mechanisms were found to be dominant.

9.2. *Ultrasound and iontophoresis*

Synergy between ultrasound and iontophoresis is expected since these enhancers enhance transdermal transport through different mechanisms. Indeed, this combination has been found to enhance transdermal transport better than each of them alone. Specifically, Le *et al.* (2000) performed an investigation of the synergistic effect of ultrasound and iontophoresis on transdermal transport using a model drug, heparin. Ultrasound was applied only once to each skin piece, along with 1% solution of dodecyl pyridinium chloride, for approximately 10 minutes prior to the application of iontophoresis. The enhancement of heparin flux due to ultrasound + iontophoresis treatment was about 56-fold (note that iontophoresis was applied only for 1 hour). This enhancement was higher than the sum of those obtained during ultrasound alone (3-fold) and iontophoresis alone (15-fold). Thus, the effect of ultrasound and iontophoresis on transdermal heparin transport is truly synergistic.

The synergistic effect of ultrasound and iontophoresis on transdermal transport was attributed to ultrasound-induced structural changes in the skin. Specifically, application of ultrasound should disorder the lipid bilayers of the skin, thereby introducing new transport pathways. The presence of these pathways decreases skin's impedance and size-selectivity. Both these effects should result in increased transdermal transport.

9.3. *Ultrasound and electroporation*

Electroporation enhances transdermal transport through enhanced diffusion (via skin poration), electrophoresis, and electroosmosis. Kost *et al.* (1996) investigated the synergistic effect of therapeutic ultrasound and electroporation on the transdermal transport of two molecules, calcein and sulforhodamine. Application of ultrasound (1 MHz, 2 W/cm^2) did not enhance transdermal calcein flux, while application of electroporation alone enhanced transdermal calcein transport to 0.1 μg/cm^2/hour. However, a simultaneous application of ultrasound and electroporation enhanced transdermal calcein transport to 0.3 μg/cm^2/hour. Application of ultrasound also reduced the threshold voltage for electroporation. The threshold electroporation voltage for electroporation (under the protocol described in Kost *et al.* (1996) is $\sim$53 $\pm$ 3 V in the absence of ultrasound and $\sim$46 $\pm$ 3 V in the presence of ultrasound. The voltage required to achieve a given transdermal flux was also smaller in the presence of ultrasound. For example, to achieve a transdermal sulforhodamine flux of 0.15 μg/cm^2/hour, the required voltage is $\sim$95 V in the absence of ultrasound and 75 V in the presence of ultrasound.

The authors suggested that ultrasound might play a two-fold role in enhancing the effect of electroporation on transdermal transport. Firstly, ultrasound may induce partial structural disordering of the skin's lipid bilayers. Since the electrical resistance of the disordered bilayers is likely to be smaller than that of the normal lipid bilayers, the applied voltage may concentrate preferentially across the normal bilayers. Secondly, ultrasound may also induce convection across the skin. Both effects were found to play important roles in the synergistic effect of ultrasound and electroporation on transdermal transport of calcein and sulforhodamine. Detailed studies are required to understand the mechanisms of this synergy further.

10. Mathematical Modeling of Sonophoresis

Substantial efforts have been undertaken to develop mathematical models of transdermal drug transport during low-frequency sonophoresis (Tezel *et al.*, 2002a; Tang *et al.*, 2001; Tezel *et al.*, 2003). Typically, a porous pathway model is used for this purpose. The fundamental underlying assumption of the porous pathway model is that both in the absence and presence of ultrasound, hydrophilic permeants migrate through the skin via tortuous cylindrical pores filled with water. Other model assumptions include (i) the permeants/ions behave as hard spheres which have no specific interactions with the pore walls, and (ii) the anions and cations in the electrolyte solution have the same valence, z, and similar diffusion coefficients.

The general expression for permeability, P_p of a hydrophilic permeant diffusing through a porous membrane (*e.g.*, skin) is given by:

$$P_p = \frac{\varepsilon D_p^{pore}}{\tau \Delta x} \tag{1}$$

where ε, τ, and Δx are the porosity, tortuosity, and thickness of the membrane respectively, and D_p^{pore} is the diffusion coefficient of the permeant in the liquid-filled, pores within the membrane. According to the hindered transport theory (Deen, 1987), D_p^{pore} is a function of both the permeant and the membrane characteristics. D_p^{pore} can be expressed as a product of the permeant diffusion coefficient at infinite dilution, D_p^{∞}, and permeant diffusion hindrance factor, $H(\lambda_p)$, where λ_p is the ratio of the hydrodynamic radius of the permeant, r_p, and the average pore radius of the membrane, r, *i.e.*, $\lambda_p = r_p/r$. With the aforementioned changes, Eq. (1) becomes as follows:

$$P_p = \frac{\varepsilon}{\tau \Delta x} D_p^\infty H(\lambda_p) \tag{2}$$

For $\lambda_p < 0.4$, the diffusion hindrance factor, $H(\lambda_p)$, is given by the following (Deen, 1987):

$$H(\lambda_p) = (1 - \lambda_p)^2 (1 - 2.104\lambda_p + 2.09\lambda_p^3 - 0.95\lambda_p^5) \tag{3}$$

An equation similar to Eq. (3) can be written for the permeability of current carrying ions. Specifically,

$$P_{ion} = \frac{\varepsilon}{\tau \Delta x} D_{ion}^\infty H(\lambda_{ion}), \tag{4}$$

where D_{ion}^∞ is the ion diffusion coefficient at infinite dilution, and $H(\lambda_{ion})$ is the hindrance factor for the ion, given by Eq. (3) with λ_p replaced by λ_{ion}, where $\lambda_{ion} = r_{ion}/r$, with r_{ion} the hydrodynamic radius of the ion. Combining Eqs. (2) and (4) gives:

$$\frac{P_p}{P_{ion}} = \frac{D_p{}^\infty H(\lambda_p)}{D_{ion}^\infty H(\lambda_{ion})} \tag{5}$$

By relating P_{ion} to skin resistivity and D_{ion}^∞ to electrochemical properties of PBS, Tang *et al.* (2001) have shown that Eq. (5) can be rewritten as follows:

$$log P_p = log C_3 - log R \tag{6}$$

where R is the skin resistivity ($k\Omega cm^2$) and C_3 is:

$$C_3 = \frac{kT}{2z^2 F c_{ion} e_0} \frac{D_p^\infty H(\lambda_p)}{D_{ion}^\infty H(\lambda_{ion})} \tag{7}$$

where k is the Boltzmann constant (1.38×10^{-23} J/K/molecule), T is the absolute temperature (298 K), z is the electrolyte valance (1), F is the Faraday constant (9.648×10^4 C/mol), c_{ion} is the electrolyte molar concentration (0.137 M) and e_0 is the electronic charge (1.6×10^{-19} C). Equation 6 indicates that a plot of $log P_p$ versus $log R$ should exhibit a linear behavior with a slope of -1. Equation 6 provides a general equation to theoretically describe the diffusion of a hydrophilic permeant across the skin under any permeation conditions, including passive control and diffusion after ultrasound treatment. However, the y-intercept ($log C_3$) may differ for the various permeation conditions, depending on the average pore radius, r, corresponding to a particular permeation condition. Accordingly, a change in r manifests itself through a change in the intercept of $log P_p - log R$ correlation, whereas changes in ε, τ, and Δx do not affect the intercept value. Once the pore size is determined, ε/τ can be determined from the following two equations.

$$\frac{\varepsilon}{\tau} = \frac{\Delta x}{\sigma_{sol} R} \frac{1}{H(\lambda_{ion})} \tag{8}$$

or

$$\frac{\varepsilon}{\tau} = \frac{\Delta x P_p}{D_p^{\infty} H(\lambda_p)} \tag{9}$$

where σ_{sol} is the conductivity of the electrolyte solution. Using these equations, the dependence of transdermal transport pathways (r, ε/τ) on ultrasound parameters has been studied. It has been shown that ultrasound frequency does not affect the average pore radius, as determined from mannitol permeability (28 ± 12Å). This value is the same as that for passive diffusion. If the passive delivery of hydrophilic permeants is hypothesized to occur through imperfections (cracks) in the skin, then LFS could be generating more of these already existing imperfections. In such case, the average pore radius will not be altered with different frequencies since ultrasound does not create different (unique) type of pathways. The enhancement of skin permeability originates from increased porosity and/or reduced tortuosity. The average ε/τ value for passive diffusion is $\sim 3.5 \times 10^{-6}$ and with the application of ultrasound, the ε/τ value could be increased up to $\sim 6.0 \times 10^{-3}$, an enhancement of approximately 1700-fold. The ε/τ value does not directly tell if the actual porosity, ε, is increased or the tortuosity, τ, is decreased or both. Still, a limiting case could be applied where it is assumed that with the application of ultrasound cylindrical channels, $i.e.$, $\tau = 1$, are created that are responsible for permeant delivery (assuming that the effects of ultrasound are strong enough to create pathways all through the lipid bilayers). Also, as the effect of ultrasound on the skin is heterogeneous, a fair assumption would be that the porosity and permeability increase mainly within the localized transport pathways (LTPs). Since the LTPs occupy approximately 5% of the sonicated skin area regardless of application frequency, with this approach, the porosity within these areas could be calculated to be approximately 12%. Using the porous pathway model, the dermis porosity, which is the most porous section of the skin, was calculated to be 18%. These values suggest that with the application of ultrasound, the SC barrier properties are reduced and LTPs which are on the order of magnitude as porous as the dermis are created.

11. Safety of Low-Frequency Ultrasound

Safety of low-frequency sonophoresis has been evaluated in several studies. Histological studies performed on the rat and pig skins indicated no structural changes in the skin on a length scale of $\sim\mu$m (Mitragotri *et al.*, 1996b). Accordingly, the structural changes in the stratum corneum appear to occur at a sub-micron scale. Singer *et al.* performed a toxicological analysis of low-frequency sonophoresis. They found a dose-dependent effect of ultrasound on the skin. They concluded that low-frequency ultrasound at low intensities appears safe for enhancing the topical delivery of medications, producing only minimal urticarial reactions. Higher-intensity ultrasound produced significant thermal effects. (Singer *et al.*, 1998) Boucaud *et al.* (2000) also performed a microstructural analysis of skin samples exposed to ultrasound. They reported no detectable changes in the skin structure of human skin at an intensity of 2.5 W/cm^2. Hairless rat skin exposed to the same intensity showed slight and transient erythema and dermal necrosis at 24 hours. Tolerance of low-frequency ultrasound by patients has been reported in a number of studies. Kost *et al.* (2000) reported that low-frequency ultrasound was well-tolerated by patients. More recently, a clinical study on the use of low-frequency ultrasound for lidocaine delivery has also been reported (Katz *et al.*, 2004). However, it must be realized that ultrasound, like any other energy source, is likely to exhibit a window of parameters within which safe application can be practised. Accordingly, a careful selection of parameters must be performed in sonophoresis studies.

A device based on low-frequency sonophoresis has recently been approved by the FDA for skin permeabilization. This device, named SonoPrep^{TM}, is manufactured by Sontra Medical Inc. (Fig. 7). Currently, the devcie is used to deliver topical anesthetics and additional applications are in the early-late clinical trials.

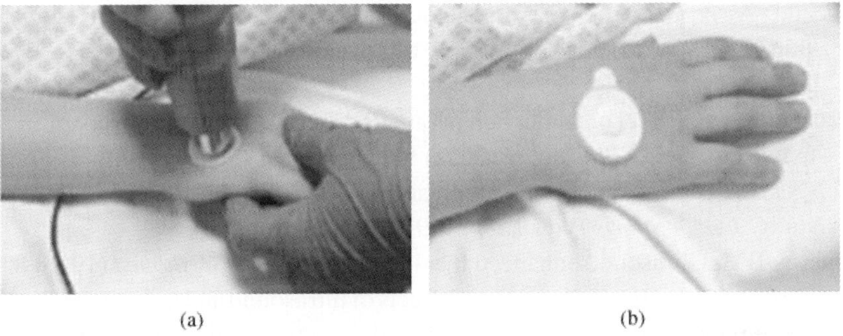

(a)   (b)

Fig. 7.   Printed with permission from Sontra Medical Inc. Use of SonoPrep™ for local anesthesia. (a) shows ultrasound application for skin permeabilization. (b) shows a patch placed on permeabilized skin for delivery of anesthesia.

References

Alexandrov AV. Ultrasound-enahnced thrombolysis for stroke: Clinical significance. *Eur J Ultrasound* (2002) **16**(1–2): 131–140.

Alvarez-Roman R *et al.* Skin permeability enhancement by low-frequency sonophoresis-Lipid extraction and transport pathways. *J Pharm Sci* (2003) **92**(6): 1138–1146.

Benjamin T, Ellis A. The collapse of cavitation bubbles and the pressures thereby produced against solid boundaries. *Philos Trans R Soc London Ser A* (1966) **260**: 221–240.

Benson HAE, McElnay JC, HJ. Influence of ultrasound on the percutaneous absorption of niicotinate esters. *Pharm Res* (1991) **9**: 1279–1283.

Benson HAE, McElnay JC, Harland R. Phonophoresis of lingocaine an prilocaine from Emla cream. *Int J Pharm* (1988) **44**: 65–69.

Benson HAE, McElnay JC, HR. Use of ultrasound to enhance percutaneous absorption of benzydamine. *Phys Ther* (1989) **69**(2): 113–118.

Black G. Interaction Between anionic surfactants and skin, in *Pharmaceutical Skin Penetration Enhancement*, Walters K, HAdgraft J, (eds.) (1993) Marcel Dekker: New York, Basel, Hong Kong, pp. 145–174.

Blake J, Gibson D. Cavitation bubbles near boundaries. *Annual Rev Fluid Mech* (1985) **19**: 99–123.

Bommannan D *et al.* Sonophoresis. I. The use of high-frequency ultrasound to enhance transdermal drug delivery. *Pharm Res* (1992a) **9**(4): 559–564.

Bommannan D *et al.* Sonophpresis. II. Examination of the mechanism(s) of ultrasound-enhanced transdermal drug delivery. *Pharm Res* (1992b) **9**(8): 1043–1047.

Boucaud A *et al.* Clinical, histologic, and electron microscopy study of skin exposed to low-frequency ultrasound. *Anatom Rec* (2001) **264**: 114–119.

Boucaud A *et al.* Effect of sonication parameters on transdemral delivery of insulin to hairless rats. *J Pharm Sci* (2002) **91**(3): 113–119.

Byl NN *et al.* The effects of phonophoresis with corticosteroids: A controlled pilot study. *J Orth Sports Phys Ther* (1993) **18**(5): 590–600.

Cameroy BM. Ultrasound enhanced local anesthesia. *Am J Orthoped* (1966) **8**: 47.

Ciccone CD, Legin BQ, Callamaro JJ. Effects of ultrasound and trolamine salicylate phonophoresis on delayed-Onset muscle soreness. *Phys Ther* (1991) **71**(9): 666–678.

Coleman AJ, Saunders JE. A review of the physical properties and biological effects of the high amplitude acoustic field used in extracorporeal lithotripsy. *Ultrasonics* (1993) **31**(2): 75–89.

Coodley GL. Bursitis and post-traumatic lesions. *Am Pract* (1960) **11**: 181–187.

Deen WM. Hindered transport of large molecules in liquid-filled pores. *AIChE J* (1987) **33**: 1409–1425.

Diederich CJ, Hynnen K. Ultrasound technology for hyperthemia. *Ultrasound Med Biol* (1999) **25**(6): 871–887.

Fellinger K, Schmidt J. Klinik and Therapies des Chromischen Gelenkreumatismus. *Maudrich Vienna, Austria* 1954.

Gockel CM, Bao S, Beagley KW. Transcutaneous immunization induces mucosal and systemic immunity: A potent method for targeting immunity to the female reproductive tract. *Mol Immunol* (2000) **37**(9): 537–44.

Goes JC, Landecker A. Ultrasound-induced lipoplasty (UAL) in breast surgery. *Aesthetic Plast Surg* (2002) **26**(1): 1–9.

Griffin JE. Physiological effects of ultrasonica energy as it is used clinically. *J Am Phys Ther Assoc* (1966) **46**: 18–26.

Griffin JE *et al.* Patients tretaed with ultrasonic driven hydrocortisone ans with ultrasound alone. *Phys Ther* (1967) **47**(7): 600–601.

Griffin JE, Touchstone JC. Low-Intensity phonophoresis of cortisol in swine. *Phys Ther* (1968) **48**(12): 1136–1344.

Griffin JE, Touchstone JC. Effects of ultrasonic frequency on phonophoresis of cortisol into swine tissues. *Am J Phys Med* (1972) **51**(2): 62–78.

Griffin JE, Touchstone J. Ultrasonic movement of cortisol in to pig tissue. *Am J Phys Med* **44**(1): 20–25.

Guzman HR *et al.* Ultrasound-mediated disruption of cell membranes. I. Quantification of molecular uptake and viability. *J Acoust Soc Am* (2001) **110**(1): 588–596.

Hadjiargyrou M *et al.* Enhancement of fracture healing by low intensity ultrasound. *Clin Orthop* (1998) **355**(Suppl): S216–S229.

Hofman D, Moll F. The effect of ultrasound on *in vitro* liberation and *in vivo* penetration of benzyl nicotinate. *J Control Rel* (1993) **27**: 187–192.

Johnson ME *et al.* Synergistic effect of ultrasound and chemical enhancers on transdermal drug delivery. *J Pharm Sci* (1996) **85**(7): 670–679.

Joshi A, Raje J. Sonicated transdermal drug transport. *J Control Rel* (2002) **83**(1): 13–22.

Kleinkort JA, Wood F. Phonophoresis with 1 percent versus 10 percent hydrocortisone. *Phys Ther* (1975) **55**(12): 1320–1324.

Kost J *et al.* Enhanced transdermal delivery: Synergistic effect of ultrasound and electroporation. *Pharm Res* (1996) **13**(4): 633–638.

Kost J *et al.* Transdermal extraction of glucose and other analytes using ultrasound. *Nat Med* (2000) **6**(3): 347–350.

Kost J, Langer R. Ultrasound-mediated transdermal drug delivery, in *Topical Drug Bioavailability, Bioequivalence, and Penetration*, Shah VP, Maibach HI, (eds.) (1993) Plennum: New York, pp. 91–103.

Kost J, Leong K, LR. Ultrasound-enhanced polymer degradation and release of incorporated substances. *Proc NAtl Acad Sci* (1989) **86**: 7663–7666.

Kost J, Mitragotri S, Langer R. Phonophoresis, in *Percutaneous Absorption*, Bronaugh R, Maibach HI, (eds.) (1999) pp. 615–631.

Katz NP *et al.* Rapid onset of cutaneous anesthesia with EMLA cream after pretreatment with a new ultrasound emitting device. *Anesth Analg* (2004) **98**(2): 371–376.

Kwok CS *et al.* Self-assembled molecular structures as ultrasonically-responsive barrier membranes for pulastile delivery. *J Biomed Mater Res* (2001) **57**(2): 151–164.

Lauterborn W, Bolle H. Experimental investigations of cavitation bubble collapse in the neighbourhood of a solid boundary. *J Fluid Mech* (1975) **72**: 391–399.

Le L, Kost J, Mitragotri S. Combined effect of low-frequency ultrasound and iontophoresis: Applications for transdermal heparin delivery. *Pharm Res* (2000) **17**(9): 1151–1154.

Levy D *et al.* Effect of ultrasound on transdermal drug delivery to rats and guinea pigs. *J Clin Invest* (1989) **83**: 2974–2078.

Linder JR. Evolving applications of contrast ultrasound. *Am J Cardiol* (2002) **90**(Suppl. 10A): 72J–80J.

Machet L, Boucaud A. Phonophoresis: Efficiency, mechanisms, and skin tolerance. *Int J Pharm* (2002) **243**(1–2): 1–15.

Machluf M, Kost J. Ultrasonically enhanced transdermal drug delivery. Experimental approaches to elucidate the mechanism. *J Biomat Sci* (1993) **5**: 147–156.

McElnay JC *et al.* The effect of ultrasound on the percutaneous absorption of lingocaine. *Br J Clin Pharmacol* (1985) **20**: 421–424.

Menon G, Bommanon D, Elias P. High-frequency sonophoresis: Permeation pathways and structural basis for enhanced permeability. *Skin Pharmacol* (1994) **7**(3): 130–139.

Merino G *et al.* Frequency and thermal effects on the enhancement of transdermal transport by sonophoresis. *J Control Rel* (2003) **88**(1): 85–94.

Merriono G *et al.* Frequency and thermal effects on the enhancement of transdermal transport by sonophoresis. *J Control Rel* (2003) **88**(1): 85–94.

Merrino G, Kalia YN, Guy RH. Ultrasound-enhanced transdermal transport. *J Pharm Sci* (2003) **92**(6): 1125–1137.

Miller D, Quddus J. Sonoporation of monolayer cells by diagnostic ultrasound activation of contrast-agent gas bodies. *Ultrasound Med Biol* (2000) **26**(4): 661–667.

Mitragotri S. Synergistic effect of enhancers for transdermal drug delivery. *Pharm Res* (2000) **17**(11): 1354–1359.

Mitragotri S. Effect of bilayer disruption on transdermal transport of low-molecular weight hydrophobic solutes. *Pharm Res* (2001) **18**: 1022–1028.

Mitragotri S. Healing sound: The use of ultrasound in drug delivery and other therapeutic applications. *Nat Rev Drug Discov* (2005) **4**(3): 255–260.

Mitragotri S *et al.* A mechanistic study of ultrasonically enhanced transdermal drug delivery. *J Pharm Sci* (1995a) **84**(6): 697–706.

Mitragotri S *et al.* Synergistic effect of low-frequency ultrasound and sodium lauryl sulfate on transdermal transport. *J Pharm Sci* (2000) **89**(7): 892–900.

Mitragotri S *et al.* Analysis of ultrasonically extracted interstitial fluid as a predictor of blood glucose levels. *J Appl Physiol* (2000a) **89**(3): 961–966.

Mitragotri S *et al.* Determination of the threshold energy dose for ultrasound-induced transdermal drug delivery. *J Control Rel* (2000b) **63**: 41–52.

Mitragotri S *et al.* Synergistic effect of low-frequency ultrasound and sodium lauryl sulfate on transdermal drug delivery. *J Pharm Sci* (2000c) **89**(7): 892–900.

Mitragotri S *et al.* Transdermal extraction of analytes using low-frequency ultrasound. *Pharm Res* (2000d) **17**(4): 466–470.

Mitragotri S, Blankschtein D, Langer R. Sonophoresis: Ultrasound mediated transdermal drug delivery, in *Encl of Pharm Tech*, Swarbrick J, Boylan J, (eds.) (1995a) Marcel Dekker.

Mitragotri S, Blankschtein SD, Langer R. Ultrasound-mediated transdermal protein delivery *Science* (1995b) **269**: 850–853.

Mitragotri S, Blankschtein D, Langer R. Sonophoresis: Enhanced transdermal drug delivery by application of ultrasound, in *Encyl Pharm TEch* SJ, J. Boylans, (eds.) (1996a) pp. 103–122.

Mitragotri S, Blankschtein D, Langer R. Transdermal drug delivery using low-frequency sonophoresis. *Pharm Res* (1996b) **13**(3): 411–420.

Mitragotri S, Blankschtein D, Langer R. An explanation for the variation of the sonophoretic transdermal transport enhancement from drug to drug. *J Pharm Sci* (1997) **86**(10): 1190–1192.

Mitragotri S, Kost J. Low-frequency sonophoresis: A non-invasive method for drug delivery and diagnostics. *Biotech Prog* (2000a) **16**(3): 488–492.

Mitragotri S, Kost J. Transdermal delivery of heparin and low-molecular weight heparin using low-frequency ultrasound. *Pharm Res* (2000b) **18**(8): 1151–1156.

Mitragotri S, Kost J. Low-frequency sonophoresis: A review. *Adv Drug Del Rev* (2004) **56**(5): 589–601.

Moll MA. New approaches to pain. *US Armed Forces Med Serv DIg* (1979) **30**: 8–11.

Morimoto Y *et al.* Elucidation of the transport pathway in hairless rat skin enhanced by low-frequency sonophoresis based on the solute-water transport relationship and confocal microscopy. *J Control Rel* (2005) **103**(3): 587–597.

Naude A. Ellis On the mechanisms of cavitation damage by non-hemispherical cavities in contact with solid boundary. *Trans ASME J Basic Eng* (1961) **83**: 648–556.

Nelson JL *et al.* Ultrasonically activated chemotherapeutic drug delivery in a rat model. *Cancer Res* (2002) **62**(24): 7280–7283.

Ogra PL *et al.* Handbook of mucosal immunology. (1994) Academic Press: New York.

Plesset M, Chapman R. Collapse of an initially spherical vapour cavity in the neighbourhood of a solid boundary. *J Fluid Mech* (1971) **47**: 283–290.

Prausnitz MR, Mitragotri S, Langer R. Current status and future potential of transdermal drug delivery. *Nat Rev Drug Discov* (2004) **3**(2): 115–124.

Price RJ, Kaul S. Contrast ultrasound targeted drug and gene delivery: An update on a new therapeutic modality. *J Cardiovasc Pharmacol Ther* (2002) **7**(3): 171–180.

Quillen WS. Phonophoresis: A Review of the literature and technique. *Athelet Train* (1980) **15**: 109–110.

Roitt I, Brostoff J, Male D. *Immunology*. 5th ed. (1998) London: Mosby.

Scharton-Kersten T *et al.* Transcutaneous immunization with bacterial ADP-ribosylating exotoxins, subunits, and unrelated adjuvants. *Infect Immun* (2000) **68**(9): 5306–5313.

Singer AJ *et al.* Low-frequency sonophoresis: Pathologic and thermal effects in dogs. *Acad Emerg Med* (1998) **5**(1): 35–40.

Smith NB, Lee S, Shung KK. Ultrasound-mediated transdermal *in vivo* transport of insulin with low-profile cymbal arrays. *Ultrasound Med Biol* (2003) **29**(8): 1205–1210.

Speed CA. Therapeutic ultrasound in soft tissue lesions. *Rheumatology* (2001) **40**(12): 1331–1336.

Suslick KS. *Ultrasound: Its Chemical, Physical and Biological Effects.* (1989) VCH Publishers.

Sundaram J, Mitragotri MB, S. An experimental analysis of ultrasound-induced permeabilization. *Biophys J* (2002).

Tachibana K. Transdermal delivery of insulin to alloxan-diabetc rabits by ultra-sound exposure. *Pharm Res* (1992) **9**(7): 952–954.

Tachibana K, Tachibana S. Transdermal delivery of insulin by ultrasonic vibration. *J Pharm Pharmacol* (1991) **43**: 270–271.

Tachibana K, Tachibana S. Use of ultrasound to enhance the local anesthetic effect of topically applied aqueous lidocaine. *Anestheiology* (1993) **78**(6): 1091–1096.

Tana *et al.* Induction of intestinal IgA and IgG antibodies preventing adhesion of verotoxin-producing Escherichia coli to Caco-2 cells by oral immunization with liposomes. *Lett Appl Microbiol* (2003) **36**(3): 135–139.

Tang H *et al.* Theoretical description of transdermal transprt of hydrophilic perme-ants: Application to low-frequency sonophoresis. *J Pharm Sci* (2001a) **90**(5): 543–566.

Tang H *et al.* Theoretical description of transdermal transport of hydrophilic perme-ants: Application to low-frequency sonophoresis. *J Pharm Sci* (2001b) **90**(5): 545–568.

Tang H *et al.* An investigation of the role of cavitation in low-frequency ultrasound-mediated transdermal drug transport. *Pharm Res* (2002) **19**(8): 1160–1169.

Tang H, Blankschtein D, Langer R. An investigation of the role of cavitation in low-ferquency ultrasound-mediated transdermal drug transport. *Pharm Res* (2002a) **19**(8): 1160–1169.

Tang H, Blankschtein D, Langer R. Effects of low-frequency ultrasound on the transdermal penetration of mannitol: Comparative studies with *in vivo* and *in vitro* studies. *J Pharm Sci* (2002b) **91**(8): 1776–1794.

Terahara T *et al.* Dependence of low-frequency sonophoresis on ultrasound parameters; Distance of the horn and intensity. *Int J Pharm* (2002) **235**(1–2): 35–42.

Terahara T, Mitragotri S, Langer R. Porous resins as a cavitation enhancer for low-frequency sonophoresis. *J Pharm Sci* (2002) **91**(3): 753–759.

Tezel A *et al.* Frequency dependece of sonophoresis. *Pharm Res* (2001) **18**(12): 1694–1700.

Tezel A *et al.* Synergistic effect of low-frequency ultrasound and surfactant on skin permeability. *J Pharm Sci* (2001) **91**(2): 91–100.

Tezel A *et al.* Topical delivery of anti-sense oligonucleotides using low-frequency sonophoresis. *Pharm Res* (2004) **21**(12): 2219–2225.

Tezel A *et al.* Low-frequency ultrasound as a transcutaneous immunization adjuvant. *Vaccine* (2005) **23**(29): 3800–3807.

Tezel A, Mitragotri S. Interactions of inertial cavitation bubbles with stratum corneum lipid bilayers during low-frequency sonophoresis. *Biophys J* (2003) **85**(6): 3502–3512.

Tezel A, Sens A, Mitragotri S. A theoretical analysis of low-frequency sonophoresis: Dependence of transdermal transport pathways on frequency and energy density. *Pharm Res* (2002) **19**(12): 1841–1846.

Tezel A, Sens A, Mitragotri S. Investigations of the role of cavitation in low-frequency sonophoresis using acoustic spectroscopy. *J Pharm Sci* (2002b) **91**(2): 444–453.

Tezel A, Sens A, Mitragotri S. A theoretical description of transdermal transport of hydrophilic solutes induced by low-frequency sonophoresis. *J Pharm Sci* (2003) **92**(1): 381–393.

Tezel A, Sens A, Mitragotri S. Description of transdermal transport of hydrophilic solutes during low-frequency sonophoresis based on a modified porous pathway model. *J Pharm Sci* (2003) **92**(2): 381–393.

Unger EC *et al.* Local drug and genen delivery through microbubbles. *Prog Cardiovasc* (2001) **44**(1): 45–54.

Walters KA. Surfactants and percutaneous absorption, in Predictions of Percutaneous Penetration, Scott RC, Guy RH, Hadgraft J, (eds.) (1990) IBC Technical Services: London. pp. 148–162.

Weimann LJ, Wu J. Transdermal delivery of poly-l-lysine by sonomacroporation. *Ultrasound Med Biol* (2002) **28**(9): 1173–1180.

Williams AR. Phonophoresis: An *in vivo* evaluation using three topical anaesthetic preparations. *Ultrasonics* (1990) **28**: 137–141.

Wu J, Ross JP, Chiu J-F. Reparable sonoporation generated by microstreaming. *J Acoustic Soc Am* (2002) **111**(3): 1460–1464.

VIII

CLINICAL APPLICATIONS OF HIGH INTENSITY FOCUSED ULTRASOUND IN THE TREATMENT OF PATIENTS WITH SOLID MALIGNANCY

Feng WU

This chapter is to introduce Chinese clinical experience of using extracorporeal ultrasound-guided high intensity focused ultrasound (HIFU) for the treatment of patients with solid malignancy. From December 1997 to March 2004, approximately 3,500 patients with solid tumors received HIFU treatment in 20 Chinese hospitals. The tumors treated with HIFU include liver cancer, malignant bone tumors, breast cancer, soft tissue sarcomas, kidney cancer, pancreatic cancer, abdominal and pelvic malignant tumors, uterine fibroid, benign breast tumors, and hepatic hemangioma. Furthermore, the same device and clinical therapy plan have been introduced into the UK, Japan, and South Korea, and so far, more than 300 patients have received the treatment outside China. In this chapter, the history and mechanism of HIFU, HIFU therapeutic plan, and three-dimensional conformal HIFU ablations are presented. Imaging techniques employed in HIFU planning, therapy procedure, and follow-up assessments, particularly ultrasound-guided HIFU technology, are described in detail. In clinical applications, clear evidence of circumscribed tumor destruction and small vascular vessel damage are detected histologically. Follow-up images reveal an absence of viable tumor as well as obvious regression of the ablated tumors. Long-term survival benefit is observed in patients with hepatocellular carcinoma, breast cancer, and osteosarcoma.

                    F. Wu

1. Introduction

Using thermal energy to treat human neoplasm dated back to that approximately five thousand years ago, where physicians in Egypt used cautery with heated implements to destroy tumors (Breasted, 1930). In the past two decades, new thermal therapies, including microwave (Matsukawa *et al.*, 1997; Sato *et al.*, 1998; Dong *et al.*, 2003), laser (Bremer *et al.*, 1998; Dowlatshahi *et al.*, 2000; Robinson *et al.*, 1998; Vogl *et al.*, 1995), cryotherapy (Dale *et al.*, 1998; Lezoche *et al.*, 1998; Staren *et al.*, 1997), and radiofrequency (Gazelle *et al.*, 2000; McGahan & Dodd, 2001; Bohm *et al.*, 2000), have been developed to ablate solid tumors by a minimally invasive route. Such therapies are attractive to both patients and physicians, as they can cause patients lesser damage than open surgery, reducing the length of hospital stay, and money. These technological advances have initiated a change from open surgery towards less invasive techniques in the treatment of tumors. However, they require at least percutaneous access to insert an instrument into the targeted tumor in the management of thermal ablation, and are usually performed in patients with tumors less than 4 cm in diameter (Dodd *et al.*, 2000).

Noninvasive, image-guided, *in situ* tumor ablation with high intensity focused ultrasound (HIFU) energy has recently received increasing interest as a promising modality for the treatment of localized solid malignancies (Kennedy, 2005). Since an ultrasound beam can be focused and transmitted through solid tissues, it is possible to use an extracorporeal ("outside-the-body") source of ultrasound for therapeutic purpose. If sufficient acoustic energy is concentrated within the focal volume, the temperature in that region may be raised to levels at which the tumors are cooked, resulting in coagulation necrosis (Fig. 1). Compared with the minimally invasive modalities, HIFU is a truly noninvasive therapy, without damaging overlying and surrounding vital structures. The thermal ablation provides a potential therapy for destroying entire tumors in a 3-dimensional conformal fashion, and it is expected to be very precise and complete with almost no limitation of tumor size and shape. As a result, these advantages make it one of the most attractive potential therapies for the localized treatment of tumor in the future.

HIFU has a different modality from conventional hyperthermia, which has been used in combination with radiotherapy or chemotherapy since

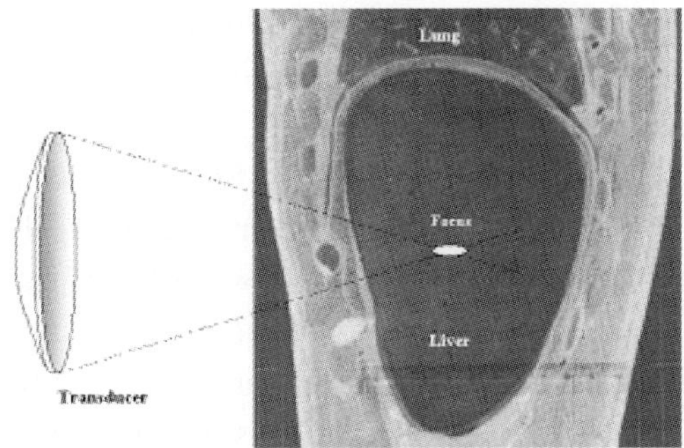

Fig. 1.   A schematic diagram of the principle of HIFU.

the 1980s. The purpose of hyperthermia is to raise the temperature of the tumor from 37°C to 42–45°C for ~30–60 minutes. However, the temperature distributions induced *in vivo* are nonuniform because of tissue cooling by blood flow, and it is extremely difficult to induce thermal exposure in a complete coagulation necrosis of a targeted tumor. With HIFU, the temperature within the focal zone is rapidly raised to a temperature above 56°C and is held for 1–3 seconds. The rapid deposition of HIFU thermal energy causes a peak in temperature rise that is unaffected by the blood flow cooling. Therefore, it is generally believed that there is no need to insert thermocouple probes into the targeted tumor to describe temperature distribution during HIFU procedure.

2. History of Extracorporeal HIFU

In 1942, Lynn and his colleagues reported for the first time using HIFU to cause tissue destruction (Lynn *et al.*, 1942). However, the Fry brothers (William and Frank Fry) at the University of Illinois, USA, did most of the early research works involved in HIFU in the 1950s. They found that the lesion induced with HIFU exposure was well circumscribed, without any destruction of overlying and surrounding tissues. William Fry and his colleagues successfully performed HIFU to produce lesions deep in the brain of animals such as cat and monkey (Fry *et al.*, 1954; Fry *et al.*, 1955). The Fry's subsequently developed techniques to treat patients with Parkinson's disease and other neurological conditions after removing a piece of skull for creating an "acoustic window" (Fry, 1958). Early reports were encouraging in the treatment of Parkinson's disease, but the Indiana team did not continue their work because the effective drug levodopa was introduced at the same time.

In the 1970s, Fred Lizzi's group at the Riverside Research Institute in New York, USA put considerable effort into applying HIFU in the field of ophthalmology. They investigated the possibility of using HIFU to treat glaucoma, choroidal melanomas and capsular tears, and clinical results looked very exciting (Lizzi, 1993; Coleman *et al.*, 1986; Coleman *et al.*, 1991). However, the advent of medical lasers for use in ophthalmology occurred simultaneously. Due to the ease of its use, the laser has superseded HIFU in most ophthalmological applications.

The developments of medical imaging modalities, such as computed tomography (CT), B-mode ultrasonography, and magnetic resonance imaging (MRI), have led to recent advances in HIFU technology in the past 2 decades. Based on their experience with extracorporeal shock-wave lithotripsy, which was used for destroying calculi of the kidney, ureter and bladder by physical forces in clinical practice, Guy Vallancien and his colleagues at the institute Mutualiste Montsouris in Paris, France constructed an extracorporeal focused ultrasound device with Dr Dory's help in the 1990s. His team used this pyrotherapy device to treat superficial bladder tumors under ultrasound imaging guidance in phase I and II clinical trials. In phase I trial, 5 patients were enrolled and cystoscopy was performed before and after treatment. The disappearance of the tumor in two cases and coagulation necrosis in the remaining patients were noted (Vallancien *et al.*, 1993). In phase II trial, a total of 25 patients with low-grade superficial bladder tumor were recruited. After treatment, 67% of the patients were tumor free at 1 year, and no invasion or metastasis was detected with follow-up of 3–21 months (Vallancien *et al.*, 1996). However, when 2 patients with metastatic liver cancer were treated with the same device prior to surgical resection, the results looked unsatisfactory. There was no visible effect in one case, and in another, there was extensive tissue laceration and patchy necrosis (Vallancien *et al.*, 1992).

Gail ter Haar and her colleagues at the Royal Marsden Hospital in London, UK built a prototype of HIFU in the 1990s. This device employed a spherical ceramic transducer of 10 cm diameter and 15 cm focal length. It was driven at a frequency of 1.7 MHz and operated at free field spatial intensities between $1000\,\text{W}\cdot\text{cm}^{-2}$ and $4660\,\text{W}\cdot\text{cm}^{-2}$ (ter Haar *et al.*, 1991). In phase I trial, a total of 68 patients were treated with this device. The results demonstrated that HIFU treatment of liver cancer was well tolerated; some moderate local pain was observed, but only in a few patients (Visioli *et al.*, 1999).

Our group at the Institute of Ultrasonic Engineering in Medicine and the Clinical Center for Tumor Therapy of Chongqing Medical University in Chongqing, China initiated the HIFU research in 1988. Laboratory and animal studies were carried out from 1988 to 1997. After finishing studies in animals such as goat, pig and monkey, we designed and constructed an extracorporeal HIFU prototype for clinical trials. Real-time ultrasound imaging was employed to guide and monitor the ablation procedure in this prototype. On December 10, 1997, my colleagues and I used it to perform the first HIFU treatment in China for a boy with tibia osteosarcoma. The treatment was very successful without any complication. Till October 2001, a total of 1038 patients with solid tumors received extracorporeal HIFU in 10 Chinese hospitals (Wu *et al.*, 2004). Solid malignancies treated with HIFU included primary and metastatic liver cancer, malignant bone tumor, breast cancer, soft tissue sarcoma, kidney cancer, pancreatic cancer, advanced local tumors and solid metastatic deposits of colorectal origin within the abdominal and pelvic cavities. Benign tumors such as uterine fibroid, benign breast tumor, and hepatic hemangioma were also treated. From November 2001 to March 2004, approximately 2500 patients underwent HIFU treatment in 20 Chinese hospitals. To date, the same device (Model-JC HIFU system, Chongqing HAIFU, China) and clinical therapeutic plans have been introduced into UK (Kennedy & Roberts, 2004; Kennedy & Phillips, 2004), Japan (Okuno *et al.*, 2004), and South Korea (Dr. Sang and Dr. Park, personal communication), and so far, more than 300 patients have received the treatment outside China.

Ultrasound imaging was used in all the HIFU devices mentioned above to guide and monitor therapeutic procedure. However, Kullervo Hynynen's group at the Brigham and Women's Hospital in Boston, USA incorporated HIFU into an MRI system, and constructed an MRI-guided HIFU device in the 1990s (Okuno *et al.*, 2004). With MRI thermometry techniques, the device can record focal temperature rises on the anatomical images during treatment procedure. Till now, this MRI-guided HIFU has been used clinically to ablate breast neoplasm and uterine fibroids, and the results indicate successful ablation of targeted tumors (Hynynen *et al.*, 2001; Tempany *et al.*, 2003).

Although the purpose of this section is to describe extracorporal HIFU treatment, it is necessary to introduce some clinical experiences of using a transrectal HIFU device in the treatment of patients with prostate cancer. Till now, two commercially available devices are reported to treat prostate cancer in clinical practice. One transrectal device (Sonablate, Focused Surgery, USA) uses a 4 MHz PZT transducer for both imaging and treatment (Madersbacher *et al.*, 1993), and another (Ablatherm, EDAP, France) uses a 2.25–3.0 MHz rectangular transducer for treatment and a retractable 7.5 MHz probe for imaging guidance (Chaussy & Thuroff, 2000). These devices have been widely used in the treatment of patients with prostate cancer, and clinical results are very exciting. Negative biopsy rates were observed in 87.2% of patients, and prostate specific antigen values remained at their nadir in 84.1% 1 year after HIFU (Thuroff *et al.*, 2003).

3. Mechanism of HIFU Ablation

Ultrasound is a form of vibrational energy. It propagates as a mechanical wave by the motion of particles in the medium. The wave propagation leads to compressions and rarefactions of the particles, so that a pressure wave is transmitted along with the mechanical movement of the particles. As an ultrasound beam propagates through the body, it loses energy due to ultrasonic attenuation in tissue, caused by both scattering and absorption. The absorption of ultrasonic energy causes a local temperature rise in tissue if the rate of heating exceeds the rate of cooling. In HIFU, the absorption is greatest in the focus, where the acoustic intensity is at its highest. Additionally, during the rarefaction of the pressure wave, gas can be drawn out of the solution, and the bubbles subsequently formed may be acted on by the acoustic wave. When they reach the size of resonance, these bubbles suddenly collapse, causing mechanical stresses on surrounding tissues.

Two main mechanisms are directly involved in the tissue damage induced by HIFU exposure. The first is a thermal effect from the conversion of mechanical energy into heat in the tissue, and the second is through cavitation. The thermal effect depends on the temperature achieved and the length of HIFU exposure. If the temperature rise is above a threshold of 56°C and the exposure time is 1 second (Hill *et al.*, 1994), irreversible cell deaths will be induced through coagulation necrosis. In fact, the temperature at a focal volume may rise rapidly above 80°C during HIFU treatments (**?**). A steep temperature gradient is detected between the focus and normal non-focal surrounding tissue, and therefore a sharp demarcation between the treated and untreated tissue is demonstrated in histological examination (Fig. 2).

The second mechanism is acoustic cavitation (Maris & Balibar, 2000). Acoustic cavitation can be defined as the interaction of a sound field with the microscopic gas bodies in a sonicated medium. The presence of small gaseous nuclei existing in subcellular organelles and fluid in tissue are the source of cavitation, which can expand and contract under the influence of the acoustic pressure. During the collapse of bubbles, the acoustic pressure is more than several thousand Pascals, and the temperatures reach several thousand degrees Celsius (Mason, 1998). Therefore, it may cause tissue damage that is less predictable than the effect to tissue shape and position caused by heating (Hill *et al.*, 1994). However, recent experimental studies have been investigating the idea of promoting cavitation for enhancing the level of ablation and reducing required exposure times (Sokka *et al.*, 2003). This is in contrast to previous approaches, where cavitation was viewed as an unpredictable damage mechanism that should be avoided (Clement, 2004).

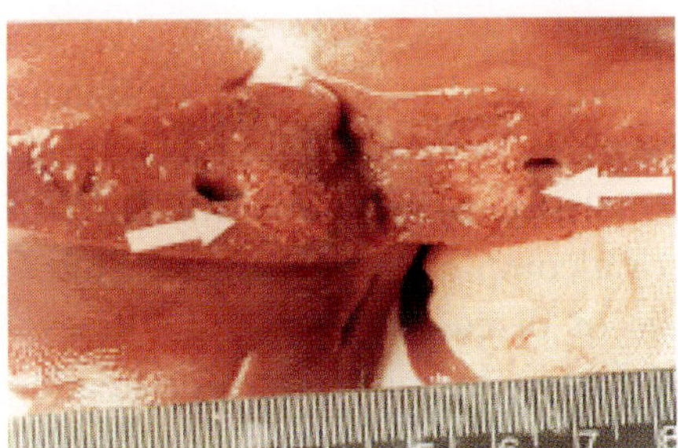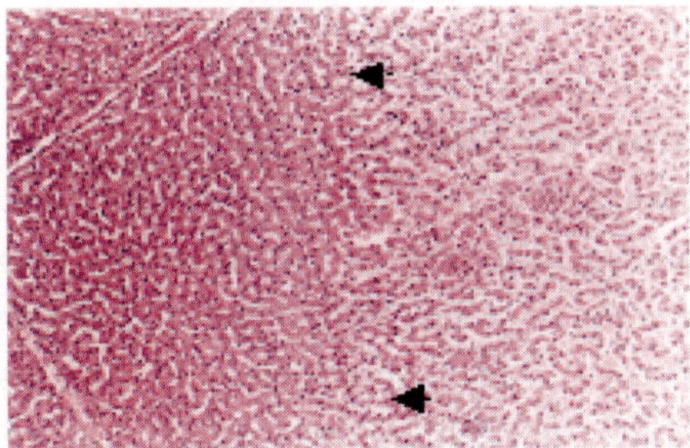

Fig. 2. A volume of coagulation necrosis induced with HIFU therapy *in vivo* in pig liver. The margin (arrows) is very clear between the treated and untreated tissue at macroscopic examination. Even under microscopy there is a very narrow boundary (arrows) between live cells and dead cells at the edges of the necrosis volume.

Furthermore, it would be impossible to identify distinctly thermal effect from mechanical effect due to acoustic cavitation in tissue during HIFU ablation, and they can simultaneously occur within tissue in practice. Therefore, the coagulation necrosis induced by HIFU can be considered as the result of biological effects from a combination of mechanical stresses and thermal damage on tissue. While the tissue is heated, gas bubbles are drawn out of solution more easily. This leads to the decreased threshold of acoustic pressure for cavitation, and a large volume of lesion can be synergistically induced in the targeted tissue (ter Haar, 2001).

4. HIFU Therapeutic Plan

The aim of HIFU treatment is to deliver extracorporeal focused ultrasound energy to a well-defined targeted volume at depth through the intact skin, and thereby induce coagulation of the tumor without causing damage to the overlying or surrounding vital structures. As tumor geometry is usually complicated, three-dimensional (3D) therapeutic planning based on images is essential in achieving a complete ablation. The spatial distribution of thermal ablation delivered depends on a well-thought available plan, therapeutic device, and doctor expertise. The processes of HIFU treatment planning and the technical considerations relative to this therapeutic planning will be described later in this chapter.

4.1. *Pre-HIFU planning*

The process of HIFU treatment for the individual patient with malignant tumor includes a number of steps, as shown in Table 1. Each of these steps requires special knowledge and close collaboration with other members of the team to ensure accurate execution of a complicated set of procedures. It begins with the pathologic diagnosis of disease and accurate assessment of the tumor using TNM classification. As modalities for treating solid malignancy are usually multiple, combining local therapies such as surgery or radiation and systemic therapy such as chemotherapy, a decision as to whether the planned treatment is curative or palliative is made from a multidisciplinary clinical meeting held with surgeons, oncologists, radiologists, radiation oncologists, and pathologists. The role and scheduling of

Table 1. Pre-HIFU planning processes.

Step 1	Diagnosis	Serum level of specific tumor markers
		Imaging examinations, such as MRI/CT and US imaging
		Tumor pathologic diagnosis
		Staging of patients (*e.g.*, TNM)
		↓
Step 2	Therapeutic aims	Cure
		Palliation
		↓
Step 3	Therapeutic modalities	Surgery
		Chemotherapy
		Radiotherapy
		HIFU
		Other treatments
		↓
		HIFU Patient

chemotherapy or vascular embolization of the tumor in relation to a session of HIFU are defined at the start. Subsequently, the location and extent of the tumor relative to the overlying and adjacent critical normal tissue are determined by a variety of imaging modalities. However, sometimes pre-HIFU adjuvant treatments may influence the site and size of the targeted volume. For instance, patients with typical osteosarcoma are treated with neo-adjuvant several circles of chemotherapy, and obvious regression of the tumor is usually observed in these patients.

4.2. *Imaging for HIFU planning*

Imaging aspects includes tumor size, shape, number, margin, and location within the organ relative to large blood vessel, nervous fiber, as well as vital structures that might be at risk of injure by the thermal ablation. Using contrast-enhanced technique, tumor vascularity is assessed to determine the acoustic energy distribution in the tumor.

Imaging taken for HIFU treatment planning is usually different from those taken for diagnostic use. Apart from imaging aspects of the tumor, adjacent organs close to the targeted volume require attention for the purpose of safety. Using available imaging techniques, the relationship between the tumor and its surrounding organs is evaluated. For instance, a hepatic tumor in the lower part of the left liver may be near to stomach, duodenum, and colon. Compared with magnetic resonance imaging (MRI) and computed tomography (CT), real-time ultrasound imaging is more important to assess the relationship between the tumor and the gastrointestinal tracts.

MRI and CT examinations include non-enhanced and contrast-enhanced scan. Either MRI or CT is selected to perform for the acquisition of tumor data. The sequences used for imaging are seen in Sec. 6 (Imaging in HIFU).

Ultrasound imaging includes B-mode imaging, color Doppler and power ultrasound imaging, and contrast ultrasound examination. Attention must be given to the characteristics of the tumor gray-scale, margin, motion and vascularity, particularly big blood vessels that are more than 2 mm in diameter in the tumor and/or surrounding the tumor. If ultrasound imaging is used for the guidance of ablative procedures, non-enhanced and contrast-enhanced MRI/CT will be performed as an essential imaging examination to compensate for some of the shortcomings of ultrasound imaging, such as less sensitivity in predicting the tumor margin, and occasional poor lesion detection as a result of overlying bone (*e.g.*, ribs). Comparing the difference between the MRI/CT and ultrasound imaging appearances before planning HIFU treatment protocol should be a routine practice.

4.3. *Tumor volume localization*

The targeted tumor volume is described as the macroscopic extent of the tumor, which is palpable, visible and detectable by available radiological examinations. If the determination of the targeted volume depends on the diagnostic techniques including CT/MRI and ultrasound imaging, it is essential to indicate which methods have been used for its determination.

Tumor cells are likely to extend beyond the actual tumor margins into the normal tissue, and recently, available image techniques may not exactly circumscribe acute tumor margins. The failure to achieve a satisfactory ablation margin will be accompanied by a high local recurrence ratio. However, available data for quantifying this margin of tumor volume are lacking. The definition of targeted volume is based on knowledge from surgical and postmortem specimens, and patterns of tumor recurrence, as well as from clinical experience. It may be the most difficult and subjective step in the HIFU planning process.

For curative treatment, the aim is to induce complete coagulation of a targeted tumor and the estimated extent of the microscopic spread surrounding the visible tumor. This is a principle that is routine in conventional surgery in order to ensure the removal of adjacent micro-satellites, and to allow for the uncertainty that frequently exists concerning the exact location of definite tumor margins. A number of factors, such as the age of the patient and considerations of normal tissue tolerance, may affect the maximum volume considered to be appropriate for treatment. For instance, hepatocellular carcinoma is frequently seen in the setting of hepatic cirrhosis with partial liver dysfunction. Definition of targeted volume is cautiously determined for each patient. If the extent of ablative tissue is the same as one of the surgical resection, including the tumor and 2 cm margin of normal tissue surrounding the tumor, HIFU may offer its equivalent effectiveness and considerably decreased risk of morbidity and mortality in this high-risk patient population.

4.4. *Acoustic path for ultrasound energy entry*

Acoustic path is defined as a direct path between HIFU transducer and a targeted volume at depth, where the focused ultrasound beam from the radiating surface can directly penetrate through the overlying tissue of the targeted volume, thereby destroying the tumor. This path is usually the shortest route of focused ultrasound beam from the skin to the targeted volume.

As the ultrasound energy is attenuated while it penetrates through the tissue, it is very important to achieve a large surface area for the acoustic path, and then ultrasound beam can sufficiently be converged through the targeted volume. This geometrical gain of focusing is necessary to overcome the attenuation loss and to induce complete coagulation of the targeted volume. However, several factors are involved to influence the extent of the path, including the diameter of HIFU transducer, frequency, tumor depth and volume, and the structure of the overlying tissue, as well as the principal method that is used to make the transducer.

4.5. *Ultrasonic properties of overlying tissues*

Although many factors can influence the energy deposition of focused ultrasound beam, the absorbed power density in the targeted volume may be estimated. One of the most important factors is attributed to the ultrasonic property of the overlying tissues between the skin and the target. The beam is attenuated by absorption and scattering, while it propagates through these overlying tissues. It is also reflected from the surfaces of various structures in the overlying tissues. Furthermore, the heterogeneity of the overlying tissues, such as ribs and muscular tendons, may change the beam propagation direction, focus location, shape and size of a focal area. Thus, it is very important to know the ultrasonic properties of the overlying tissues, and a precise analysis of the acoustic properties of the overlying tissues during the treatment planning for an individual patient may avoid undesirable effects, thereby achieving a successful HIFU ablation.

Tissue ultrasound amplitude attenuation is a sum of the losses from absorption and scattering of ultrasonic energy in tissue. Each tissue has an attenuation value of its own. For instance, the amplitude attenuation values in lung and bone tissue are approximately 430–480 $\mathrm{Npm}^{-1}\,\mathrm{MHz}^{-1}$ and 150–350 $\mathrm{Npm}^{-1}\,\mathrm{MHz}^{-1}$ respectively, which are the highest among the living tissues (Dunn, 1974; Wells, 1977; Hill *et al.*, 2004). Fatty tissue has lower values, ranging from 5 to 9 $\mathrm{Npm}^{-1}\,\mathrm{MHz}^{-1}$, the soft tissue values are generally about 10 $\mathrm{Npm}^{-1}\,\mathrm{MHz}^{-1}$ (Goss *et al.*, 1979; Goss *et al.*, 1978; Goss *et al.*, 1980). Compared with normal tissue, the attenuation in the tumor is usually higher. The attenuation in brain tumor is higher than that in the normal brain (Kikuchi *et al.*, 1957), and a similar difference is also detected between breast cancer and normal breast (Calderon *et al.*, 1976). However, the definition of the attenuation in the overlying tissue and the tumor is relative. While the deep part of a targeted tumor is treated with HIFU, it also includes the normal tissues between the skin and the superficial margin of the tumor and the neoplastic tissue in the front of the focus.

Images taken from the treatment planning can provide useful information about the overlying tissues. By using a HIFU device they are reassessed under the guidance of real-time ultrasound imaging when the patient lies on the treatment bed in a correct therapy position. The composition, interface, and thickness of the overlying tissue are carefully recorded. Then, ultrasound attenuation in the overlying tissue may be simply estimated and should be documented in writing with a diagram. These data may obviously vary due to the tumor location and patient position for treatment. Acoustic properties of the overlying tissues, the interfaces between the tissues, and incident angle of ultrasound beam can obviously affect the ultrasound attenuation. A large amount of energy reflection occurs when a focused ultrasound beam propagates from muscle layer to the bone surface such as ribs. This can cause the loss of energy deposition in the targeted volume, and may increase local temperature of muscle-bone interface because the amplitude attenuation coefficient of ultrasound is about 10–20 times higher in bone than in soft tissue (Wells, 1977; Hill *et al.*, 2004). Furthermore, attention must be given to the large variations in the overlying tissue thickness among individual patients (*e.g.*, thin or overweight patient).

It is believed that there is only a small amount of energy reflection between the soft tissue interfaces because of small variations in the acoustic impedance of soft tissues. The largest one is the interface between fat and muscle tissues, but it causes only 1–2% of the beam intensity to be reflected (Wells, 1977; Hill *et al.*, 2004). It must be noted that some exceptional cases are observed in clinical application. For instance, the beam reflection is very low theoretically on the interface between subcutaneous tissue and rectus abdominis. As fibrous tissue forms a strong layer of connective tissue on the surface of the rectus abdominis, it can cause a higher reflection of ultrasound beam on this interface.

4.6. *Therapeutic planning using HIFU device*

Using a HIFU device, the position of a patient is decided with the help of an imaging system equipped in the device. This position must be comfortable, reproducible, and suitable for acquisition of imaging for planning and subsequent treatment. It is technically ideal to achieve either the shortest way or enough surface extent of the acoustic path for the treatment of a targeted volume. The choice of position for treatment is dependent on the tumor location, size and shape, which are shown on both MRI/CT and ultrasound imaging before the planning process, though palpation is important to the superficial tumors such as breast cancer. It is necessary that the patient be treated in one position during the entire process of the procedure. The change of patient position may result in alterations in internal and external anatomy and risk of mis-target. However, if the patients require a change of position for the purpose of treatment during the procedure, it must be technically designed in advance and carefully recorded, so that the over- or under-dosage of the acoustic energy within the targeted volume can be avoided.

The position of the patient, all positioning aids and anatomical measurements should be accurately documented in writing with a diagram and digital photos to ensure reproducibility through all the stages of the planning process and subsequent treatment. However, sometimes the position may be constrained by equipment limitations. For instance, the arm position may be restricted by the limited size of the treatment bed. Attention should be given when the patient's position is selected.

Immobilization is required during the HIFU procedure. It varies according to the technique being used and the location of the tumors. Total physical restraint is essential to protect the patients who are receiving a particular kind of anesthesia method. Appropriate immobilization can be achieved with the various fixing aids such as hanging belts of sponge, pillows, leg restraints, and foot rests. It must be ascertained that the respiration of patients is free while the fixation is performed, without any pressure effect on the chest and the abdomen.

Clinical studies have reported that there is organ motion occurring in the body. Either diaphragm movement during respiration or the pulsating of large arteries usually causes this motion. Furthermore, organ movement may not be uniform, but dependent on the individual patient. It is recommended that this variation be previously estimated, and then measured using real-time ultrasound imaging during the planning session for each patient. The movement of the diaphragm caused by respiration can obviously move some internal organs such as liver, pancreas and kidney. It is very important to control the large movement of these organs during the HIFU procedure, particularly for the small volume tumor. An alternative technique of active breathing control involves immobilized breathing using general anesthesia; this method may be used for treatment of the liver and kidney, where excursions of up to 3 cm may occur.

Once the patient is correctly positioned and secured, the skin overlying the tumor is brought in contact with degassed water or a plastic bag filled with degassed water via acoustic gel, so that the ultrasound beam can transmit from the water into the tissue. The positions of the entire targeted tumor and surrounding vital structures are determined using the real-time diagnostic ultrasound imaging. With the movement of the diagnostic probe from one side of the tumor to the other, images of the targeted volume are achieved (Fig. 3). Then, 3D ultrasound imaging of the tumor can be done by using sequential scans of the treatment volume.

For therapeutic purposes, the entire tumor is segmented into slices for ultrasound imaging; the spacing between slices depends on the size, shape, and location of the region of tumor and acoustic window. The extent of the separation is usually about 5–10 mm, although it varies with different tumors. The targeted volume is defined as the volume of tissue that includes the tumor visualized on the ultrasound imaging and regions considered to be at risk for microscopic extension. If the margin of the tumor is not clear enough, MRI or CT scans are available to make it clearer. By using a tracker ball or mouse with interactive software program, the contours of the targeted volume can be manually outlined at the planning computer on each ultrasound slice (Fig. 4), and then transferred to the planning system. Finally,

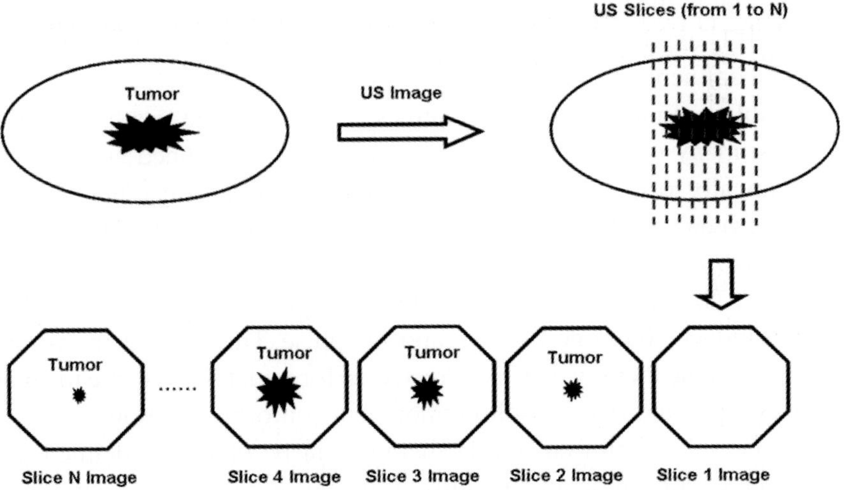

Fig. 3.   Schematic diagram showing that the entire tumor can be segmented into slices on ultrasound imaging.

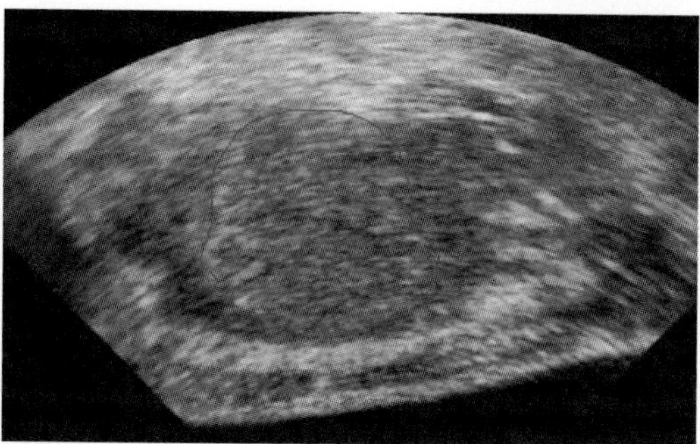

Fig. 4. The contour of the targeted volume on one ultrasound slice is manually outlined at the planning system.

the targeted volume that includes the margin with appropriate margins at all levels is built into the computer memory.

5. HIFU 3-D Conformal Therapy

The volume of tissue ablation induced with one HIFU exposure can be regarded as a lesion. The focal volume of HIFU transducer is usually ellipsoid or cigar-shaped, with dimensions of 8–15 mm along the beam axis and 1–3 mm in the transverse direction. Therefore, the lesion induced with single HIFU exposure is usually very small. While lesions are placed side by side, confluent volumes of ablation can be achieved.

To ablate clinically relevant volumes of tissue for the treatment of carcinomas, many of these small lesions should be positioned side by side systematically to "paint out" a targeted volume, without any remaining live tissue between each lesion. Figure 5 shows that multiple-pulse HIFU exposures *in vitro* in ox liver can produce coagulation necrosis, which spells out HIFU. The line-necrosis in each letter consists of many necrotic dots, which is induced by a one-by-one exposure pulse. This result demonstrates that, if a suitable therapy plan is correctly performed, HIFU is able to ablate various shapes and sizes of solid tumors in a conformal fashion.

As a result, conformal HIFU therapy can be clinically defined as a precise procedure to ablate an entire tumor by moving high-energy concentrated focus side by side in a 3-D fashion. At the beginning of the HIFU procedure, the targeted tumor is identified and divided into parallel slices

Fig. 5. Multiple-pulse HIFU exposures can achieve coagulation necrosis that spells out HIFU *in vitro* in ox liver, indicating that HIFU ablation is a 3-D conformal treatment.

of 5 mm separation by moving the diagnostic probe. Using HIFU exposure regimes, the tumor on each slice is completely ablated, and this process is repeated slice by slice to achieve complete coagulation of the targeted tumor, as shown as Fig. 6. There are four exposure regimes that are usually used in the HIFU procedure. They include single exposure for a cigar-shaped lesion, either multiple or single exposures or linear scan exposures for a line-shaped lesion, and a convergent scan for the lesion of deep tumor.

A single exposure can be made to induce a cigar-shaped lesion when the location of the focal volume is immoveable (Fig. 7). The exposure time for each pulse ranges from one second to several seconds. The single exposure can be repeated at predetermined intervals in the same position. Multiple single exposures can produce a line-shaped lesion through placing single-exposure lesions side by side with a present overlap and with a predetermined time interval between exposures (Fig. 8). The multiple single exposures can be repeated in the perpendicular direction to form a slice-shaped lesion (Fig. 9). A line-shaped lesion can also be achieved by a linear

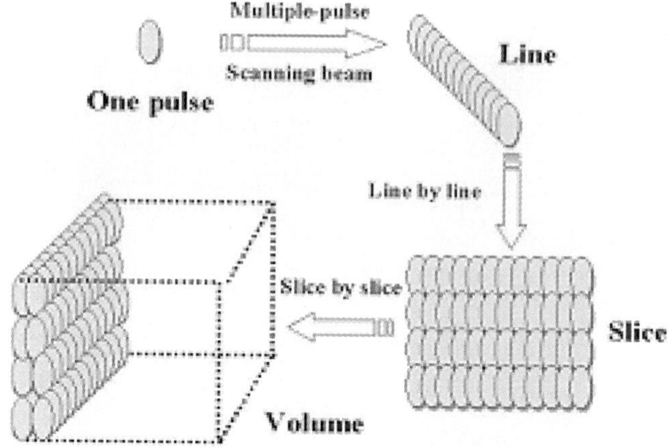

Fig. 6. Schematic diagram showing the HIFU conformal therapeutic plan, which is used to ablate the whole volume of solid tumor.

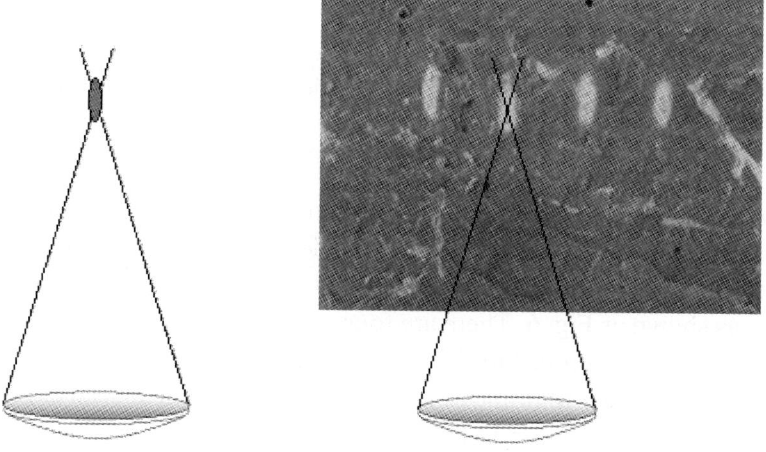

Fig. 7. Schematic diagram showing single exposure regime used in HIFU procedure.

track exposure in which the activated transducer is moved at a constant speed over a line (Fig. 8). This may be made by traversing one or more times in one direction only, or by scanning in both directions ("there and back") without pausing at the furthest extremity. Several of these tracks may be superimposed in one exposure period at chosen (preset) time intervals. Superimposition of tracks leads to an increase in the extent of ablation

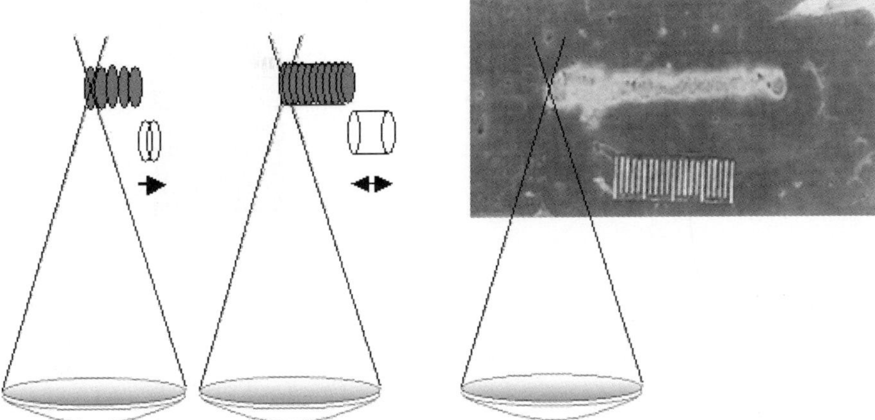

Fig. 8. Schematic diagram showing a line-shaped lesion induced by either multiple single exposures or a linear scan exposure.

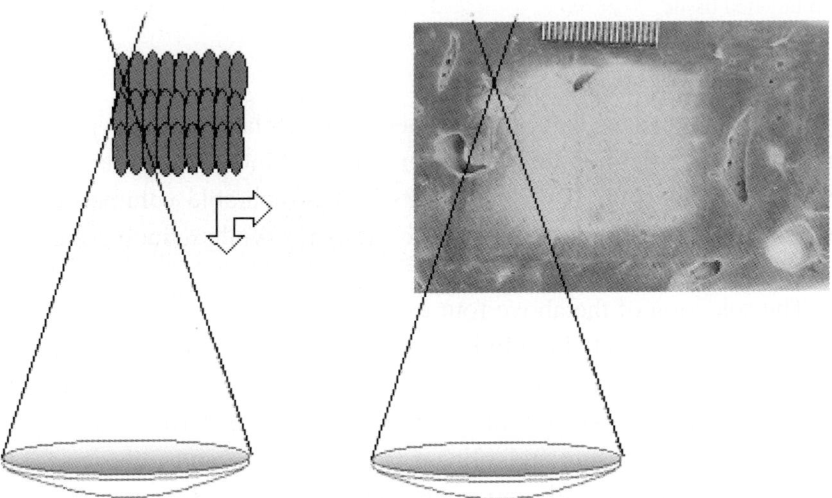

Fig. 9. Schematic diagram showing a slice-shaped lesion induced by either assorted multiple single exposures or assorted linear scan exposures.

in the direction perpendicular to the direction of motion due to thermal conduction. As a result, a slice-shaped lesion can be induced in this way, as shown in Fig. 9. From one slice-shaped lesion to the next, confluent volumes of ablation can be achieved.

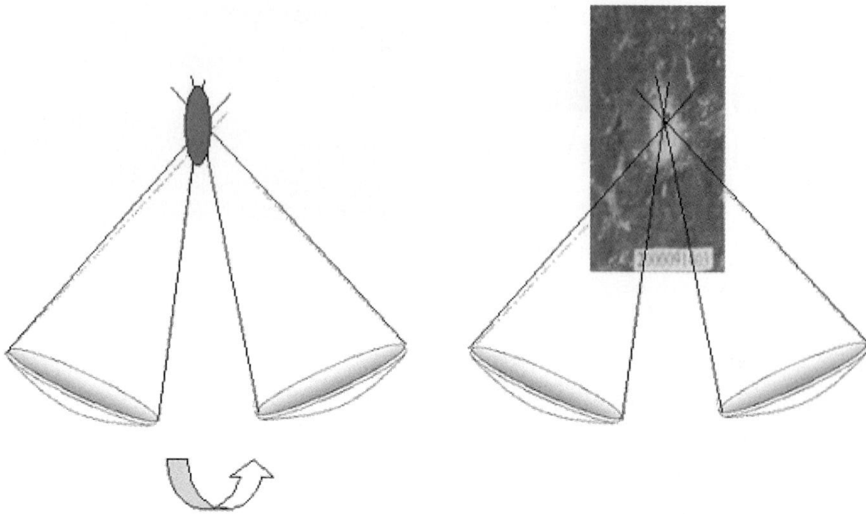

Fig. 10. Schematic diagram showing a convergent scan exposure used for the ablation of deep-targeted tissue.

A convergent scan can be performed for the ablation of a deep-targeted volume. In this regime, the transducer is moved in an arc centered on the geometric focus (Fig. 10). This results in a comparable volume of tissue ablation to that given by a single static exposure, while reducing the exposure to the skin.

The selection of the above four exposure regimes during HIFU procedure is very complicated in clinical practice. It depends on the component of overlying tissue structure, acoustic window, the depth of tumor from the skin, vital structures surrounding tumor, tumor vascularity and size. For instance, single exposure and a linear scan exposure can be chosen for the treatment of a superficially, poor vascularized tumor. However, a convergent scan exposure and multiple single exposures are usually used in the treatment of deep vasculiarized tumors. In clinics, they can be separately used for an individual patient simultaneously. Therefore, only doctors with a knowledge base from a specialized training course could perform this treatment. The experience that doctors have and the reasonable judgment that they can make during the HIFU procedure are important at the early stage of HIFU clinical application. As therapeutic data are extensively collected for each type of solid malignancy, improvement is expected in the near future.

6. Imaging in HIFU

Recent developments of imaging modalities such as CT and MRI have dramatically led to significant advances in HIFU technology. Accurate anatomical information is an essential precondition for planning and implementing HIFU procedure to the entire extent of the malignancy. In fact, radiological and medical images of various types are employed at each step of the HIFU treatment process, including diagnosis, assessment of the extent of disease, treatment planning, treatment and assessment of tumor response, follow-up, and outcome evaluation. Therefore, radiological and medical images are of utmost importance in HIFU treatment. With the help of new imaging modalities, doctors are now able to define treatment volumes and critical structures with great precision, thus reducing marginal misses and energy exposure to normal tissues. Such capabilities may permit a higher rate of complete tumor ablation, potentially leading to improvement in local tumor treatment.

Medical images are classified into two types: anatomic and physiologic images. The former category usually include CT, MRI, ultrasonography, digital subtraction angiography (DSA);, the latter are single photon emission computed tomography (SPECT), and positron emission tomography (PET). Anatomic images can provide accurate anatomical information about tumor extent, whereas physiologic images can provide physiologic information on the function of tumors. They are both acquired as digital data, and can be mathematically processed.

6.1. *Medical images used in HIFU*

CT is an X-ray imaging technique used to visualize thin slices of the body. Early CT scanners employed a translate-rotate motion and required long durations ranging from 20 seconds to 5 minutes to acquire a complete set of data for one image. Modern scanners are much faster, acquiring the data for one image in only 1 to 3 seconds. Faster and more accurate CT examination has recently become possible with a new device, the helical scanner.

When contrast agents are used, enhanced CT can provide improved visualization of certain tumors. CT images can be used in various areas of HIFU treatment, including the delineation of the targeted volume, the determination of relative geometry of critical structures, and follow-up evaluation of treatment response. However, the majority of CT images can only provide cross-sectional anatomy images. Even though sagittal or coronal images can be reconstructed from sequential and preferably contiguous axial images, the resolution of such reconstructed images is generally much inferior to that of axial images.

MRI usually presents unique anatomical information and tumor detail. It can offer excellent discrimination of certain tumors with high contrast and good resolution, as well as the ability to select arbitrary planes such as transversal, sagittal and coronal directions for imaging. When contrast agents such as gadolinium compounds are injected, the appearance of the resulting enhanced MRI image is much better than that of its non-enhanced counterpart. The utilization of MRI in HIFU treatment is the same as that with CT. However, in thermometry techniques, MRI can be used as an imaging-guided device to record focal temperature rises on anatomic images during HIFU procedures (Cline *et al.*, 1992; Cline *et al.*, 1994; Hynynen *et al.*, 1993; Hardy *et al.*, 1994).

Due to its extensive availability, real-time visualization, flexibility, non-ionization and low cost, ultrasonography is widely used in clinical practice. It can show tomographic views in almost any orientation. Compared with CT/MRI, ultrasonography produces images with poor resolution. Furthermore, as ultrasound beams cannot penetrate bone or gas-filled cavities such as the lung and gastrointestinal tract, the application is limited. Medical ultrasound imaging systems can be employed as a real-time imaging guided device to identify, to target the tumor to be treated, and to monitor HIFU procedure (Coleman *et al.*, 1991; Gelet *et al.*, 1996; Foster *et al.*, 1993; Coleman *et al.*, 1985; ter Haar *et al.*, 1998; Wu *et al.*, 2002). It is also used to assess the tissue response through gray-scale changes caused by cavitation in focal volume, which is an indication of ablation following each exposure (Wu *et al.*, 1998).

DSA is a standard part of the evaluation of patients with a suspicious malignant tumor. It demonstrates the tumor vascularity and stain, the extent of tumor mass, and the anatomic variants of the regional arterial supply. The use of this technique yields satisfactory diagnostic and anatomic details in most cases of solid malignancies. Since it is an interventional examination, extensive applications of DSA are relatively limited in clinical practice.

SPECT is a radionuclide scanning technique that uses a radioisotope as a tracer to assess abnormal tumor function, rather than to provide simple anatomy. The radioisotopes, such as ^{99m}Tc sestamibi and ^{99m}Tc methylene diphosphate, usually have a high extraction rate at the malignant tumors. It can provide physiological imaging information through tomographic images of the radioactivity distribution within tumor tissue.

PET can determine the level of localized radioactivity by detecting a sufficient number of the two 180-degree opposed photos and using imaging reconstruction algorithms. It is another functional type of imaging that can provide localized physiological information on the presence of tumors.

6.2. *Medical imaging for HIFU planning*

Diagnostic images used in the preparation of HIFU ablation have been described in Sec. 4.2, *Imaging for HIFU planning*. Most anatomic image modalities can be employed to provide anatomical information for determining the location, number and size of tumors and the surrounding vital structures. For instance, in the treatment of liver cancer, it is very important preoperatively to know the relationship between the tumor and its surrounding structures, such as bile ducts, gallbladder, gastrointestinal tract, diaphragm, and large blood vessels. These pre-HIFU images are fundamental images on which the suitability of a patient for HIFU ablation is assessed. In addition, physiological imaging may be used as a pre-HIFU image for the purpose of assessing tumor response to the ablation.

6.3. *Medical imaging for HIFU procedure*

To optimize the ablation of a tumor, it is fundamental to use precise and dependable imaging techniques for ascertaining the adequacy of the treatment. This imaging can be used as an imaging-guided device to identify and target the tumor to be treated, monitor the therapy procedure, and to assess therapy response within targeted tissue. In particular, recent studies involved with the development of imaging procedures enable rapid assessment of the extent of targeted tissue destruction caused by HIFU ablation.

As a result, either ultrasonography or MRI is employed to guide extracorporeal HIFU procedure. Individual preferences or personal research interests may dictate the selection of imaging technique.

There are advantages and disadvantages in both ultrasonography and MRI when each type of device is incorporated into a HIFU system. Clinical ultrasound imaging device is inexpensive, extensively available, flexible, capable in real-time visualization, and valuable in the treatment of organs such as the liver and kidney, which are moved by respiration. The main disadvantage of ultrasonography is poorer imaging resolution than MRI, particularly in predicting tumor margins. It may provide occasional poor lesion detection through lack of inherent tissue contrast or because of overlying bone structures such as ribs. MRI can provide three-dimensional imaging with better resolution. Using indirect thermometry technique it can measure focal temperature rises following HIFU exposure. However, high cost, long treatment time, and problems in tracking a moving target such as the liver may limit extensive application of MRI-guided HIFU devices in clinics.

Due to ultrasonography's poor resolution, good-quality MRI is effectively used to compensate for some of the shortcomings of diagnostic ultrasound imaging, if an ultrasound-guided HIFU device has a problem in predicting the tumor margin. A combined utilization of MRI and ultrasonography before HIFU treatment can fully provide accurate imaging information for determining the number, sizes of tumors, and their relationship to surrounding vital structures. While the ultrasound-guided HIFU device is used in our clinical application, we feel that preoperative MR imaging is very helpful in establishing the 3-D coordinates of the targeted tumor in HIFU planning session. We routinely compare the difference between the MRI and US image appearances in creating a HIFU treatment plan for the complete ablation of a tumor.

When MRI is used in a HIFU procedure, the temperature rises are recorded in the targeted region. On the other hand, ultrasonography can provide significant changes in imaging information within the focal volume during a HIFU procedure. These changes are made evident by increased levels of tissue grey-scale on ultrasound imaging immediately after HIFU exposure, and most of them become gradually less evident and sometimes disappear within several minutes after the ablation. In our animal studies, both *in vivo* and *in vitro*, we find that hyperechoic zones in the targeted tissue correspond mainly to the extent of the coagulation necrosis. There is a close relationship between the extent of necrosis as measured by gross examination and the hyperechoic extent measured immediately after HIFU on the ultrasound image in pig liver. As HIFU exposures consist of single exposures, multiple-single-exposures and scan track exposures, a cigar-shaped lesion and a line-shaped lesion, as well as a slice-shaped lesion, can be obviously detected on real-time ultrasound imaging following relative HIFU exposures, as shown in Figs. 11–13.

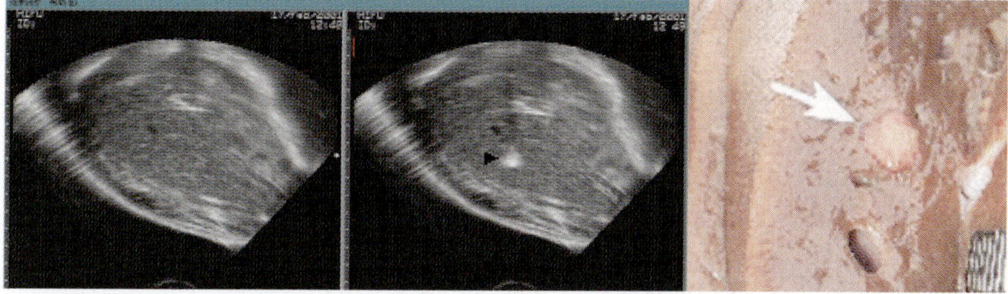

Ultrasonography before HIFU   Ultrasonography immediately after HIFU   Macroscopic change in histology

Fig. 11.   Grey-scale change *in vivo* in pig liver cancer obtained on real-time ultrasonography immediately after HIFU single exposure. Compared to imaging before HIFU, hyperechogenic region (arrow) is seen in targeted region, and conformed to an end-view of the cigar-shaped lesion (arrow) induced by HIFU single exposure.

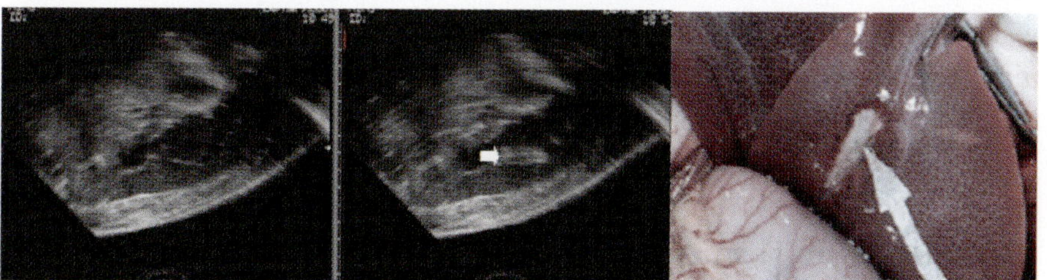

Ultrasonography before HIFU   Ultrasonography immediately after HIFU   Macroscopic change in histology

Fig. 12.   Grey-scale change *in vivo* in pig liver cancer obtained on real-time ultrasonography immediately after a scan track exposure. Compared to imaging before HIFU, hyperechogenic region (arrow) is seen in targeted region, and conformed to the line-shaped lesion (arrow) induced by a scan track exposure.

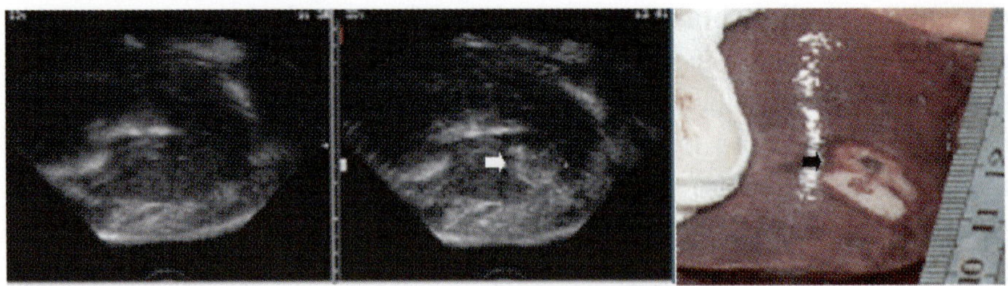

Ultrasonography before HIFU   Ultrasonography immediately after HIFU   Macroscopic change in histology

Fig. 13. Grey-scale change *in vivo* in pig liver cancer obtained on real-time ultrasonography immediately after 2 scan track exposures. Compared with imaging before HIFU, hyperechogenic region (arrow) is seen in targeted region, and conformed to the slice-shaped lesion (arrow) induced by 2 scan track exposures.

These grey-scale changes observed during HIFU procedure are of importance in the treatment of solid malignancy. They provide feed-back control imaging information, monitor therapeutic effects, and control ultrasound energy deposition in the focal volume during the ablation procedure. Figure 14 shows the process of grey-scale changes on real-time ultrasound imaging during the ablation for a patient with big hepatocellular carcinoma. While the focus of HIFU is moved along one slice of the tumor in a scanning fashion from deep to superficial, a hyperechogenic region is clearly detected on ultrasound imaging in this slice of tumor.

Although the mechanism involved in tissue grey-scale changes during HIFU procedure is not clear, to date, it is generally considered that gas bubbles that originate from acoustic cavitation and the vaporization of tissue water are the main factors. The development of ultrasound contrast agents may improve the accuracy of ultrasound imaging for evaluating the final therapeutic effect of vascularized tumor, immediately after the treatment is finished. To our knowledge, however, there is no previous experience of real-time evaluation of the therapeutic effects with ultrasound contrast agents during HIFU procedures.

6.4. *Follow-up imaging for assessment of HIFU ablation*

It is important to detect untreated regions of a targeted tumor that require immediate retreatment, and to demonstrate complete ablation of treated

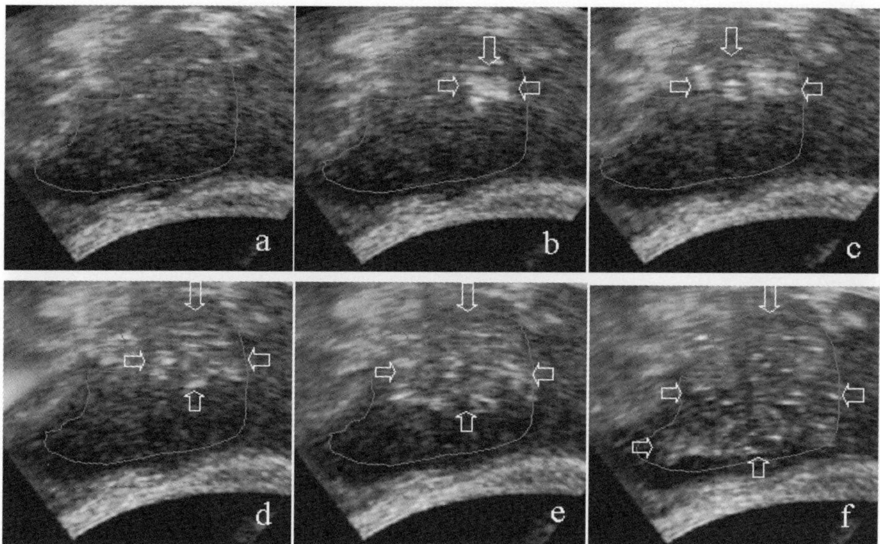

Fig. 14.   HIFU procedure. Compared to tumor imaging (outlined) before HIFU (a), hyper-echogenic region (arrows) is seen in targeted region (b)–(e), until complete ablation achieved in this slice of the tumor (f).

tumors as early as possible, following HIFU thermal ablation. As postpro-cedural core biopsy does not provide pathologic results for the entire treated tumor, follow-up imaging is essential to evaluate the short-term efficacy of *in situ* HIFU ablation. It is generally believed that, if untreated, residual viable tumor foci will regrow and result in therapeutic failure. The failure to detect focal areas of viable tumor in the treated regions early after thermal ablation can lead to local recurrence and to long distance metastases.

Prior to and following each treatment episode, enhanced-CT and enhanced-MRI, ultrasonography, DSA, SPECT, and PET can be employed to evaluate the response of targeted tumors after HIFU procedure is fin-ished. These modalities, anatomical or physiological, can provide imaging information in determining the therapeutic effects on both tumor vascular-ity and on cellular functions immediately after HIFU, as well as changes in tumor size during long-term follow-up period.

Using color and power Doppler methods, ultrasonography can assess changes in tumor vascularity after HIFU ablation (Fig. 15). However, in some cases, especially in the tumors with poor blood supply, ultrasound

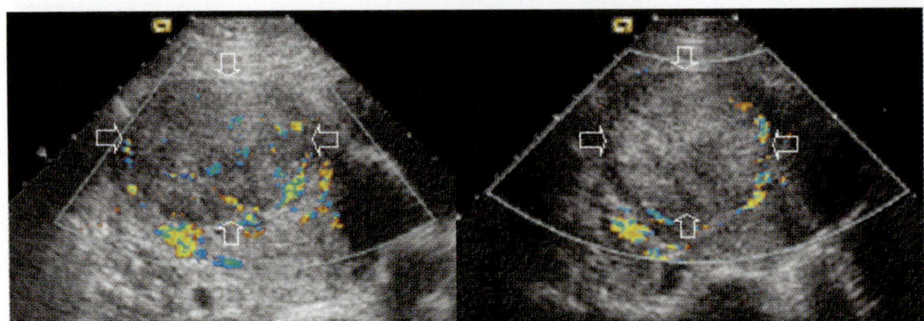

Color Doppler ultrasound imaging before HIFU Color Doppler ultrasound imaging 5 days after HIFU

Fig. 15. Doppler signal changes in human uterine fibroid (arrows) treated with HIFU *in situ*. Compared to imaging before HIFU, Doppler signals (blue or red color) are obviously decreased in the tumor after HIFU, indicating the destruction of tumor vascularity (images provided by courtesy of Prof. Wei Wang at Beijing 307 Hospital, China).

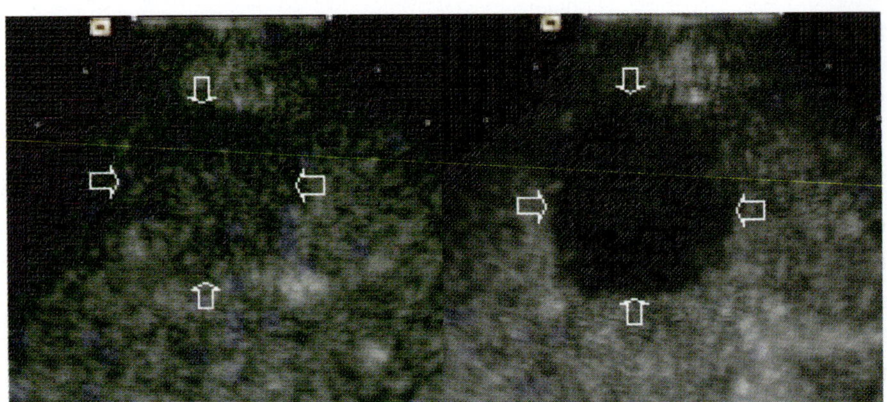

Contrast ultrasound imaging before HIFU Contrast ultrasound imaging 1 day after HIFU

Fig. 16. Microbubble-contrast ultrasound images in a patient with metastatic liver cancer before and after HIFU treatment. Before HIFU, perfusion could be identified within the targeted tumor. After HIFU, there was no evidence of perfusion.

imaging is not sufficiently sensitive for the detection of damage to tumor blood vessels. Using ultrasound contrast agents, ultrasonography can provide imaging information to evaluate the therapeutic response of non-vascularized tumors after HIFU treatment (Fig. 16). Furthermore, DSA can clearly show variants of regional blood supply in the treated tumor after

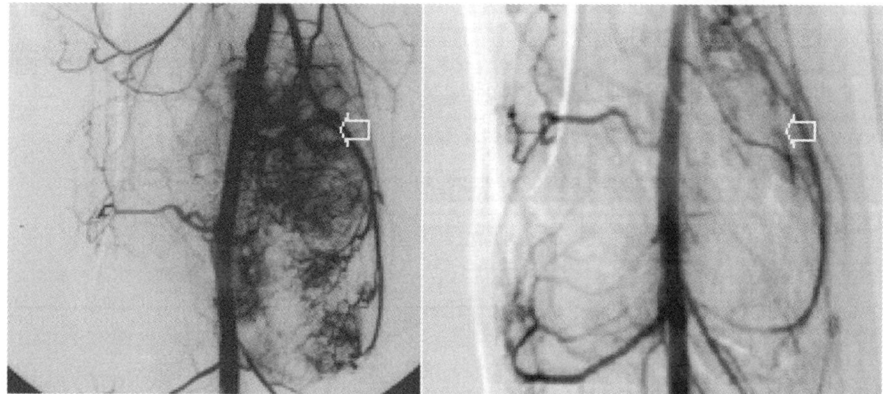

DSA imaging before HIFU　　　　　　　　DSA imaging 3 months after HIFU

Fig. 17. DSA images obtained in a patient who underwent HIFU treatment for distal femur osteosarcoma. Before HIFU persistence of tumor vascularity and capillary stain (arrow) is clear within tumor tissue. But, 3 months after HIFU, complete disappearance of tumor vascularity and stain is seen within the treated tumor (arrow).

HIFU ablation (Fig. 17). Due to interventional examination, applications of DSA are relatively limited. As a physiological imaging, SPECT can provide tomographic images of the radioactivity distribution in a small number of tumors such as osteosarcoma (Fig. 18) and breast cancer (Fig. 19). However, it does not clearly identify the therapeutic response in most tumors, particularly in patients with liver cancer. Theoretically, PET can be employed to detect physiological function in almost solid malignancies. Unfortunately, until now, no data are available in HIFU ablation.

Non-enhanced CT obtained 1–2 weeks after HIFU ablation are not sufficiently sensitive to assess therapeutic response, especially in encapsulated lesions such as those of hepatocellular carcinoma, and of osteosarcoma lesions located in the long bone marrow cavity. Compared with non-enhanced CT, non-enhanced MRI may characteristically reveals varied signals of ablated tumors on both T1- and T2-weighted images after HIFU ablation. Contrast-enhanced CT is useful for demonstrating changes in tumor vascular perfusion, and for distinguishing the difference between nonviable and residual viable tumor directly in the treated regions. The most striking changes are seen in contrast-enhanced MRI, where it is common to observe the absence of contrast enhancement in the treated tumors

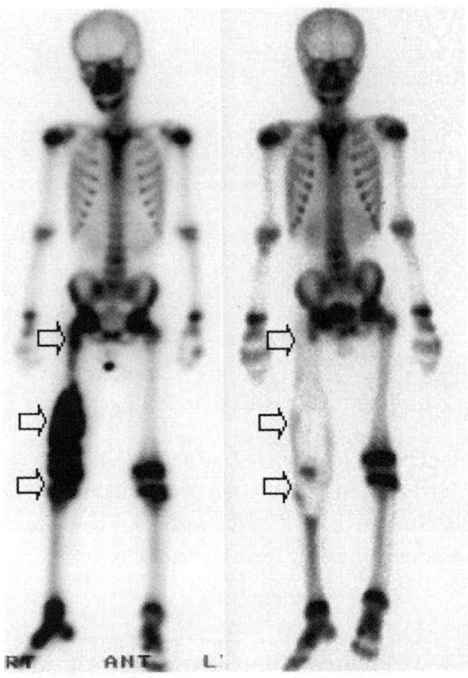

SPECT imaging before HIFU   SPECT imaging 2 weeks after HIFU

Fig. 18. [99m]Tc methylene diphosphonate SPECT images obtained in a patient who underwent HIFU ablation for treatment of a 46 cm long right femoral and tibial osteosarcoma. Before HIFU an increased uptake of the radioisotope is detected in local abnormality (arrows). However, 2 weeks after HIFU the tracer uptake of treated tumor disappeared completely in the treated region (arrows), indicating a positive therapeutic response and an absence of viable tumor.

that originate from liver, pancreas, kidney, breast, bone, soft tissue, and uterine (Figs. 20–26). Areas of hypoattenuation, shown on MRI or CT, that did not enhance after contrast material administration were considered to represent necrotic tissue. Still-enhancing areas were assumed to reveal residual viable tumor. In addition, a thin peripheral rim of enhancement may be detected surrounding the coagulation necrosis. This densely enhancing peripheral rim on delayed contrast imaging should not be misconstrued as residual tumor. In fact, this rim represents an inflammatory reaction to thermal ablation. However, a thick irregular rim at the edge of a treatment site is the most common feature of partial thermal ablation. In conclusion, among

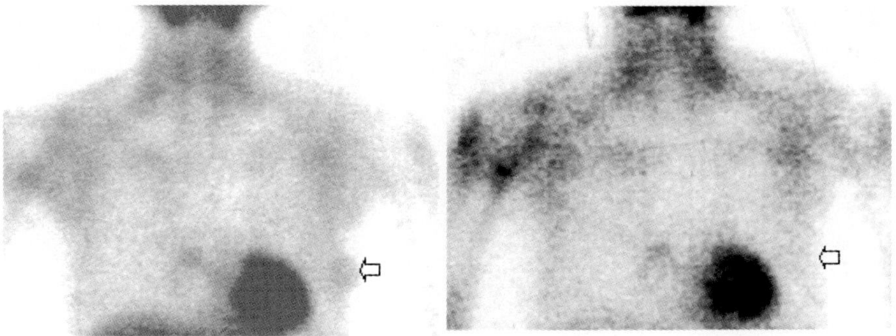

Fig. 19. ^{99m}Tc sestamibi SPECT images in a patient who underwent HIFU ablation for breast cancer. Before HIFU an increased uptake of the radioisotope is detected in left breast (arrow). However, 2 weeks after HIFU the tracer uptake of treated tumor disappeared completely in the treated region (arrow), indicating a positive therapeutic response and an absence of viable tumor.

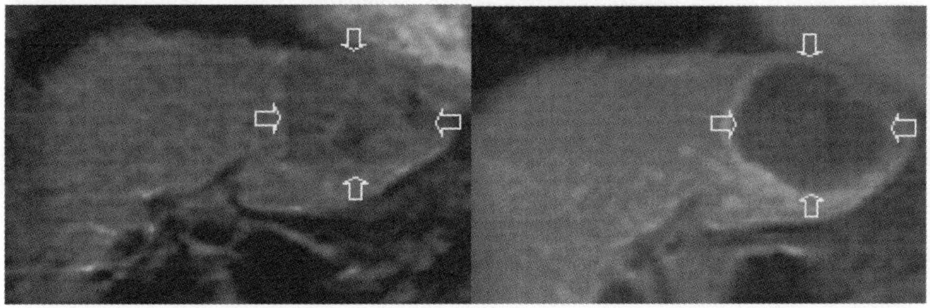

Fig. 20. Contrast-enhanced MRI in a patient who received HIFU ablation for hepatocellular carcinoma. Before HIFU contrast enhancement is detected within the tumor in the left liver (arrows). However, 2 weeks after HIFU there is no enhancement in the treated region (arrows), indicating a positive therapeutic response.

the follow-up images, enhanced CT or MRI would be standard imaging criteria for response assessment of treated tumors after HIFU ablation.

There is a lack of consensus on a standard regimen for follow-up imaging. Our clinical experience shows that diagnostic images, particularly enhanced MRI or CT, can be used to assess the efficacy of HIFU therapy

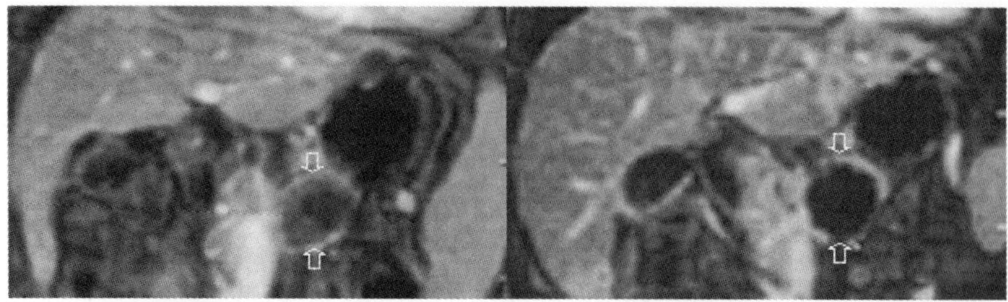

Enhanced-MRI before HIFU   Enhanced-MRI 2 weeks after HIFU

Fig. 21. Contrast-enhanced MRI in a patient who received HIFU ablation for pancreatic carcinoma. Before HIFU contrast enhancement is detected within the tumor in the body of the pancreas (arrows). However, 2 weeks after HIFU there is no enhancement in the treated region (arrows), indicating a positive therapeutic response.

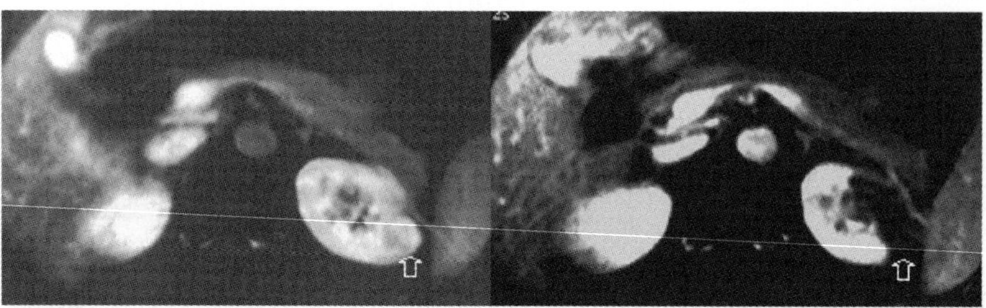

Enhanced-MRI before HIFU   Enhanced-MRI 2 weeks after HIFU

Fig. 22. Contrast-enhanced MRI in a patient who received HIFU ablation for renal cell carcinoma. Before HIFU contrast enhancement is detected within the tumor in the left kidney (arrow). However, 2 weeks after HIFU there is no enhancement in the treated region (arrow), indicating a positive therapeutic response.

1–2 weeks afterwards. In addition to reporting tumor size and the diameter of the ablation volume, assessment of contrast enhancement or lack of it in the treated tumor can provide imaging information about tumor response and residual live tumor cells after HIFU ablation. Follow-up imaging at 3 months is necessary to detect new-growth tumors in untreated regions. Imaging at 6–12 months can show obvious regression of the lesion and the region of coagulation necrosis. Most frequently, the treated volume without blood supply shrinks by less than 20–50% in volume.

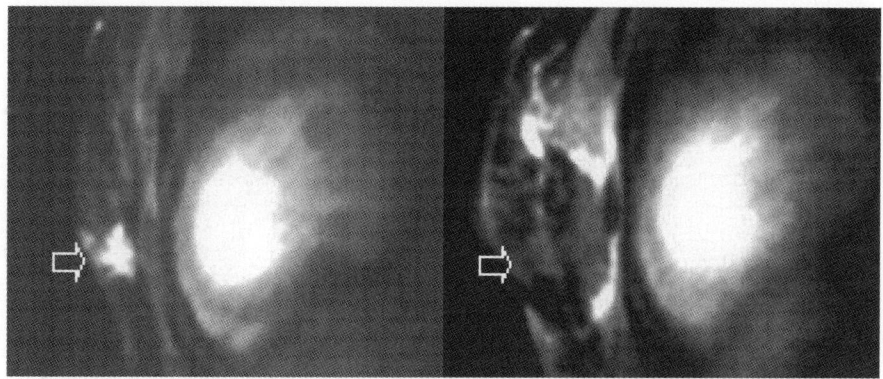

Enhanced-MRI before HIFU   Enhanced-MRI 2 weeks after HIFU

Fig. 23.   Contrast-enhanced MRI in a patient who received HIFU ablation for breast cancer. Before HIFU contrast enhancement is detected within the tumor in the left breast (arrow). However, 2 weeks after HIFU there is no enhancement in the treated region (arrow), indicating a positive therapeutic response.

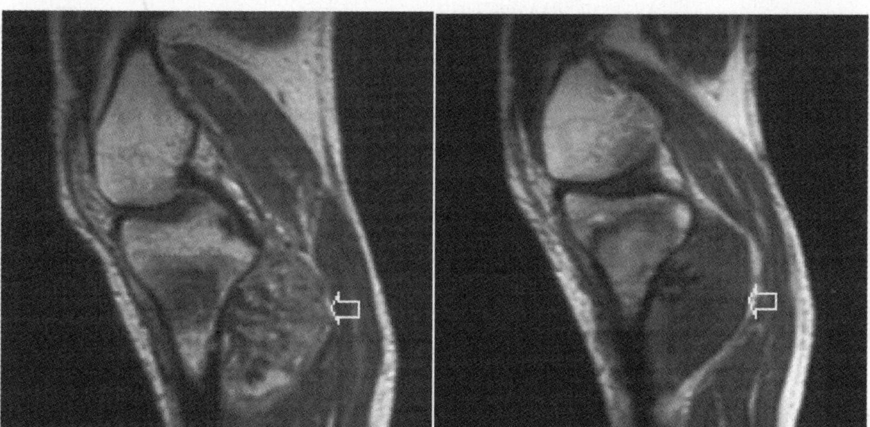

Enhanced-MRI before HIFU   Enhanced-MRI 2 weeks after HIFU

Fig. 24.   Contrast-enhanced MRI in a patient who received HIFU ablation for osteosarcoma. Before HIFU contrast enhancement is detected within the tumor in the tibia (arrow). However, 2 weeks after HIFU there is no enhancement in the treated region (arrow), indicating a positive therapeutic response.

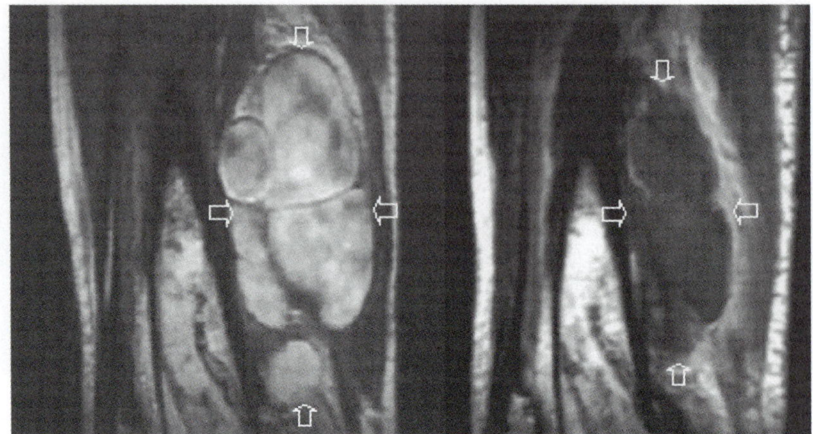

Enhanced-MRI before HIFU   Enhanced-MRI 2 weeks after HIFU

Fig. 25. Contrast-enhanced MRI in a patient who received HIFU ablation for soft tissue sarcoma. Before HIFU contrast enhancement is detected within the tumor in the leg (arrows). However, 2 weeks after HIFU there is no enhancement in the treated region (arrows), indicating a positive therapeutic response.

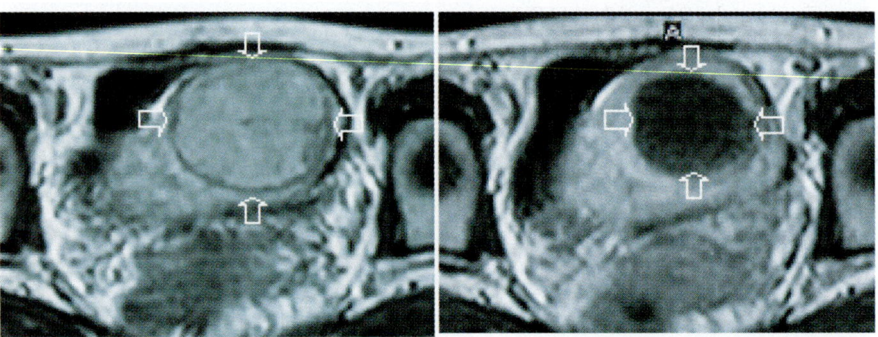

Enhanced-MRI before HIFU   Enhanced-MRI 2 weeks after HIFU

Fig. 26. Contrast-enhanced MRI in a patient who received HIFU ablation for uterine fibroid. Before HIFU contrast enhancement is detected within the tumor in the uterine (arrows). However, 2 weeks after HIFU there is no enhancement in the treated region (arrows), indicating a positive therapeutic response (images provided by courtesy of Prof. Yong-Jian Zhou at Guangzhou 1st Municipal Hospital, China).

7. Clinical Applications of Extracorporeal HIFU

Since HIFU was first used in the 1950s for patients with neurological disease during surgical procedure, it has been studied in the laboratory to treat normal tissue and implanted tumors in animals for a long time (Linke *et al.*, 1973; Lee *et al.*, 1979; Adams *et al.*, 1996; Chapelon *et al.*, 1992; Chen *et al.*, 1993; Sibille *et al.*, 1993; Watkin *et al.*, 1996; Rowland *et al.*, 1997; Wang *et al.*, 2003; Vykhodtseva *et al.*, 1995; Yang *et al.*, 1993; Wang *et al.*, 1997). The recent resurgence of this non-invasive therapy is driven by the advances in the development of medical imaging techniques, which makes it possible to target HIFU extracorporeally and precisely ablate a tumor at depth. Thus far, except for transrectal HIFU, which has been utilized for prostate cancer therapy, only two extracorporeal HIFU devices have been clinically used in the centers worldwide. They incorporate either MRI or B-mode ultrasonography to monitor the therapeutic procedure. The advantages and limitations of both imaging modalities used in HIFU have been described in Sec. 6, *Imaging in HIFU*. Clinical applications of these two extracorporeal HIFU devices are described below.

To date, MRI-guided HIFU has only been used to treat breast neoplasm and uterine fibroids (Hynynen *et al.*, 2001; Tempany *et al.*, 2003). Several clinical trials, phase I and phase II, have been performed in small numbers of patients with breast cancer, and results indicate that MRI-guided HIFU is safe, effective, and feasible in the treatment of this cancer (Hynynen *et al.*, 2001; Gianfelice *et al.*, 2003; Huber *et al.*, 2001). To my knowledge, no long-term follow-up survival rate is available yet. In the treatment of patients with uterine fibroids, pathological examination showed clear evidence of coagulation necrosis induced with HIFU exposure, and complete or partial ablation was identified using contrast-enhanced MR imaging (Stewart *et al.*, 2003). Uterine fibroid symptoms are obviously improved after HIFU treatment (Hindley *et al.*, 2004).

Extracorporeal ultrasound-guided HIFU has been widely used in China since 1999, and more than 3500 patients with various types of solid malignancy have now received this treatment for the purpose of either cure or palliation. The malignancies treated with HIFU include those of the liver, breast, kidney, pancreas, soft tissue, and bone; the benign tumors treated include uterine fibroid, breast fibroadenomas and hepatic hemangioma

(Wu *et al.*, 2004). Most of these clinical applications present encouraging short-term outcomes; long-term follow-up survival data are now emerging for the treatment of hepatocellular carcinoma, breast cancer and osteosarcoma. As large numbers of patients with solid malignancy are treated in China, the clinical experiences with extracorporeal ultrasound-guided HIFU are very important, and should be shared worldwide.

Much of the material of Sec. 7 is about the clinical knowledge and practice of HIFU in China. It should be appreciated that it is not intended to be exhaustive, but serve as an illustration of our clinical experience. Much of the clinical application is very recent, and detailed survival data will follow in subsequent publications. Any available clinical trial and survival data from the second affiliated hospital of Chongqing Medical University, China are included in the relevant sections below.

7.1. *Purposes of HIFU treatment*

In practice, cancer therapy usually needs to have multiple treatment methods for long-term survival benefit in addition to local therapy such as surgery. For instance, in the treatment of patients with breast cancer, surgery, chemotherapy, radiotherapy and endocrine therapy must be provided in tandem, because many clinical results indicate that the combination of these modalities can provide better survival benefit than one in isolation. HIFU is a local therapy for non-invasive destruction of the tumor, and it is essential to combine it with other therapies in clinical applications.

There are two goals of HIFU in the treatment of patients with solid malignancy. One goal of this ablation in patients with early-stage cancer is to effect a cure. In order to achieve this purpose, HIFU can be used as a local treatment to induce complete necrosis of the targeted tumor. Additional treatments such as chemotherapy, radiotherapy and endocrine therapy are essential to patients with breast cancer for conservation of the diseased breast, if HIFU is used locally in patients with early-stage breast cancer. In surgical oncology, it is necessary to resect the entire tumor along with an adequate tumor-free margin, to prevent local recurrence. In the same way, HIFU treatment should adopt a similar principle and aim to kill the entire malignant focus along with tumor-free margin of healthy tissue. However, the definition of an adequate tumor-free margin varies with the type of malignant tumor. For instance, the surgical margin in hepatic resection for colorectal metastasis was defined as 2 cm preferably, but no less than 1 cm of normal liver (Cady *et al.*, 1998). If the objective of HIFU is to replicate the success of liver resection, the same tumor free margin should be treated.

The other goal of HIFU treatment is palliative for patients with advanced-stage cancer. They are usually those who have an unresectable tumor and for whom conventional tumor therapies, including chemotherapy and radiotherapy, have failed to control tumor growth. HIFU can be clinically used to impede tumor growth and to improve the quality of life for such patients. Among those treated with HIFU in China, most are advanced-stage patients who are beyond the scope of conventional treatments. In the circumstances, HIFU can be successfully performed as a palliative method using partial or complete ablation. Symptoms such as pain caused by tumor disappear after HIFU, and survival time can be extended.

7.2. *Anesthesia selection for HIFU procedure*

Almost all patients have an uncomfortable sense of pain originating from the targeted tissue during HIFU procedure. Also, it is almost impossible for them to tolerate one fixed position without any motion for a long time. Therefore, either local or general anesthesia, as well as sedation is essential to HIFU treatment. The selective standard of anesthesia is dependent on two factors: (1) The most important is the patient's general condition that decides which kind of anesthesia is suitable, and how far the targeted organ can move. (2) If clinical examinations show that the patient is able to receive any kind of anesthesia, the movement of the targeted organ becomes the dominant factor to influence the decision made by an anesthetist, experienced in collaborating with HIFU doctors.

The anesthetist selects the anesthetic, primarily on the basis of targeted organ motion, ablation time, patient position, tumor location, and therapeutic ultrasound exposure. General anesthesia is usually used to ensure immobilization of targeted organs such as liver, kidney and pancreas during the HIFU procedure. Endotracheal intubation and mechanical ventilation enables single lung ventilation on one side, and therefore controls the movement of these organs caused by respiration. Furthermore, it has the supplementary benefit of permitting temporary suspension of respiration with controlled pulmonary inflation, necessary to ablate a liver or kidney tumor behind the ribs.

7.3. *HIFU treatment for liver cancer*

From March 1998 to October 2001, a total of 474 patients with liver cancer, including primary and metastatic liver cancer, have received HIFU treatment at ten hospitals in China (Wu *et al.*, 2004). Almost all patients had unresectable hepatocellular carcinoma (HCC) ranging from 4 cm to 15 cm in diameter. The diagnosis of HCC was determined by means of either US-guided biopsy or from the combination of diagnostic images that show classic manifestations of this tumor and an abnormal α-fetoprotein (AFP) level ($>200\,\mu$g L^{-1}).

Among them, most patients were advanced-stage patients with hepatic cirrhosis, and HIFU was used as a palliative therapy in clinical practice. After the treatment, clinical symptoms, such as loss of appetite, weight loss, discomfort or pain in the liver region, were obviously relieved in 86.6% patients. Serum AFP level was decreased by more than 50% in 65.3% patients. Compared with pre-HIFU images, follow-up MRI or CT examinations showed partial or complete coagulation necrosis of the targeted tumors (Li *et al.*, 2004).

A prospective, nonrandomized clinical trial was performed in Chongqing Medical University, China (Wu *et al.*, 2004). A total of 55 patients with HCC with cirrhosis were enrolled in this trial. Among them, 51 patients had unresectable HCC. Tumor size ranged from 4 to 14 cm in diameter with a mean diameter of 8.14 cm. According to TNM classification (6th ed.), 15 patients corresponded to stage II, 16 to stage III$_A$, and 24 to III$_C$. All patients had HIFU, and the median number of HIFU sessions was 1.69. The results showed that HIFU was safe, and no severe side effect was observed after the treatment. Follow-up imaging indicated an absence of tumor vascular supply and the shrinkage of treated lesions (Fig. 27). Serum AFP returned to normal level in 34% of patients. The overall survival rates at 6, 12, and 18 months were 86.1%, 61.5%, and 35.3%, respectively. The survival rates were significantly higher in patients in stage II than those in stage III$_A$ ($P < 0.0132$) and in stage III$_C$ ($P < 0.0265$), as shown in Fig. 28.

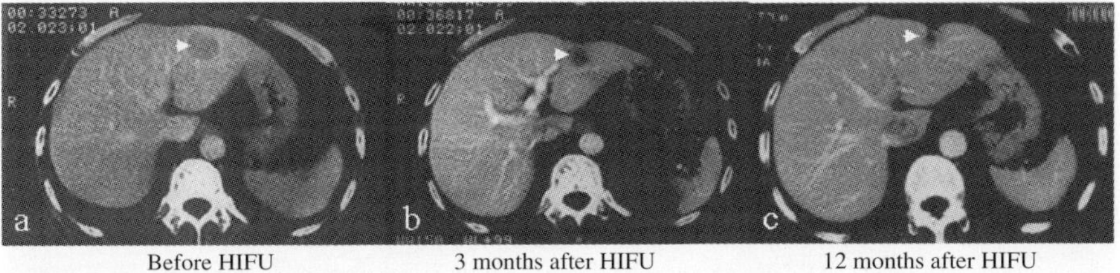

Fig. 27. Enhanced CT scans obtained in a patient who had HIFU treatment alone for HCC. Before treatment, the lesion, 4 cm in diameter, is located in the left lobe of the liver (arrow). 3 months after HIFU, no tumor blood supply is seen in targeted region (arrow). 12 months after HIFU, an obvious shrinkage of treated lesion is seen with an absence of blood supply (arrow).

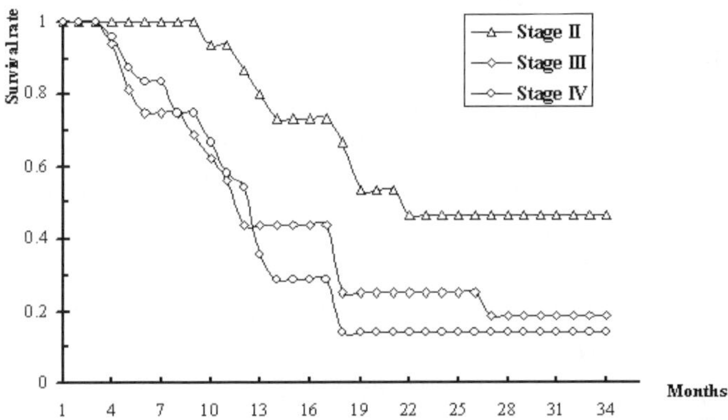

Fig. 28. Cumulative survival curves for 55 patients with HCC according to TNM stage.

A randomized, controlled clinical trial was also performed to assess the local therapeutic efficacy of HIFU therapy combined with transcatheter arterial chemoembolization (TACE), and TACE alone for 50 patients with stage-IV_A HCC (TNM classification, 5th ed.) at our tumor center in Chongqing, China (Wu *et al.*, 2005). Of these, 26 patients underwent TACE alone and the remaining 24 patients underwent TACE, followed by HIFU ablation within 2 to 4 weeks. The tumor size was 4 to 14 cm in diameter (mean = 10.5 cm). Immediate therapeutic effects were assessed by follow-up Doppler ultrasound, CT or MRI. All patients were followed from 3 to 24 months (mean 8 months) to observe long-term therapeutic efficacy and complications in both groups. Tumor reduction rates, median survival

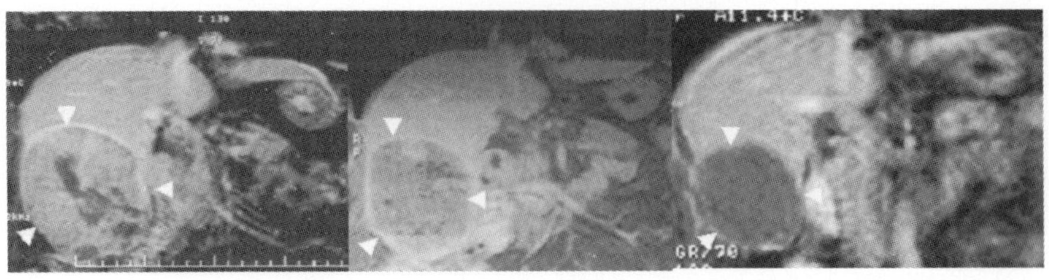

Before TACE   4 weeks after TACE   2 weeks after HIFU

Fig. 29. Enhanced-MR images obtained in a patient who underwent the combination of TACE and HIFU ablation for HCC. Before TACE, rich blood supply was observed in HCC lesion (arrows); 4 weeks after TACE, just before HIFU, tumor blood supply was reduced, but contrast enhancement still remained in some areas within the tumor (arrows); 2 weeks after HIFU, no evidence of contrast enhancement was observed in the treated HCC (arrows), indicative of complete coagulation necrosis in the treated region.

time, and cumulative survival rates in both groups were calculated using unpaired Student t test and Kaplan-Meier method. The results indicated that no severe complication was observed after HIFU. Follow-up imaging showed absence or reduction of blood supply in the lesion when compared with TACE alone (Fig. 29). The median survival times for patients were 11.3 months in group 2, and 4 months in group 1 ($P = 0.0042$). The 6-month survival rate of patients was 80.4–85.4% in group 2 and 13.2% in group 1 ($P = 0.0029$), and 1-year survival rate was 42.9% and 0% respectively (Fig. 30). The median reductions in tumor size as a percentage of the initial tumor volume at 1, 3, 6, 12 months postoperatively were 28.6%, 35%, 50%, and 50% in group 2, while the median reduction were 4.8%, 7.7%, 10% and 0% in group 1 respectively ($P < 0.01$).

Prospective non-randomized clinical trials are being performed to evaluate the safety and effectiveness in the treatment of metastatic liver cancer. They are phase I and II trials in which the same Chinese ultrasound-guided HIFU is used at the Churchill Hospital in Oxford, UK. From November 2002 to August 2004, a total of 22 patients with metastatic liver cancer were treated with HIFU. Using either radiological images such as MRI and contrast ultrasound, or histological examinations, 20 of 22 patients were assessed. The result indicated that HIFU exposure resulted in discrete ablation zones of liver tumors in all evaluable patients (100%) (Rowland *et al.*, 2004).

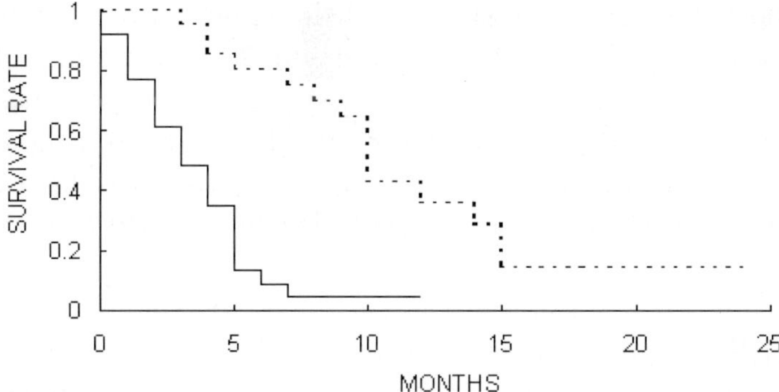

Fig. 30.   Cumulative survival curves, calculated with the Kaplan-Meier method, for patients treated with either TACE alone or combined TACE and HIFU (… combined TACE and HIFU group; — TACE group).

The adverse event profile was favorable when compared with open or minimally invasive techniques.

As HCC is frequently seen in the setting of hepatic cirrhosis, local therapies such as surgery and minimally invasive modalities (radiofrequency, laser, microwave), can be performed only in 10% to 20% of patients with HCC (Farmer *et al.*, 1994; Lin *et al.*, 1997; Lin *et al.*, 1987; Zibari *et al.*, 1998; Goldberg *et al.*, 2000). Most of the HCC patients lose the chance to be treated with these modalities due to the presence of multiple bilateral lesions, tumor invasion of the portal vein and the underlying advanced liver cirrhosis. For these patients, HIFU may have the potential to change the patient outcome dramatically. The experiences achieved in China for the treatment of unresectable HCC indicate that HIFU may be used as an alternative modality for patients unsuitable for conventional therapies.

7.4. *HIFU treatment for breast cancer*

Breast cancer is the most common malignancy in women, and annually, more than 1 million new cases of breast cancer are diagnosed worldwide. Radical and modified radical mastectomy, including axillary lymph node dissection, have long been regarded as appropriate therapies. During the last two decades, significant advances have been made in the development of early detection modalities and therapeutic methods. Breast conservation surgery, combined with radiotherapy, chemotherapy and hormonal therapy, is performed with increasing frequency in patients with early-stage breast cancer. The move from the mastectomy toward breast conservation therapy has not changed long-term survival rates of patients with breast cancer (Curran *et al.*, 1998; Fisher *et al.*, 1995; Jacobson *et al.*, 1995; Veronesi *et al.*, 1993).

A randomized clinical trial was performed to explore the possibility of using HIFU for the treatment of patients with localized breast cancer at the Chongqing Medical University in China (Wu *et al.*, 2003). A total of 48 women with biopsy-proven breast cancer (T_{1-2}, N_{0-2}, M_0) were randomized into the control group in which modified radical mastectomy was performed, and the HIFU group in which an extracorporeal HIFU ablation of breast cancer was followed by modified radical mastectomy. Short-term follow-up, pathologic and immunohistochemical stains were performed to assess the therapeutic effects on the tumor and the complications of HIFU. The results showed that no severe side effect was observed in the HIFU-treated patients. Pathologic findings revealed that HIFU-treated tumor cells underwent complete coagulation necrosis, and tumor vascular vessels were severely damaged. Immunohistochemical staining showed that no expression of proliferating cell nuclear antigen (PCNA), matrix metalloproteinase-9 (MMP-9), and cell surface glycoprotein CD44v6 was detected within the treated tumor cells in the HIFU group, indicating that the treated tumor cells lost the abilities of proliferation, invasion and metastasis (Wu *et al.*, 2003). As a result, HIFU could be effective, safe, and feasible in the extracorporeal treatment of localized breast cancer.

Furthermore, long-term survival data were obtained in a non-randomized prospective trial, in which 22 breast cancer patients received breast conservation treatment with HIFU (Wu *et al.*, 2005). Disease TNM stage was classified as stage I in 4 patients, stage II_A in 9 patients, stage II_B in 8 patients, and stage IV in 1 patient. Tumor size ranged from 2 to 4.8 cm in diameter (mean = 3.4 cm). All patients received chemotherapy, radiation and tamoxifen after HIFU for the primary lesions. Outcome measures included radiological and pathological assessment of the treated tumor, cosmesis, and local recurrence. A cumulative survival rate was calculated by using the Kaplan–Meier method. The results indicated that no

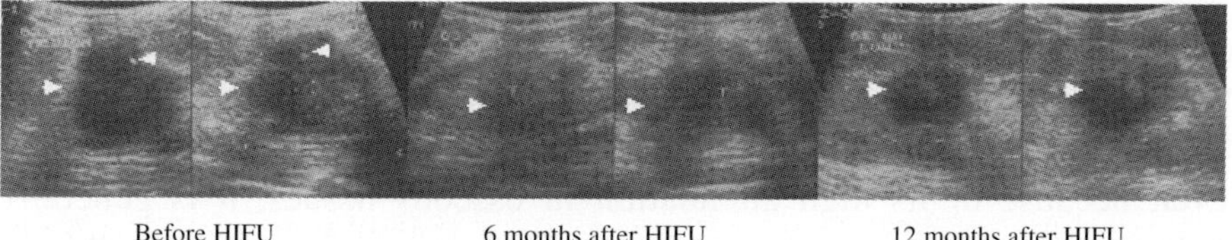

Fig. 31.   Color Doppler US imaging of a left breast cancer (arrows) in a patient before and after HIFU ablation. Before HIFU the breast lesion is circumscribed, and blood supply is observed (arrowhead); 6 and 12 months after HIFU ablation an obvious regression of treated lesion is seen with an absence of blood supply (arrows).

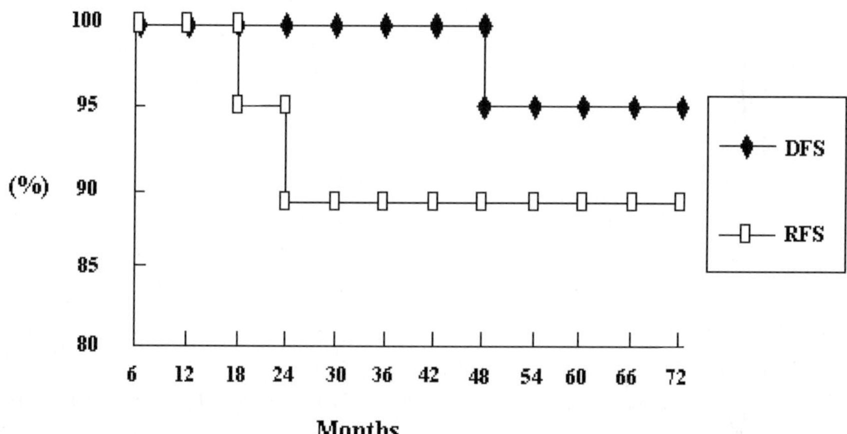

Fig. 32.   Disease-free survival (DFS) curve and recurrence-free survival (RFS) curve for patients with breast cancer treated by HIFU ablation.

severe complications were encountered after HIFU. Post-operative imaging demonstrated positive response and regression of all treated lesions (Fig. 31). Follow-up biopsy revealed coagulation necrosis of the targeted tumor and subsequent replacement by fibroblastic tissue. After a median follow-up of 54.8 months, 1 patient died, 1 was lost during follow-up, and 20 were still alive. Two of 22 patients developed local recurrence. Five-year disease-free survival and recurrence-free survival were 95% and 89%, respectively (Fig. 32). Cosmetic result was judged as good to excellent in 94% of patients.

7.5. *HIFU treatment for osteosarcoma*

An ultrasound beam is easily transmitted through soft tissues and parenchymatous organs *in vivo*, except air-containing organs such as lungs. However, because of its high attenuation in osseous tissues, it is generally believed that US propagation through the bone is almost impossible in the diagnosis and treatment of bone disease. However, recent transcranial ultrasound techniques, such as transcranial color-coded real-time sonography and transcranial Doppler, have allowed noninvasive imaging of brain parenchyma and color flow imaging of intracranial vessels, and have become reliable methods for the examination of patients with stroke (Becker *et al.*, 1993; Bogdahn *et al.*, 1990; Kimura *et al.*, 1996; Kushner *et al.*, 1991; Martin *et al.*, 1995; Smith *et al.*, 1986). These studies imply that, despite the anatomical obstacle, US beams have been transmitted through bones. In the field of HIFU, it has been discovered that focused US can cause thermal lesions in animal brains through the skull (Fry, 1977; Fry & Barger 1978). As an aggressive malignant neoplasm, most osteosarcomas may be lytic, despite the limited production of mineralized osteiod or bone tissue (Weis, 1998). Slight to complete cortical destruction within tumor lesions makes possible ultrasound beam propagation through the damaged osteogenic structure into the medullary space in which osteosarcoma originates. Therefore, HIFU can be used as a noninvasive therapy to treat patients with osteosarcoma through the bone containing soft tissue of tumor and the weakened bone.

For the purpose of conserving the diseased-limb, HIFU has been used as a non-invasive approach in the treatment of patients with malignant bone neoplasm, in tandem with chemotherapy (Wu *et al.*, 2005). In a perspective clinical trial, 44 patients with biopsy-proven malignant bone tumors were treated with HIFU (osteosarcoma: 32; chondrosarcoma: 3; periosteal osteosarcoma: 2; Ewing sarcoma: 1; other malignant bone tumor: 3; and unclassified tumor: 2). These tumors were situated as follows: distal femur: 20; proximal tibia: 7; mid-shaft of femur: 6; ilium: 2; shaft of fibula: 2; others: 4. HIFU was given as a noninvasive limb-salvage treatment in combination with neoadjuvant chemotherapy (methotrexate, adriamycin, cisplatin and ifosfamide) in 34 patients (Enneking's Stage II$_b$). Ten patients with stage III$_b$ (9 patients with lung metastasis) were treated with HIFU alone with palliative intent. The largest dimension of the tumors ranged from

5 to 46 cm. Postoperative biopsy, follow-up imaging (DSA, CT or MRI, and ECT), and functional evaluation were performed, and median survival time was calculated using the Kaplan–Meier method. After HIFU treatment, histopathological examination demonstrated clear evidence of tumor destruction and regrowth of normal bone in the treated region (Fig. 33). When compared with baseline, follow-up imaging indicated complete coagulative necrosis of the treated tumors. Enneking's functional scores were >20, 15–20, and <15 in 20, 14 and 5 cases respectively. Median follow-up was 23 months (ranging from 10 to 40 months). Total survival rate was 85% (38/44). One patient with stage II_b disease, and five patients with stage III_b disease died as a result of distant metastases after HIFU treatment. Five

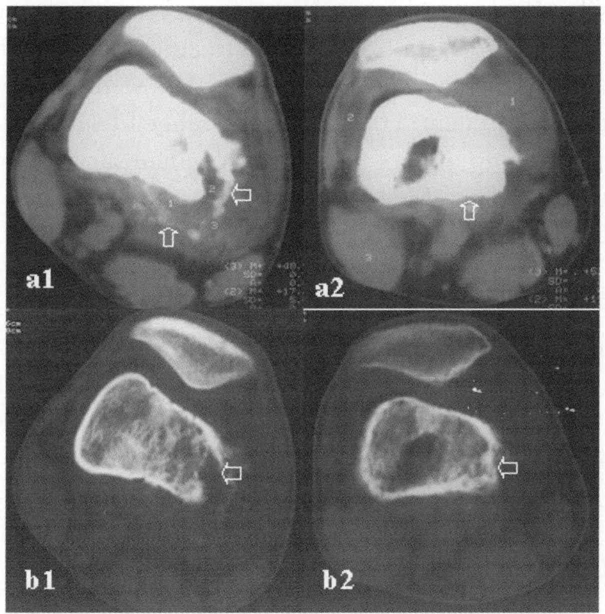

Fig. 33.   Non-enhanced CT in a patient with femoral osteosarcoma before and after HIFU treatment. (a1) Before HIFU, as the tumor invades soft tissue, tumor mass containing bone tissue is detected on CT imaging (arrows); (b1) it is also seen that the cortex of the femur is completely destroyed (arrow), and "acoustic window" formed can let ultrasound beams penetrate the weakened bone to treat the tumor in the medulla. (a2) Three years after HIFU, the tumor in soft tissue disappears (arrow); (b2) the destroyed cortex is repaired by normal bone tissue (arrow).

patients underwent amputation after local recurrence. Few complications were observed during follow-up. These were limited to 3 pathological fractures, 2 cases of peripheral nerve damage, case of restricted joint movement, and 1 case of epiphyseal separation. As a result, it is concluded that HIFU is safe, effective, and feasible in the treatment of patients with malignant bone tumors.

Recently, a non-randomized clinical trial using HIFU for the treatment of osteosarcoma patients has been completed in the Chongqing Medical University, China (Chen *et al.*, 2004). A total of 71 patients with biopsy-proven osteosarcoma were recruited in the trial. Among them, 64 patients were diagnosed as typical osteosarcoma, 3 as juxtacortical osteosarcoma, 2 as telangiectasis osteosarcoma, 1 as parosteal osteosarcoma, and 1 as osteoblastoma. According to surgical classification, 57 patients corresponded to stage II_b, and 14 to stage III_b. Fifty-seven patients with stage-IIb were treated with HIFU as a limb-salvage treatment, in combination with neoadjuvant chemotherapy, and 14 with stage III_b were treated with HIFU alone with palliative intent. Follow-up time ranged from 2 to 64 months, with a mean follow-up time of 22 months. Median survival time was calculated using the Kaplan–Meier method. The results indicated that overall survival rates at 1, 2, 3, 4 and 5 years were 83.3%, 66.0%, 63.2%, 59.0% and 59.0% respectively. Median survival rates at 1, 2, 3, 4 and 5 years were 92.4%, 83.2%, 79.6%, 74.3% and 74.3% in stage II_b patients, while the median survival rates at 1, 2 and 3 year were 47.6%, 7.9% and 0% in stage III_b patients respectively ($P < 0.0001$). These results are very encouraging, concluding that HIFU can be used as a locally limb-salvage therapy in the treatment of patients with localized osteosarcoma.

7.6. *HIFU treatment for other malignancies*

From December 1997 to October 2001, a total of 77 patients with soft tissue sarcoma received HIFU treatment in China (Wu *et al.*, 2004). Most of the patients had recurrent soft tissue sarcoma after surgery. Among them, 18 patients were treated with HIFU in the Chongqing Medical University. Before treatment, pathological examination showed liposarcoma in 6 patients, synovial sarcoma, fibrosarcoma and malignant peripheral nerve sheath tumor in 2 patients each and other soft tissue sarcomas in 5 patients.

The tumor size ranged from 5.5 to 16 cm in diameter (mean = 8.6 cm), and follow-up time varied from 11 to 39 months (median = 21 months). After HIFU treatment, contrast-enhanced MRI showed the complete ablation of the targeted tumor. Of the total, 16 patients are still alive (survival rate of 90%), and 2 patients died of metastasis after HIFU treatment. Three patients had local recurrence and then underwent a second HIFU treatment for the purpose of control.

HIFU treatment was performed in 12 patients with advanced stage renal cell carcinoma and 1 patient with colon cancer metastasized to kidney (Wu *et al.*, 2003). Patients were followed after treatment to observe complications and long-term therapeutic efficacy. Complications and changes in symptoms seen at presentation were recorded. Mid stream urine specimens were sent for microscopy and serum creatinine was measured postoperatively. Follow-up radiological examinations were performed to detect tumor response to the ablation. The results showed that 13 patients received HIFU treatment safely, including 10 who had partial ablation and 3 who had complete tumor ablation. After HIFU, hematuria disappeared in 7 of 8 patients and flank pain of presumed malignant origin disappeared in 9 of 10 patients. Postoperative images showed a decrease in or absence of tumor blood supply in the treated region and significant shrinkage of the ablated tumor. Of the 13 patients, 7 died (median survival of 14.1 months, range of 2 to 27) and 6 were still alive with a median follow-up of 18.5 months (range of 10 to 27). This clinical experience reveals that HIFU is safe, effective and feasible in the treatment of patients with advanced renal malignancy.

From December 2000 to September 2002, HIFU treatment was performed in 8 patients with advanced pancreatic cancer (Wu *et al.*, 2005). The tumor ranged from 4.5 to 8 cm in diameter (mean = 5.89 cm), and was mainly located in the pancreatic body and tail. Serum amylase and bilirubin were measured daily after HIFU to assess the safety. Postoperative radiological examinations, including CT, MRI and ultrasonography, were performed to evaluate tumor response. Complications and changes in symptoms seen at presentation were recorded. Patients were followed up after treatment to observe long-term therapeutic efficacy. Eight patients received HIFU treatment safely, including 2 cases undergoing thermal ablation of hepatic metastases simultaneously. No complications were observed postoperatively. After HIFU, pre-existing severe back pain of presumed malignant origin disappeared in each patient. Follow-up images showed reduction or absence of tumor blood supply in the treated region and significant shrinkage of the ablated tumor. Four of the 8 patients died (median survival time $= 11.25$ months, range of 2–17 months), and the remaining 4 patients were still alive with a median follow-up time of 11.5 months (range of 9 to 16 months). Therefore, it is concluded that HIFU is safe, effective and feasible in the treatment of patients with pancreatic cancer.

For the purpose of analgesia, HIFU treatment can be performed alone for the treatment of advanced cancer patients who had severe pain caused directly by their cancers. Most of the patients are provided with appropriate pain medications, including anti-neoplastic therapy and pharmacological approaches, but the cancer pain was still not well controlled before HIFU. Our clinical experiences indicate that HIFU is able to control the pain successfully, without any local complication. After HIFU treatment, severe cancer pain was significantly relieved, and patients' daily activities, quality of life, and psychological status were markedly improved.

7.7. *Complications of HIFU treatment*

Among 1038 patients treated with HIFU from December 1997 to October 2001, an extremely low major complication rate has been observed. 5–10% of the patients had low-grade fever up to 38.5°C that persisted for approximately 5–7 days after HIFU ablation. The severity and time of fever seems to be directly related to the amount of destroyed tissue.

At the beginning of the HIFU clinical trial, 10–20% patients had HIFU-induced skin burns, but these were not severe. The reason for this is largely the lack of experience in performing HIFU ablation and in evaluating damaged-skin changes on real-time US imaging. However, at the present moment, the rate of skin burn has significantly decreased ($<5\%$). Either tumor bleeding or large blood vessel rupture has never been detected following HIFU ablation.

Some treated patients (20–30%) experience slight and mild local pain within 1 week after HIFU ablation, with only 5–10% of the patients who were given 3–5 days of prescription for oral analgesics.

Six of 474 patients with liver cancer had hepatic abscesses within 2–3 weeks of HIFU treatment. Four of 153 patients with malignant bone tumors had local infection within 1–3 months of HIFU treatment. Four patients with malignant tumors had bowel perforation because of severe abdominal cohesion induced by a previous operation. It caused HIFU mistargeting, such that the treated- region included the tumor and the cohesive bowel. Four patients with primary malignant tumor had complete bone fracture in the treated region. Fortunately, 2 recovered and new normal bone has grown, and it was united with new normal bone tissue 3 months after damage. Nerve fiber damage has been caused by HIFU in 4 patients with malignant bone tumor. However, nerve functions including sensation and motion recovered completely in 2 patients, and the other 2 patients partially recovered within 1 year after HIFU.

8. Future of HIFU

Multiple-central, long-term follow-up results of HIFU in the treatment of patients with solid malignancy are scant because this is a fairly new technique. Controlled clinical trials are ongoing, and detailed results will be published in due course. More extensive survival data is also being collected for each specific clinical application, and this will follow in future publications. Clinical experiences in China demonstrate that HIFU is safe, effective and feasible in the treatment of malignant solid tumors. However, HIFU technology is still being developed, and its clinical applications for the treatment of solid malignancies is currently in the infant stage. It is very important to summarize the indications and contra-indications for HIFU treatment in each solid malignancy. The close cooperation between radiologists, oncologists and oncology surgeons will guarantee careful selection of the therapeutic options suited to individual patients. Till now, the clinical results achieved are exciting and encouraging, but long-term follow-up results of randomized clinical trials in the centers worldwide is necessary to fully determine the true efficacy of this non-invasive therapeutic modality.

However, much supplementary investigation is necessary to further evaluate the HIFU treatment plans, the relationship between HIFU dosage and the extent of coagulation necrosis, and factors that can influence focused ultrasound energy deposition in target tissue including tissue structure, movement, function and perfusion. For instance, in our animal studies, it has been indicated that when mechanical and pharmacological means were used to manipulate tissue perfusion, perfusion-mediated tissue cooling could directly affect the shape and size of tissue necrosis induced by HIFU ablation. On the basis of these important findings, it seems that reduced tissue perfusion causes an increase in the volume of coagulation necrosis. Therefore, a better understanding of perfusion effects and a new method of controlling its cooling forces are essential in improving results.

Beyond optimization of technical and physiological parameters, it is obvious that HIFU ablation must be performed with exact knowledge, not only of the number and location of the lesions, but also the biological characteristics and natural history of the tumor being treated. Despite successful destruction of primary lesions, patients with distant metastases in multiple organs are unlikely to be treated with local therapy such as surgical techniques and thermal ablation. Therapeutic failure in these patients is mainly due to uncontrolled growth of new and earlier undetected metastases.

The goal of tumor therapy is that all cancer cells in the patient's body must be completely killed. For patients with cancer, the therapeutic plan for the disease must be a multiple treatment plan, which includes local treatments such as surgery and radiotherapy, and systemic therapy such as chemotherapy and immunotherapy. A similar multidisciplinary approach including other modalities is important in the treatment of solid malignancies. Like surgery, HIFU is a local ablation. Therefore, it is essential to combine HIFU with other therapies including chemotherapy and radiotherapy. However, there are many questions needing to be answered, such as how to select the sequence of the combination, and what types of standards are employed in the multidisciplinary therapies for each cancer, if HIFU is to be widely used in clinical practice. Thus, success achieved in the application of HIFU treatment is mainly dependent on the HIFU technique, but also on a better understanding of the natural characteristics of tumors.

Appendix–Glossary

Ablation: The therapeutic use of cold or thermal effect to induce the selective destruction of a targeted tissue such as tumor.

Attenuation: Process by which a beam of ultrasound is reduced in intensity when passing through material — combination of absorption and scattering processes.

Calculus: A solid concretion or stone which forms within the urinary tract (kidney).

Cavitation: The production of small vapor-containing bubbles or cavities in a liquid or tissue by ultrasound.

Choroid: Middle layer of the vertebrate eye, between retina and sclera.

Confluent: Joining; running together.

Cortical: Pertaining to or of the nature of a cortex or bark.

Cosmesis: A concern in therapeutics, especially in surgical operations, for the appearance of the patient; *i.e.*, a resort to an operation which will improve the appearance.

Cryotherapy: The selective destruction of tissue by extreme cold or freezing.

CT: Computerized tomography

DSA: Digital subtraction angiography

Endotracheal: Within the trachea.

Extracorporeal: Situated or occurring outside the body.

Fibroadenoma: A benign solid growth, usually found in the breast.

Gadolinium: A supposed rare metallic element, with a characteristic spectrum, found associated with yttrium and other rare metals.

Glaucoma: A group of eye diseases characterised by an increase in intraocular pressure which causes pathological changes in the optic disk and typical defects in the field of vision.

Gray scale: The various shades of gray or luminance values in a video picture. As industrial test standards, gray wedges are used with discrete steps incrementing in brightness by factors of ~ 7.3.

Helical CT: Computed tomography in which the X-ray tube continuously revolves around the patient, who is simultaneously moved longitudinally; computer interpolation allows reconstruction of standard transverse scans or images in any preferred plane.

Hematuria: The finding of blood in the urine.

Hepatic: Pertaining to the liver.

Hepatocellular: Pertaining to or affecting liver cells.

HIFU: High intensity focused ultrasound

Histology: The study of cells and tissue on the microscopic level.

Hyperechogenic: In ultrasonography, pertaining to material that produces echoes of higher amplitude or density than the surrounding medium.

Hyperechoic: Denoting a region in an ultrasound image in which the echoes are stronger than normal or than surrounding structures

Hyperthermia: Abnormally high body temperature (from 42 to 45 degree centigrades), especially that induced for therapeutic purposes.

Immunohistochemistry: Histochemical localization of immunoreactive substances using labelled antibodies as reagents.

In vivo: Within the living body.

In vitro: Within a glass, observable in a test tube, in an artificial environment.

Liposarcoma: A malignant tumour derived from primitive or embryonal lipoblastic cells.

Lithotripsy: Known as extracorporeal shock wave lithotripsy, this procedure uses sound waves delivered inside a water bath to pulverize kidney stones painlessly inside the body.

Lytic: Pertaining to lysis or to a lysin.

Melanoma: A tumour arising from the melanocytic system of the skin and other organs. When used alone the term refers to malignant melanoma.

Metastasis: The transfer of disease from one organ or part to another not directly connected with it. It is due to transfer of cells, as in malignant tumors. The capacity to metastasize is a characteristic of all malignant tumors.

MRI: Magnetic resonance imaging

Necrosis: The sum of the morphological changes indicative of cell death and caused by the thermal ablation.

Neoplasm: New and abnormal growth of tissue, which may be benign or cancerous.

Osteosarcoma: Malignant tumour of bone (probably neoplasia of osteocytes).

Palliative: An alleviating medicine that affording relief, but not cure.

Percutaneous: Performed through the skin, as injection of radiopacque material in radiological examination or the removal of tissue for biopsy accomplished by a needle.

Perfusion: The act of pouring over or through, especially the passage of a fluid through the vessels of a specific organ.

PET: Position emission tomography

Pyrotherapy: Treatment of disease by inducing an artificial fever in the patient.

Rarefaction: The process of becoming light or less dense; the condition of being light; opposed to condensation.

Real-time ultrasonography: Rapid serial ultrasound images produced using a phased array or scanning transducer; produces a video display of organ motion, such as heart valve or fetal motion.

Rectus abdominis: A long flat muscle that extends along the whole length of both sides of the abdomen. It flexes the vertebral column, particularly the lumbar portion; it also tenses the anterior abdominal wall and assists in compressing the abdominal contents.

Sonicate: To expose a suspension of cells or microbes to the disruptive effect of the energy of high frequency sound waves.

SPECT: Single photon emission computed tomography.

Telangiectasis: Dilatation of the capillary vessels.

Target volume: An object volume fixed as goal or point of treatment.

Tomography: The recording of internal body images at a predetermined plane by means of the tomograph, also called body section roentgenography.

Transducer: A device that transforms one type of energy to another.

Vascularized tumor: Growth of blood vessels into a tumor with the result of a prelude to more rapid growth and often to metastasis.

References

Adams JB, Moore RG, Anderson JH, Strandberg JD, Marshall FF, Davoussi LR. High-intensity focused ultrasound ablation of rabbit kidney tumors. *J Endourol* (1996) **110**: 71–75.

Becker G, Winkler J, Hofmann E, Bogdahn U. Differentiation between ischemic and hemorrhagic stoke by transcranial color-coded realtime sonography. *J Neuroimag* (1993) **3**: 41–47.

Bogdahn U, Becker G, Winkler J, Greiner K, Perez J, Meurers B. Transcranial color-coded real-time sonography in adults. *Stroke* (1990) **21**: 1680–1688.

Bohm T, Hilger I, Muller W, Reichenbach JR, Fleck M, Kaiser WA. Saline-enhanced radiofrequency ablation of breast tissue: An *in vitro* feasibility study. *Invest Radiol* (2000) **35**: 149–157.

Breasted JH. (ed.), *The Edwin Smith Surgical Papyrus*. (1993) Chicago University Press, Chicago.

Bremer C, Allkemper T, Menzel J, Sulkowski U, Rummeny E, Reimer P. Preliminary clinical experience with laser-induced interstitial thermotherapy in patients with hepatocellular carcinoma. *J Magn Reson Imag* (1998) **8**: 235–239.

Cady B, Jenkins RL, Steele GD, Lewis WD, Stone MD, McDermott WV, Jessup JM, Bothe A, Lalor P, Lovett EJ, Lavin P, Linehan DC. Surgical margin in hepatic resection for colorectal metastasis: A critical and improvable determinant of outcome. *Ann Surg* (1998) **227**: 566–571.

Calderon C, Vilkomerson D, Mezrich R, Etzold KF, Kingsley B, Haskin M. Differences in the attenuation of ultrasound by normal, benign, and malignant breast tissue. *J Clin Ultrasound* (1976) **4**: 249–254.

Chapelon JY, Margonari J, Theillere Y, Gorry F, Vernier F, Blane E, Gelet A. Effects of high-intensity focused ultrasound on kidney tissue in the rat and the dog. *Eur Urol* (1992) **22**: 147–153.

Chaussy C, Thuroff S. High-intensity focused ultrasound: Complications and adverse effects. *Molec Urol* (2000) **4**: 183–187.

Chen L, Rivens I, ter Haar GR, Riddler S, Hill CR, Bensted JP. Histological changes in rat liver tumours treated with high-intensity focused ultrasound. *Ultrasound Med Biol* (1993) **19**: 67–74.

Chen W, Wang W, Zhu H, Li K, Sue H, Bai L, Bai J, Zou J, Wu F, Wang Z. Clinical follow-up reports on high-intensity focused ultrasound treatment of osteosarcoma, in *Proc 4th International Symposium on Therapeutic Ultrasound*, Tachibana K, ter Haar GR (eds.), ISTU, Kyoto (2004) pp. 162.

Clement GT. Perspectives in clinical uses of high-intensity focused ultrasound. *Ultrasonics* (2004) **42**: 1087–1093.

Cline HE, Schenek JF, Hynynen K, Watkins RD, Schenek JF, Jolesz FA. MR-guided focused ultrasound surgery. *J Comput Assist Tomogr* (1992) **16**: 956–965.

Cline HE, Schenek JF, Watkins RD, Hynynen K, Jolesz FA. Magnetic resonance-guided thermal surgery. *Magn Reson Med* (1993) **30**: 98–106.

Coleman DJ, Lizzi FL, Driller J, Rosado AL, Chang S, Iwamoto T, Rosenthal D. Therapeutic ultrasound in the treatment of glaucoma. I. Experimental model. *Ophthalmology* (1985) **92**: 339–336.

Coleman DJ, Lizzi FL, Silverman RH, Dennis PH, Driller J, Rosado A, Iwamoto T. Therapeutic ultrasound. *Ultrasound Med Biol* (1986) **12**: 633–638.

Coleman DJ, Silverman RH, Iwamoto T, Lizzi FL, Rondeau MJ, Driller J, Rosado A, Abramson DH, Ellsworth RM. Treatment of glaucoma with high-intensity focused ultrasound. *Ophthalmology* (1986) **93**: 831–833.

Curran D, van Dongen JP, Aaronson NK, Kiebert G, Fentiman IS, Mignolet F, Bartelink H. Quality of life of early-stage breast cancer patients treated with radical mastectomy or breast-conserving procedure: Results of EORTC trial 10801. The European Organization for Research and Treatment of Cancer

(EORTC), Breast Cancer Co-operative Group (BCCG). *Eur J Cancer* (1998) **34**: 307–314.

Dale PS, Souza JW, Brewer DA. Cryosurgical ablation of unresectable hepatic metastases. *J Surg Oncol* (1998) **68**: 242–245.

Dong B, Liang P, Yu X, Su L, Yu D, Cheng Z, Zhang J. Percutaneous sonographically guided microwave coagulation therapy for hepatocellular carcinoma: Results in 234 patients. *Am J Roentgenol* (2003) **180**: 1547–1555.

Dodd III GD, Soulen MC, Kane RA, Livraghi T, Lees WR, Yamashita Y, Gillams AR, Karahan OI, Rhim H. Minimally invasive treatment of malignant hepatic tumors: At the threshold of a major breakthrough. *RadioGraphics* (2000) **20**: 9–27.

Dowlatshahi K, Fan M, Gould VE, Bloom KJ, Ali A. Stereotactically guided laser therapy of occult breast tumors: Work-in-progress report. *Arch Surg* (2000) **135**: 1345–1352.

Dunn F. Attenuation and speed of ultrasound in lung. *J Acoust Soc Am* (1974) **56**: 1638–1639.

Farmer DG, Rosove MH, Shaked A, Busuttil RW. Current treatment modalities for hepatocellula carcinoma. *Ann Surg* (1994) **219**: 236–247.

Fisher B Anderson S, Redmond CK, Wolmark N, Wickerham DL, Cronin WM. Reanalysis and results after 12 years of follow-up in a randomized clinical trial comparing total mastectomy with lumpectomy with or without lumpectomy with or without irradiation in the treatment of breast cancer. *N Engl J Med* (1995) **333**: 1456–1461.

Foster RS, Bihrle R, Sanghvi NT, Fry FJ, Donohue JP. High-intensity focused ultrasound in the treatment of prostatic disease. *Eur Urol* (1993) **23**(Suppl. 1): 29–33.

Fry FJ. Precision high intensity focusing ultrasonic machines for surgery. *Am J Phys Med* (1958) **37**: 152–156.

Fry FJ. Transskull transmission of an intense focused ultrasonic beam. *Ultrasound Med Biol* (1977) **3**: 179–184.

Fry FJ, Barger JE. Acoustic properties of the human skull. *J Acoust Soc Am* (1978) **63**: 1576–1590.

Fry WJ, Barnard JW, Fry FJ, Krumins RF, Brennan JF. Ultrasonic lesions in the mammalian central nervous system. *Science* (1955) **122**: 517–518.

Fry WJ, Mosberg WH, Barnard JW, Fry FJ. Production of focal destructive lesions in the central nervous system with ultrasound. *J Neurosurg* (1954) **11**: 471–478.

Gazelle GS, Goldberg SN, Solbiati L, Livraghi T. Tumor ablation with radio-frequency energy. *Radiology* (2000) **217**: 633–646.

Gelet A, Chapelon JY, Bouvier R, Souchon R, Pangaud C, Abdelrahim AF, Cathignol D, Dubernard JM. Treatment of prostate cancer with transrectal focused ultrasound: Early clinical experience. *Eur Urol* (1996) **29**: 174–183.

Gianfelice D, Khiat A, Boulanger Y, Amara M, Belblidia A. Feasibility of magnetic resonance imaging-guided focused ultrasound surgery as an adjunct to tamoxifen therapy in high-risk surgical patients with breast carcinoma. *J Vasc Interv Radiol* (2003) **14**: 1275–1282.

Goldberg SN, Gszelle GS, Mueller PR. Thermal ablation therapy for focal malignancy: A unified approach to underlying principles, techniques, and diagnostic imaging guidance. *Am J Roentgenol* (2000) **174**: 323–331.

Goss SA, Frizzell LA, Dunn F. Ultrasonic absorption and attenuation in mammalian tissues. *Ultrasound Med Biol* (1979) **5**: 181–186.

Goss SA, Johnson RL, Dunn F. Comprehensive compilation of empirical ultrasonic properties of mammalian tissues. *J Acoust Soc Am* (1978) **64**: 423–457.

Goss SA, Johnson RL, Dunn F. Compilation of empirical ultrasonic properties of mammalian tissues. II. *J Acoust Soc Am* (1980) **68**: 93–108.

Hardy CJ, Cline HE, Watkins RD. One-dimensional NMR thermal mapping of focused ultrasound surgery. *J Comput Assist Tomogr* (1994) **18**: 476–483.

Hill CR, Rivens I, Vaughan M, ter Haar G. Lesion development in focused ultrasound surgery: A general model. *Ultrasound Med Biol* (1994) **20**: 259–269.

Hill CR, ter Haar GR. Review article: High intensity focused ultrasound-potential for cancer treatment. *Br J Radiol* (1995) **68**: 1296–1303.

Hill CR, Bamber JC, ter Haar GR. (eds.), *Physical Principles of Medical Ultrasound* (2004) John Wiley & Sons Ltd, Chichester.

Hindley J, Gedroyc WM, Regan L, Stewart E, Tempany C, Hynyen K, Mcdannold N, Inbar Y, Itzchak Y, Rabinovici J, Kim HS, Geschwind JF, Hesley G, Gostout B, Ehrenstein T, Hengst S, Sklair-Levy M, Shushan A, Joleszm F. MRI guidance of focused ultrasound therapy of uterine fibroids: Early results. *Am J Roentgenol* (2004) **183**: 1713–1719.

Huber PE, Jenne JW, Rastert R, Simiantonakis I, Sinn HP, Strittmatter HJ, von Fournier D, Wannenmacher MF, Debus J. A new noninvasive approach in breast cancer therapy using magnetic resonance imaging-guided focused ultrasound surgery. *Cancer Res* (2001) **61**: 8441–8447.

Hynynen K, Darkazanli A, Unger E, Schenck JF. MRI-guided noninvasive ultrasound surgery. *Med Phys* (1993) **20**: 107–115.

Hynynen K, Pomeroy O, Smith DN, Huber PE, McDannold NJ, Kettenbach J, Baum J, Singer S, Jolesz FA. MR imaging-guided focused ultrasound surgery of fibroadenomas in the breast: A feasibility study. *Radiology* (2001) **219**: 176–185.

Jacobson JA, Danforth DN, Cowan KH, d'Angelo T, Steinberg SM, Pierce L, Lippman ME, Lichter AS, Glatstein E, Okunieff P. Ten-year results of a comparison of conservation with mastectomy in the treatment of stages I and II breast cancer. *N Engl J Med* (1995) **332**: 907–911.

Kennedy JE. High-intensity focused ultrasound in the treatment of solid tumours. *Nature Reviews Cancer* (2005) **5**: 321–327.

Kennedy JE, ter Haar GR, Wu F, Gleeson FV, Roberts IS, Middleton MR, Cranston D. Contrast-enhanced ultrasound assessment of tissue response to high-intensity focused ultrasound. *Ultrasound Med Biol* (2004) **30**: 851–854.

Kennedy JE, Wu F, ter Haar GR, Gleeson FV, Phillips RR, Middleton MR, Cranston D. High-intensity focused ultrasound for the treatment of liver tumours. *Ultrasonics* (2004) **42**: 931–935.

Kikuchi Y, Uchida R, Tanaka K, Wagai T. The localization of brain tumors by ultrasonic techniques. A clinical review of 111 cases. *J Neurosurg* (1965) **23**: 135–147.

Kimura K, Hashimoto Y, Hirano T, Uchino M, Ando M. Diagnosis of middle cerebral artery occlusion with transcranial color-coded realtime sonography. *AJNR* (1996) **17**: 895–899.

Kushner MJ, Zanette EM, Bastianello S, Mancini G, Sacchetti ML, Carolei A, Bozzao L. Transcranial Doppler in acute hemispheric brain infarction. *Neurology* (1991) **41**: 109–113.

Lee AJ, Taberner PV, Halliwell M. Split-brain preparation by ultrasonic lesions in the rat. *Physiol Behav* (1980) **24**: 123–129.

Lezoche E, Paganini AM, Feliciotti F, Guerrieri M, Lugnani F, Tamburini A. Ultrasound-guided laparoscopic cryoablation of hepatic tumors: Preliminary report. *World J Surg* (1998) **22**: 829–835.

Li CX, Xu GL, Jiang ZY, Li JJ, Luo GY, Shan HB, Zhang R, Li Y. Analysis of clinical effect of high-intensity focused ultrasound on liver cancer. *World J Gastroenterol* (2004) **10**: 2201–2204.

Lin D, Lin SM, Liaw YF. Non-surgical treatment of hepatocellular carcinoma. *J Gastroenterol Hepa* (1997) **12**: S319–S328.

Lin TY, Lee CS, Chen KM, Chen CC. Role of surgery in the treatment of primary carcinoma of the liver: A 31-year experience. *Br J Surg* (1987) **74**: 839–842.

Linke CA, Carstensen EL, Frizzell LA, Elbadawi A, Fridd CW. Localized tissue destruction by high-intensity focused ultrasound. *Arch Surg* (1973) **107**: 887–891.

Lizzi FL. High-precision thermotherapy for small lesions. *Eur Urol* (1993) **23**(Suppl. 1): 23–28.

Lynn JG, Zwemer RL, Chick AJ, Miller AG. A new method for the generation and use of focused US in experimental biology. *J Gen Physiol* (1942) **26**: 179–193.

Madersbacher S, Kratzik C, Szabo N, Susani M, Vingers L, Marberger M. Tissue ablation in benign prostatic hyperplasia with high-intensity focused ultrasound. *Eur Urol* (1993) **23**(Suppl 1): 39–43.

Maris H, Balibar S. Negative pressures and cavitation in liquid helium. *Physics Today* (2000) **53**: 29–32.

Martin PJ, Pye IF, Abbott RJ, Naylor AR. Color-coded ultrasound of vascular occlusion in acute ischemic stroke. *J Neuroimage* (1995) **5**: 152–156.

Mason TJ. A sound investment. *Chem Ind* (1998) 878–882.

Matsukawa T, Yamashita Y, Arakawa A, Nishiharu T, Urata J, Murakami R, Takahashi M, Yoshimatsu S. Percutaneous microwave coagulation therapy in liver tumors: A 3-year experience. *Acta Radiol* (1997) **38**: 410–415.

McGahan JP, Dodd GD. Radiofrequency ablation of the liver: Current status. *Am J Roentgenol* (2001) **176**: 3–16.

Okuno T, Ganaha F, Lee CO, Shimizu T, Osako K, Oka S, Lee KH, Chen WZ, Zhu H, Park SH, Qi Z, Shi D, Song HS. Feasibility of extracorporeal HIFU using Chongqing Haifu-knife as an adjunct to the endovascular therapy for breast conservation particularly in patients with recurrent breast carcinoma, in *Proc 4th International Symposium on Therapeutic Ultrasound*, Tachibana K, ter Haar GR (eds.), ISTU, Kyoto (2004) pp. 66.

Robinson DS, Parel JM, Denham DB, Gonzalez-Cirre X, Manns F, Milne PJ, Schachner RD, Herron AJ, Comander J. Interstitial laser hyperthermia model development for minimally invasive therapy of breast carcinoma. *J Am Coll Surg* (1998) **186**: 284–292.

Rowland IJ, Rivens I, Chen L, Lebozer CH, Collins DJ, ter Haar GR, Leach MO. MRI study of hepatic tumours following high intensity focused ultrasound surgery. *Br J Radiol* (1997) **70**: 144–153.

Rowland RO, Kennedy JE, Wu F, ter Haar GR, Phillips RR, Protheroe AS, Middleton MR, Cranston DW. Preliminary experience using high-intensity focused ultrasound for the treatment of kidney and liver tumours. *Br J Cancer* (2004) **91**: S21.

Sato M, Watanabe Y, Kashu Y, Nakata T, Hamada Y, Kawachi K. Sequential percutaneous microwave coagulation therapy for liver tumor. *Am J Surg* (1998) **175**: 322–324.

Sibille A, Prat F, Chapelon JY, Abou el Fadil F, Henry L, Theillere Y, Ponchon T, Cathignol D. Extracorporeal ablation of liver tissue by high-intensity focused ultrasound. *Oncology* (1993) **50**: 375–379.

Smith SW, Trahey GE, von Ramm OT. Phased array ultrasound imaging through planner tissue layers. *Ultrasound Med Biol* (1986) **12**: 229–243.

Sokka SD, King R, Hynynen K. MRI-guided gas bubble enhanced ultrasound heating in *in vivo* rabbit thigh. *Phys Med Biol* (2003) **48**: 223–241.

Staren ED, Sabel MS, Gianakakis LM, Wiener GA, Hart VM, Gorski M, Dowlastshahi K, Corning BF, Haklin MF, Koukoulis G. Cryosurgery of breast cancer. *Arch Surg* (1997) **132**: 28–33.

Stewart EA, Gedroyc WM, Tempany CM, Quade BJ, Inbar Y, Ehrenstein T, Shushan A, Hindley JT, Goldin RD, David M, Sklair M, Rabinovici J. Focused ultrasound treatment of uterine fibroid tumors: Safety and feasibility of a non-invasive thermoablative technique. *Am J Obstet Gynecol* (2003) **189**: 48–54.

Tempany CMC, Stewart EA, McDannold N, Quade BJ, Jolesz FA, Hynynen K. MR imaging-guided focused ultrasound surgery of uterine leiomyomas: A feasibility study. *Radiology* (2003) **226**: 897–905.

ter Haar GR, Clarke RL, Vaughan MG, Hill CR. Trackless surgery using focused ultrasound: Technique and case report. *Min Inv Ther* (1991) **1**: 13–15.

ter Haar GR. Acoustic surgery. *Phys Today* (2001) **54**: 29–34.

ter Haar GR, Rivens IH, Moskovic E, Huddart R, Visioli AG. *SPIE* (1998) **270**.

Thuroff S, Chaussy C, Vallancien G, Wieland W, Kiel HJ, Le Duc A, Desgrandchamps F, De La Rosette J, Gelet A. High-intensity focused ultra-sound and localized prostate cancer: Efficacy results from the European mul-ticentric study. *J Endourol* (2003) **17**: 673–677.

Vallancien G, Chartier-Kastler E, Harouni M, Chopin D, Bougaran J. Focused extracorporeal pyrotherapy: Experimental study and feasibility in man. *Semin Urol* (1993) **11**: 7–9.

Vallancien G, Harouni M, Guillonneau B, Veillon B, Bougaran J. Ablation of superficial bladder tumors with focused extracorporeal pyrotherapy. *Urology* (1996) **47**: 204–207.

Vallancien G, Harouni M, Veillon B, Mombet A, Brisset J, Bougaran J. Focused extracorporeal pyrotherapy. *Eur Urol* (1993) **23**(Suppl 1): 48–52.

Veronesi U, Luini A, Del Vecchio M, Greco M, Galimberti V, Merson M, Rilke F, Saccozzi R, Savio T. Radiotherapy after breast-preserving surgery in women with localized cancer of the breast. *N Engl J Med* (1993) **328**: 1587–1591.

Visioli AG, Rivens IH, ter Haar GR, Horwich A, Huddart RA, Moskovic E, Padhani A, Glees J. Preliminary results of a phase I dose escalation clin-ical trial using focused ultrasound in the treatment of localized tumours. *Eur J Ultrasound* (1999) **9**: 11–18.

Vogl TJ, Muller PK, Hammerstingl R, Weinhold N, Mack MG, Philipp C, Deimling M, Beuthan J, Pegios W, Riess H. Malignant liver tumors treated with MR imaging-guided laser-induced thermotherapy: Technique and prospective results. *Radiology* (1995) **196**: 257–265.

Vykhodtseva NI, Hynynen K, Damianou C. Histologic effects of high intensity pulsed ultrasound exposure with subharmonic emission in rabbit brain *in vivo*. *Ultrasound Med Biol* (1995) **21**: 969–979.

Wang Z, Bai J, Li F, Du Y, Wen S, Hu K, Xu G, Ma P, Yin N, Chen W, Wu F, Feng R. Study of a "biological focal region" of high-intensity focused ultrasound. *Ultrasound Med Biol* (2003) **29**: 749–754.

Wang ZB, Wu F, Wang ZL, Zhang Z, Zou JZ, Liu C, Liu YG, Cheng G, Du YH, He ZC, Gu ML, Wang ZG, Feng R. Targeted damage effects of high intensity focused ultrasound (HIFU) on liver tissues of Guizhou Province miniswine. *Ultrason Sonochem* (1997) **4**: 181–182.

Watkin NA, Morris SB, Rivens IH, Woodhouse CRJ, ter Haar GR. A feasibility study for non-invasive treatment of superficial bladder tumours with focused ultrasound. *Br J Urol* (1996) **78**: 715–721.

Weis L. Common malignant bone tumors: Osteosarcoma, in *Surgery for Bone and Soft-tissue Tumors*. Simon MA, Springfield D (eds.) (1998) Lippincott-Raven, Philadelphia, pp. 265–274.

Wells PNT (ed.), *Biomedical Ultrasound.* (1977) Academic, London.

Wu F, Chen WZ, Bai J, Zou JZ, Wang ZL, Zhu H, Wang ZB. Tumor vessel destruction resulting from high-intensity focused ultrasound in patients with solid malignancies. *Ultrasound Med Biol* (2002) **28**: 535–542.

Wu F, Wang ZB, Cao YD, Chen WZ, Bai J, Zou JZ, Zhu H. A randomised clinical trial of high-intensity focused ultrasound ablation for the treatment of patients with localised breast cancer. *Br J Cancer* (2003) **89**: 2227–2233.

Wu F, Wang ZB, Cao YD, Chen WZ, Zou JZ, Bai J, Zhu H, Li KQ, Jin CB, Xie FL, Su HB, Gao GW. Changes in biologic characteristics of breast cancer treated with high-intensity focused ultrasound. *Ultrasound Med Biol* (2003) **29**: 1487–1492.

Wu F, Wang ZB, Chen WZ, Bai J, Zhu H, Qiao TY. Preliminary experience using high intensity focused ultrasound for the treatment of patients with advanced stage renal malignancy. *J Urol* (2003) **170**: 2237–2240.

Wu F, Wang ZB, Chen WZ, Wang W, Gui YZ, Zhang M, Zheng GQ, Zhou YJ, Xu GL, Li M, Zhang CW, Ye HY, Feng R. Extracorporeal high intensity focused ultrasound ablation in the treatment of 1038 patients with solid carcinomas in China: An overview. *Ultrasonics Sonochem* (2004) **11**: 149–154.

Wu F, Wang ZB, Chen WZ, Zhu H. Non-invasive ablation of high intensity focused ultrasound for the treatment of patients with malignant bone tumors. *J Bone Joint Surg Br* (2005) **87B**: S4.

Wu F, Wang ZB, Chen WZ, Zou JZ, Bai J, Zhu H, Li KQ, Xie FL, Jin CB, Su HB. Extracorporeal high intensity focused ultrasound ablation in the treatment of patients with large hepatocellular carcinoma. *Ann Surg Oncol* (2004) **11**: 1061–1069.

Wu F, Wang ZB, Chen WZ, Zou JZ, Bai J, Zhu H, Li KQ, Jin CB, Xie FL, Su HB. Advanced hepatocellular carcinoma: Treatment with high intensity focused ultrasound ablation combined with transcatheter arterial embolization. *Radiology* (2005) **235**: 659–667.

Wu F, Wang ZB, Chen WZ, Zou JZ, Bai J, Zhu H, Li KQ, Xie FL, Jin CB, Su HB, Gao GW. Extracorporeal focused ultrasound surgery for treatment of human solid carcinomas: Early Chinese clinical experience. *Ultrasound Med Biol* (2004) **30**: 245–260.

Wu F, Wang ZB, Chen WZ, Zou JZ, Bai J, Zhu H, Li KQ, Xie FL, Jin CB, Su HB. Feasibility of ultrasound-guided high intensity focused ultrasound treatment for patients with advanced pancreatic cancer: Initial experience. *Radiology* (2005) **236**: 1034–1040.

Wu F, Wang ZB, Wang ZL. Changes in ultrasonic image of tissue damaged by high intensity ultrasound *in vivo*. *J Acoustic Soc Am* (1998) **103**: 2869.

Wu F, Wang ZB, Zhu H, Chen WZ, Zou JZ, Bai J, Li KQ, Jin CB, Xie FL, Su HB, Gao GW. Extracorporeal high intensity focused ultrasound treatment for patients with breast cancer. *Breast Cancer Res Treatment* (2005) **92**: 51–60.

Yang R, Sanghvi NT, Rescorla FJ, Kopecky KK, Grosfeld JL. Liver cancer ablation with extracorporeal high-intensity focused ultrasound. *Eur Urol* (1993) **23**(Suppl 1): 17–22.

Zibari GB, Riche A, Zizzi HC, McMillan RW, Aultman DF, Boykin KN, Gonzalez E, Nandy I, Dies DF, Gholson CF, Holcombe RF, McDonald JC. Surgical and nonsurgical management of primary and metastatic liver tumors. *Am Surg* (1998) **64**: 211–221.

Index